ASQ:SE-2™ User's Guide

ASQ:SE-2
Ages & Stages Questionnaires®
Social-Emotional
SECOND EDITION

ASQ:SE-2™ User's Guide

ASQ:SE-2™
Ages & Stages Questionnaires®
Social-Emotional
SECOND EDITION

by

Jane Squires, Ph.D.

Diane Bricker, Ph.D.

and

Elizabeth Twombly, M.S.

Early Intervention Program
Center on Human Development
University of Oregon, Eugene

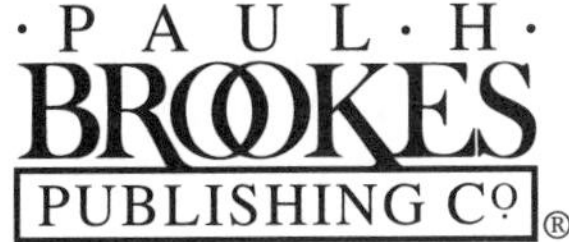

Baltimore • London • Sydney

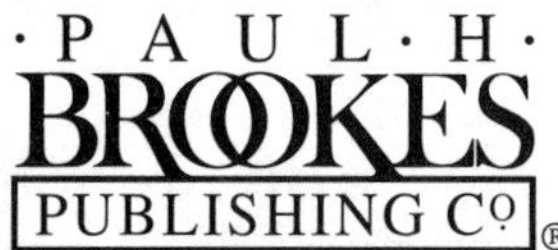

Paul H. Brookes Publishing Co.
Post Office Box 10624
Baltimore, Maryland 21285-0624
www.brookespublishing.com

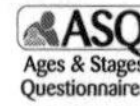

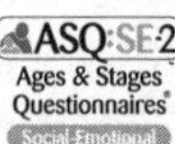

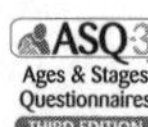

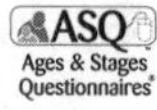

Visit www.agesandstages.com to learn more about the complete ASQ system.

Typeset by Scribe Inc., Philadelphia, Pennsylvania.
Manufactured in the United States of America by Sheridan Books, Inc., Chelsea, Michigan.

Library of Congress Cataloging-in-Publication Data

The Library of Congress has cataloged the print edition of the *ASQ:SE-2™ User's Guide* as follows:

Squires, Jane.
ASQ:SE-2 user's guide / by Jane Squires, Ph.D., Diane Bricker, Ph.D., Elizabeth Twombly, M.S., Early Intervention Program, Center on Human Development, University of Oregon, Eugene. — Second edition.
pages cm
Includes bibliographical references and index.
ISBN 978-1-59857-958-1 (paperback)
1. Child development—Testing. 2. Infants—Development—Testing. 3. Child development deviations—Diagnosis. I. Bricker, Diane D. II. Twombly, Elizabeth. III. Title.
RJ51.D48S64 2015
618.92'0075—dc23 2015013634

British Library Cataloguing in Publication data are available from the British Library.

2019 2018 2017

10 9 8 7 6 5 4

Contents

ASQ:SE-2™

Appendixes

List of Tables and Figures

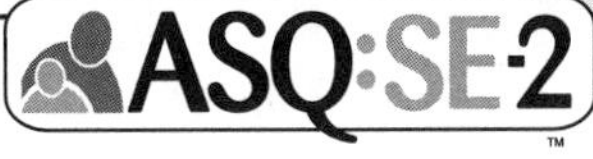

APPENDIX C

About the Authors

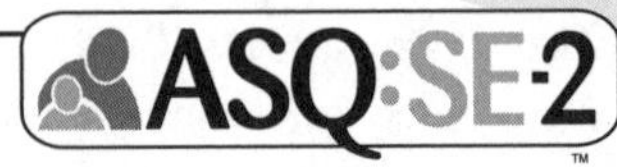

The ASQ:SE-2 system, including *Ages & Stages Questionnaires®: Social-Emotional, Second Edition* (ASQ:SE-2™) (English and Spanish), and the *ASQ:SE-2™ User's Guide,* was developed by the following authors:

Jane Squires, Ph.D., Professor, Early Intervention/Special Education; Director, Early Intervention Program; and Director, University Center for Excellence in Developmental Disabilities/Center on Human Development, College of Education, University of Oregon, Eugene

Dr. Squires is Professor of Special Education, focusing on the field of early intervention/early childhood special education. She oversees research and outreach projects in the areas of developmental screening, implementation of screening systems, early identification of developmental delays, and the involvement of parents in monitoring their young children's development. She is lead author of the *Ages & Stages Questionnaires®, Third Edition* (*ASQ-3™*; with D. Bricker; Paul H. Brookes Publishing Co., 2009), and the *Social-Emotional Assessment/Evaluation Measure* (*SEAM™*)*, Research Edition* (with D. Bricker, M. Waddell, K. Funk, J. Clifford, & R. Hoselton; Paul H. Brookes Publishing Co., 2014), and she has authored or coauthored more than 90 books, chapters, assessments, videotapes, and articles on developmental screening and early childhood disabilities. In 2013, she coauthored the book *Developmental Screening in Your Community: An Integrated Approach for Connecting Children with Services* (Paul H. Brookes Publishing Co., 2013). Dr. Squires currently teaches doctoral-level courses in early intervention/special education and conducts research on comprehensive early identification and referral systems for preschool children.

Diane Bricker, Ph.D., Professor Emerita and Former Director, Early Intervention Program, Center on Human Development, and Associate Dean for Academic Programs, College of Education, University of Oregon, Eugene

Dr. Bricker served as Director of the Early Intervention Program at the Center on Human Development, University of Oregon, from 1978 to 2004. She was a professor of special education, focusing on the fields of early intervention and social-communication.

Her professional interests have addressed three major areas: early intervention service delivery approaches, curricula-based assessment and evaluation, and developmental-behavioral screening. Dr. Bricker's work in early intervention approaches has been summarized in two volumes: *An Activity-Based Approach to Early Intervention, Fourth Edition* (with J. Johnson & N. Rahn; Paul H.

Brookes Publishing Co., 2015) and *An Activity-Based Approach to Developing Young Children's Social Emotional Competence* (with J. Squires; Paul H. Brookes Publishing Co., 2007). Her work in curricula-based assessment/evaluation has focused on the development of the *Assessment, Evaluation, and Programming System for Infants and Children, Second Edition* (*AEPS*®; with B. Capt, K. Pretti-Frontczak, J. Johnson, K. Slentz, E. Straka, & M Waddell; Paul H. Brookes Publishing Co., 2004). This measure and curricula provides intervention personnel with a system for the comprehensive assessment of young children with results that link directly to curricular content and subsequent evaluation of child progress.

Dr. Bricker has been a primary author of the *Ages & Stages Questionnaires*® (*ASQ*; with J. Squires; Paul H. Brookes Publishing Co., 1995, 1999, 2009) and directed research activities on the ASQ system starting in 1980. *Developmental Screening in Your Community: An Integrated Approach for Connecting Children with Services* (Bricker, Macy, Squires, & Marks; Paul H. Brookes Publishing Co., 2013) offers a comprehensive system for creating and operating community-wide developmental-behavioral screening programs for young children.

Dr. Bricker's distinctions include the Division of Early Childhood, Council for Exceptional Children Service to the Field Award, December 1992, and the Peabody College Distinguished Alumna Award, May 1995.

Elizabeth Twombly, M.S., Senior Researcher/Instructor, Early Intervention Program, Center on Human Development, University of Oregon, Eugene

For more than 20 years, Ms. Twombly has been involved in *Ages & Stages Questionnaires*® (*ASQ*) research projects, including renorming for the *Ages & Stages Questionnaires*®*: Social-Emotional, Second Edition* (*ASQ:SE-2*™), and the *Ages & Stages Questionnaires*®*, Third Edition* (*ASQ-3*™; Squires & Bricker; Paul H. Brookes Publishing Co., 2009). She has conducted trainings on ASQ and ASQ:SE nationally and internationally and has provided technical assistance to states on the development of early identification and referral systems for young children. Ms. Twombly is a contributing author of ASQ-3 and an author of ASQ:SE-2, the *ASQ-3*™ *Learning Activities,* and the *ASQ:SE-2*™ *Social-Emotional Learning Activities* (in press). She has special interests in helping underserved populations, including families with young children living in transition, and in developing systems of care for substance-exposed newborns. She currently is working on a team to develop a universal system of screening and referral for families with young children in the state of Oregon.

Robert Hoselton, B.S., Research Assistant, Early Intervention Program, Center on Human Development, University of Oregon, Eugene

Mr. Hoselton received a bachelor of science degree in computer science from the University of Oregon in 2004. He has been involved in several research studies on the *Ages & Stages Questionnaires*® (*ASQ*) and the *Social-Emotional Assessment/Evaluation Measure* (*SEAM*™; with J. Squires, D. Bricker, M. Waddell, K. Funk, & J. Clifford; Paul H. Brookes Publishing Co., 2014). Mr. Hoselton also develops and operates the Oregon Screening Project's research web site. He is mainly responsible for web application development, database management, and data analysis.

Kimberly Murphy, Research Assistant, Early Intervention Program, Center on Human Development, University of Oregon, Eugene

Ms. Murphy has coordinated several research studies involving both the *Ages & Stages Questionnaires*® (*ASQ*) and the *Ages & Stages Questionnaires*®*: Social-Emotional (ASQ:SE),* including data recruitment, collection, and analyses for the renorming studies of *Ages & Stages Questionnaires*®*: Social-Emotional, Second Edition* (*ASQ:SE-2*™), and *Ages & Stages Questionnaires*®*, Third Edition* (*ASQ-3*™; Squires & Bricker; Paul H. Brookes Publishing Co., 2009). She also contributes to related

ASQ materials and serves as the web content editor/coordinator for the research site designed for national ASQ and ASQ:SE data collection. She currently serves as Project Coordinator for the Oregon Screening Project, developing and operating its research web site. Ms. Murphy also works as part of a team providing statewide trainings and developing a universal system of screening and referral for families with young children in the state of Oregon.

Jill Dolata, M.A., CCC-SLP, Assistant Professor, Speech Language Pathology, Institute on Development & Disability, Oregon Health & Science University, Portland

Ms. Dolata is a Ph.D. candidate in special education and clinical sciences at the University of Oregon (Early Intervention/Early Childhood Special Education Leadership Program). Her primary clinical and research interests include the foundations of social language development and early identification of developmental delays. She participates in multidisciplinary developmental assessments and investigates early development for children born prematurely and children who may have autism spectrum disorder.

Suzanne Yockelson, Ph.D., Assistant Professor, Special Education, Brandman University, San Diego Campus

Dr. Yockelson earned her doctorate from the University of Oregon in 1999 and remained on faculty in the College of Education until 2007. Immediately following her move to California, Dr. Yockelson was the Educating Providers in the Community Coordinator at Help Me Grow in Orange County, where she worked within the county's system of health care and early childhood systems to promote developmental screening. She currently develops curriculum and teaches in the Early Childhood Special Education, Early Childhood Education, and Special Education programs at Brandman University. She also consults and trains in the United States and Canada. Her professional interests include early identification and referral of young children with special needs, social-emotional development of young children, inclusion in early childhood systems, and personnel preparation.

Maura Schoen Davis, Ph.D., Professor, Department of Education, Warren Wilson College, Asheville, North Carolina

Dr. Davis earned her doctorate from the University of Oregon, where she investigated the concurrent validity of the *Ages & Stages Questionnaires®: Social-Emotional (ASQ:SE).* She is currently a professor in the Education Department at Warren Wilson College. She teaches early childhood education courses and supervises Warren Wilson students in training at Verner Center for Early Learning.

Younghee Kim, Ph.D., Professor/Coordinator, Early Childhood Development Program, School of Education, Southern Oregon University, Ashland

Dr. Kim teaches in the Early Childhood Development, Elementary Education, and Master of Arts in Teaching Programs at Southern Oregon University. After graduating from Sogang University in Seoul, Korea, in 1985, she received her master's degree in 1992 and her doctorate in 1996 from the University of Oregon in the area of early intervention/early childhood special education. Her special research interests include alternative assessment for young children with special needs, family collaboration in early intervention, young children with emotional and social challenges, whole child development, and holistic education, as well as multicultural education for individuals with diverse backgrounds.

ABOUT THE TRANSLATORS OF ASQ:SE-2 SPANISH

Ellen McQuilkin, M.A., Professional Translator (English<>Spanish), Eugene, Oregon

Ms. McQuilkin grew up in San Diego, California, and later lived in México for 7 years, where she began to practice the art of translation. She received a bachelor's degree in music and Spanish from California State University, Chico (1984), and a master's degree in Spanish from the University of Oregon (1991), where she taught classes in Spanish language and literature for nearly a decade. Her primary areas of expertise include education, music, and the arts. She has provided numerous translations to nonprofit and social service organizations in Oregon and has collaborated on educational projects such as the Spanish version of Dynamic Indicators of Basic Early Literacy Skills (DIBELS; Indicadores Dinámicos del Éxito en la Lectura [IDEL]), a set of procedures and measures for assessing the acquisition of early literacy skills of children learning to read in Spanish. Ms. McQuilkin is a member of the American Translators Association.

Paulina Romo Villaseñor, M.A., Professional English-to-Spanish Translator, Eugene, Oregon

Ms. Romo Villaseñor, a native of Guadalajara, México, has been a translator and interpreter for more than 23 years. She currently serves as Executive Director of Downtown Languages, a nonprofit organization that offers English and life-skills classes for immigrants. She worked as a Spanish and literature teacher for more than 10 years and holds bachelor's degrees in business administration and general science (1999) as well as a master's degree in romance languages from the University of Oregon (2004). She worked closely with Ms. McQuilkin on the translation of ASQ-3™ and ASQ:SE-2™. She is the co-translator of the English–Spanish version of Indicadores Dinámicos del Éxito en la Lectura (IDEL; Dynamic Indicators of Basic Early Literacy Skills [DIBELS]) and many other projects in social services, medicine, education, and the arts.

Preface

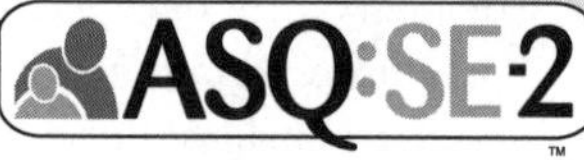

We initially began the development of the *Ages & Stages Questionnaires®: Social-Emotional (ASQ:SE™)* in the mid-1990s, at the insistence of early childhood and early intervention providers who regularly called and wrote, requesting that we expand the *Ages & Stage Questionnaires®* (ASQ; Bricker & Squires, 1999; Bricker, Squires, & Mounts, 1995; Squires & Bricker, 2009) to include the critical social and emotional domains. Practitioners working with very young children had no screening tools for assessing social and emotional problems yet were required to identify children whose social-emotional competence was not developing in a typical fashion. Practitioners wanted a tool like ASQ—one that was parent friendly, had clear assessment and scoring procedures, and had psychometric integrity.

We began with the realization that developing a screening tool for the social and emotional domains would be challenging. We were aware of the complexities involved in accurate assessment of social-emotional competence due to environmental, cultural, individual, and family variables. When is the crying of a 3-year-old "too much"? Are Lien's tantrums out of control, or are they within what is expected for a 2-year-old? Is it appropriate for Dante, a 4-year-old, to constantly cling to his mother and have difficulty separating each morning at preschool?

The development of ASQ:SE was rooted in our firm belief that parents can be accurate assessors of their young children's behaviors and development. The strong conviction that most parents can accurately evaluate their child's behaviors provided the necessary foundation for us to undertake this important task. Also compelling to us was the knowledge that the same needs that provided the impetus for the development of the ASQ remained. That is, parents and family members need to be genuinely involved in assessment, intervention, and evaluation; tests and procedures are needed to monitor the development of infants and young children at high risk for developmental and behavioral problems because of medical, biological, or environment factors or a combination; and resources remain limited, with continued pressure to find effective yet economical means to serve growing numbers of children who are at risk.

Our work in developmental screening made us aware of the growing need to examine and assess the social-emotional competence of infants and preschool children. The numbers of children living in poverty and who are more likely to show signs of anxiety, depression, and antisocial behavior are growing (Campbell et al., 2014; Children's Defense Fund, 2001; Sawhill & Karpilow, 2014; Yoshikawa, 2013). Brain research has revealed the interplay between early brain development and the quality of environmental experiences and has shown the huge impact that environmental experiences have on the developing structure of the brain (Shore, 1997). We began our original work on ASQ:SE in 1996 at the University of Oregon, where as part of a doctoral seminar we read widely and across disciplines about social and emotional competence and disability. The variety of approaches, definitions, and philosophies that we found was staggering.

After reviewing research and texts and talking with colleagues and experts, we arrived at a foundations model to undergird our development. In line with our philosophical views, a transactional approach to development (Sameroff, 2000, 2009; Sameroff & Chandler, 1975), with an ecological emphasis (Bronfenbrenner, 1977, 2009), formed the conceptual underpinnings for ASQ:SE. The social learning model (Bandura, 1977; Patterson, Reid, & Dishion, 1992), which posits that social learning occurs as a function of the child's daily social interactions, was also deemed important. In addition, the developmental organization theory of Cicchetti (1993) and the marginal deviation model (Dishion, French, & Patterson, 1995; Reid, 1993) provided useful complements. These models established that disturbances or inappropriate social learning at the earlier levels will likely cause continuing and more serious disturbances at later ages. Finally, development theory (Fischer & Rose, 1994; Gesell, 1933; Piaget, 1950) provided the foundations for the range and span of behaviors.

We generated an initial series of seven questionnaires appropriate for infants (6 and 12 months), toddlers (18 and 24 months), and preschool children (30, 36, and 48 months) that parents and caregivers could read and understand. We grouped questions into the areas that our extensive survey of literature had told us are critical for social-emotional competence—self-regulation, compliance, social-communication, adaptive functioning, autonomy, affect, and interaction with people. We followed the format of ASQ as closely as possible; however, we learned from early field trials that different answering and scoring formats are necessary to fit the assessment of social-emotional competence. Our first efforts were piloted with parents and providers across the United States, including in Healthy Start Hawaii, Early Head Start of Southern Oregon, and Oregon Migrant Head Start. We revised the questionnaire, added a 60 month interval, and in 1997 began conducting psychometric studies across the United States. From the beginning, we sought and incorporated feedback from parents and service providers. We believe this feedback has been vital to the successful development and testing of ASQ:SE.

The first edition of ASQ:SE became commercially available in 2002 (Squires, Bricker, & Twombly, 2002). In the nearly 15 years since ASQ:SE was published, its scope and audiences have grown exponentially. From early on, ASQ:SE was recognized as a parent-friendly and evidence-based tool that could measure the social, emotional, and behavioral competence of young children and provided useful information for parents and practitioners regarding a child's profile and next steps that could be taken.

Over the years, we have gathered feedback from programs and families using ASQ:SE and have become aware of additions and revisions that would improve the validity and utility of the tool. In developing ASQ:SE-2, we had six main objectives that required data collection on a large sample of children and families.

1. *To establish new cutoff scores based on a more representative normative sample than was available for the first edition:* To meet this objective, it was necessary to update the normative sample to better reflect current U.S. Census demographics.
2. *To examine selected psychometric properties of the revised measure, including its validity, reliability, and utility*
3. *To improve existing items or add items to address assessment limitations we knew existed:* For example, new questionnaire items related to autism and other social-emotional delays

have been added. These new items target early social-communication, adaptive, and autonomous behaviors. In addition, items on the first edition that parents reported were unclear were rewritten or deleted.

4. *To expand the age range of the questionnaire intervals:* The age range is extended in both directions—to include children from 1 month to 72 months of age (6 years). These changes were made based on feedback from program personnel who wanted a questionnaire to give to parents of newborns in order to bring them into to the ASQ:SE system early on, as well as to extend the upper age range of the intervals to 6 years. With this new edition, the ASQ:SE-2 can now be used throughout a child's kindergarten year. A new 2 month ASQ:SE-2 interval was developed and tested to become the initial questionnaire in a series of nine ASQ:SE-2 intervals.
5. *To modify and clarify the scoring system:* The questionnaire format has been changed to include new response options (i.e., *often or always, sometimes, rarely or never*), and a new Information Summary sheet was created.
6. *To add a monitoring zone similar to the one used with ASQ-3:* This change was undertaken to aid in score interpretation and follow-up decision-making.

We are hopeful that the expansion of the ASQ system will improve screening and monitoring efforts of programs throughout the United States and elsewhere. Photocopying is permitted according to the guidelines outlined the photocopying release on page xx.

Early identification of children with social and emotional difficulties is of paramount importance for improving outcomes for children and families. Improving screening procedures that involve parents and caregivers should result in improved early identification and timelier referral to intervention for children and families.

Jane Squires, Ph.D.
Diane Bricker, Ph.D.
Elizabeth Twombly, M.S.

REFERENCES

Bandura, A. (1977). *Self-efficacy: The exercise of control.* New York: W.H. Freeman.

Bricker, D., & Squires, J. (with Mounts, L., Potter, L., Nickel, R., Twombly, E., & Farrell, J.). (1999). *Ages & Stages Questionnaires®, Second Edition (ASQ): A parent-completed, child-monitoring system.* Baltimore, MD: Paul H. Brookes Publishing Co.

Bricker, D., Squires, J., & Mounts, L. (with Potter, L., Nickel, R., & Farrell, J.). (1995). *Ages & stages questionnaires® (ASQ): A parent-completed, child-monitoring system.* Baltimore, MD: Paul H. Brookes Publishing Co.

Bronfenbrenner, U. (1977). Toward an experimental ecology of human development. *American Psychologist, 32,* 513–531.

Bronfenbrenner, U. (2009). *The ecology of human development: Experiments by nature and design.* Cambridge, MA: Harvard University Press.

Campbell, F., Conti, G., Heckman, J., Moon, S., Pinto, R., Pungello, E., & Pan, Y. (2014). Early childhood investments substantially boost adult health. *Science, 343*(6178), 1478–1485.

Children's Defense Fund. (2001). *Child welfare and mental health division.* Retrieved from http://www.childrensdefense.org/news_stats.htm

Cicchetti, D. (1993). Developmental psychopathology. *Developmental Review, 13,* 471–502.

Dishion, T., French, D., & Patterson, G. (1995). The development and ecology of antisocial behavior. In D. Cicchetti & D. Cohen (Eds.), *Developmental psychology: Vol. 2. Risk, disorder, and adaptation.* New York, NY: Wiley.

Fischer, K.W., & Rose, S.P. (1994). Dynamic development of coordination of components in brain and behavior: A framework for theory. In G. Dawson & K.W. Fischer (Eds.), *Human behavior and the developing brain* (pp. 3–66). New York, NY: Guilford Press.

Gesell, A. (1933). Maturation and patterning of behavior. In C. Murchison (Ed.), *A handbook of child psychology.* Worcester, MA: Clark University Press.

Patterson, G.R., Reid, J., & Dishion, T. (1992). *Antisocial boys.* Eugene, OR: Castalia.

Piaget, J. (1950). *The psychology of intelligence.* (M. Piercy, & D. E. Berlyne, Trans.) London: Kegan Paul, Trench, & Trubner.

Reid, J. (1993). Prevention of conduct disorder before and after school entry: Relating intervention to developmental findings. *Development and Psychology, 5,* 243–262.

Sameroff, A.J. (2000). Ecological perspectives on developmental risk. In J.D. Osofsky & H.E. Fitzgerald (Eds.), *WAIMH handbook of infant mental health: Vol 4. Infant mental health in groups at high risk* (pp. 1–33). New York, NY: Wiley & Sons.

Sameroff, A.J. (Ed.). (2009). *The transactional model of development: How children and contexts shape each other.* Washington, DC: American Psychological Association.

Sameroff, A.J., & Chandler, M.J. (1975). Reproductive risk and the continuum of caretaking casualty. In F. Horowitz, M. Hetherington, S. Scarr-Salapatek, & G. Siegel (Eds.), *Review of child development research.* Chicago, IL: University of Chicago Press

Sawhill, I., & Karpilow, Q. (2014). *How much could we improve children's life changes by intervening early and often* (Brief #54). Washington, DC: Brookings Institute, Center on Children and Families.

Shore, R. (1997). *Rethinking the brain: New insights into early development.* New York, NY: Families and Work Institute. Retrieved from http://developingchild.harvard.edu/key_concepts/brain_architecture/

Squires, J., & Bricker, D. (2009). *Ages & Stages Questionnaires®, Third Edition (ASQ-3™): A parent-completed child monitoring system.* Baltimore, MD: Paul H. Brookes Publishing Co.

Squires, J., Bricker, D., & Twombly, L. (2002). *Ages & Stages Questionnaires®: Social-Emotional (ASQ:SE): A parent-completed, child-monitoring system for social-emotional behaviors.* Baltimore, MD: Paul H. Brookes Publishing Co.

Yoshikawa, H., Weiland, C., Brooks-Gunn, J., Burchinal, M., Espinosa, L., . . . Zaslow, M.J. (2013). *Investing in our future: The evidence base on preschool education.* New York, NY: Foundation for Child Development and Ann Arbor, MI: Society for Research in Child Development.

Acknowledgments

ASQ:SE-2

As with *Ages & Stages Questionnaires®, Third Edition* (*ASQ-3*™), the development of *Ages & Stages Questionnaires®: Social-Emotional, Second Edition* (*ASQ:SE-2*™) evolved as a result of a multitude of efforts by a myriad of people. Many individuals assisted in the development of new items for this second edition as well as helped with the process of planning, reviewing, collecting, and analyzing data.

In particular, we would like to thank our friends and colleagues who were instrumental in gathering and analyzing data over the past 7 years. Thanks to Rob Hoselton, our longtime data analyst on the ASQ project, for countless hours and unlimited patience with endless data analysis requests. Thanks to Kimberly Murphy, who coordinated the data collection and management of the project, for keeping track of numerous revisions of ASQ:SE and mountains of data on the second edition. In addition, thank you to Annette Tognazzini for clerical and technical support and more throughout the project period.

We would like to acknowledge the time and work of numerous colleagues and faculty members in our community who participated in this project. First, we thank pediatrician Dr. Kevin Marks, who has advised us on using ASQ and ASQ:SE in busy pediatric medical practices. His input on physician use, suggested modifications, and what works in real life settings has been invaluable. In addition, Dr. Robert Nickel, a developmental pediatrician who has been involved in the ASQ project since its inception, has been generous with his time and expertise for improving the second edition of ASQ:SE. Dr. Karen Lawrence participated in the initial development by helping gather data for several new items for ASQ:SE-2. Thanks to Dr. Jantina Clifford for her ongoing guidance and expertise in tool development during research meetings.

Thank you to the early intervention doctoral students who attended ASQ:SE research meetings and provided input on every aspect of this new edition. Thanks to Allison Baker for her initial help in recruiting subjects through social media, Chieh-Yu (Tom) Chen for his thoughtful analysis of gender differences, as well as Jill Dolata for her specific expertise and input on items related to autism. A big thank you for contributions over the years goes to Ching-I Chen, Kathy Moxley, Serra Acar, Sarah Hansen, Ruby Batz, Rebecca Frantz, Khaled Alkherainej, and Huichao Xie. Research meetings were greatly enhanced through their participation.

Thousands of families of infants and children, representative of every state in this country, have completed and returned questionnaires. Many of these parents have been willing to participate in a range of testing with a variety of instruments. Without the data generated by these families, we would have been unable to examine the reliability, validity, and utility of the second edition.

In addition to parents and children, we have received valuable feedback and data from professionals across the country who are using ASQ:SE with families. We thank a variety of individuals and families representing health, early childhood, early intervention, and mental health agencies. Special appreciations are given to Elaine Harrison, Sandra Stephens, and Maureen Markey of Albina Head Start/Early Head Start in Portland, Oregon, and Dr. Suzanne Bells-McManus from Head Start of Lane County for piloting the research versions of the questionnaires. Thank you to our colleagues at the Oregon Health & Science University Child Development and Rehabilitation Clinic and Early Childhood CARES, both housed at the University of Oregon, who are always generous with their time and knowledge. Thank you to Catherine Wright and colleagues in Minnesota who carried out research on ASQ:SE for several years and shared data and ideas for improvement. Thank you to those individuals at agencies who provided data, including Looking Glass Mental Health, Moss Street Child Development Center, and the Relief Nursery in Eugene, Oregon; Ohio Help Me Grow; and Families Matter in Alberta, Canada. In addition, numerous professionals from all over the country have participated in focus groups to provide feedback on new items, features, and formatting changes to ASQ:SE. We strongly believe the input from all of these professionals has resulted in a tool that is reliable and valid, easier to use, and provides new features that will enhance its utility in work with families with young children.

A group of experts, including Ellen McQuilken, Paulina Romo Villaseñor, Theresa Arellano, Ruby Batz, Evette B. Callahan, Maria Pilar Pomés Correa, Cardina Esparza, Donna Jackson-Maldonado, Isabel Piza, and Josefina Sapriza, gave feedback on the second edition Spanish translation and assisted in the development of new items for the ASQ:SE-2 Spanish. Ellen McQuilken and Paulina Romo Villaseñor translated the questionnaires and *ASQ:SE-2™ Quick Start Guide* as well as associated activities, letters, and forms that can be used to administer the tools with families. Finally, Drs. Kay Heo, Xiaoyan Bian, Hollie Hix-Small, Carmen Dionne, J. Landeira Fernandez, and Harris Huberman are among our many valuable international partners who have gathered data on adaptations and translations of ASQ:SE in international settings. They continue to devote their prodigious research skills to adaptations of ASQ:SE around the world.

ASQ:SE-2 would not exist were it not for our long-time editors and now friends at Paul H. Brookes Publishing Co., Melissa Behm, Heather Shrestha, Amy Shillady, Amy Perkins Clause, and Heather Lengyel, who have been at our side as we developed and expanded ASQ:SE to include intervals that cover ages from 1 month up to 72 months as well as electronic and web-based options. We know that ASQ:SE is a high quality, widely used screening tool because of their guidance.

The success of any complex long-term project is dependent upon an array of factors, including consistent financial support, commitment from project staff, subjects' good faith participation, ideas with merit, reasonable and practical plans of action, and luck. We have been fortunate to have had all of these.

Jane Squires, Ph.D.
Diane Bricker, Ph.D.
Elizabeth Twombly, M.S.

Photocopying Release

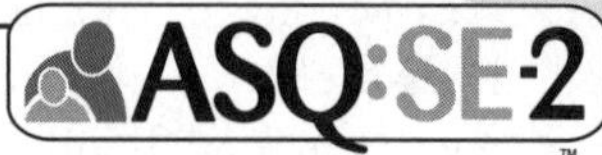

Purchasers of *Ages & Stages Questionnaires®:Social-Emotional, Second Edition (ASQ:SE-2™): A Parent-Completed Child Monitoring System for Social-Emotional Behaviors* are granted permission to photocopy the ASQ:SE-2 questionnaires, as well as the letter templates and forms from the *ASQ:SE-2™ User's Guide,* solely in the course of their agency's or practice's service provision to families. Purchasers may also photocopy the supplemental materials provided with the ASQ:SE-2 questionnaires. Photocopies may only be made from a set of original ASQ:SE-2 questionnaires and/or an original User's Guide.

Each branch office or physical site that will be using the ASQ:SE-2 system must purchase its own set of original ASQ:SE-2 questionnaires; master forms cannot be shared among sites.

Electronic reproduction and distribution of the questionnaires, letter templates and forms, and supplemental materials are prohibited except as otherwise explicitly authorized (see Frequently Asked Questions on pp. xxi–xxiv and the End User License Agreement included with the ASQ:SE-2 CD-ROM).

None of the ASQ:SE-2 materials may be reproduced to generate revenue for any program or individual. Programs are prohibited from charging parents, caregivers, or other service providers who will be completing and/or scoring the questionnaires fees in excess of the exact cost to photocopy the master forms. This restriction is not meant to apply to reimbursement of usual and customary charges for developmental, behavioral, or mental health screening when performed with other evaluation and management services.

The ASQ:SE-2 materials are meant to be used to facilitate screening and monitoring and to assist in the early identification of children who may need further social-emotional behavior assessment. Materials may not be used in a way contrary to the family-oriented philosophies of the ASQ:SE-2 developers.

Unauthorized use beyond this privilege is prosecutable under federal law. You will see the copyright protection line at the bottom of each photocopiable form.

Go to www.agesandstages.com for more information about ASQ use or to contact Brookes Publishing's Subsidiary Rights Department.

Frequently Asked Questions

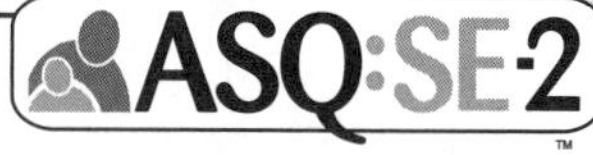

The following are some of the frequently asked questions that users pose to Brookes Publishing. The information that follows is primarily focused on rights and permissions associated with using ASQ:SE-2™.

PHOTOCOPYING

Can the ASQ:SE-2 questionnaires be photocopied?
Yes, the ASQ:SE-2 questionnaires as well as the letter templates and forms in the *ASQ:SE-2™ User's Guide* may be photocopied for use at a single physical site with all the children served by that site at no additional charge. Purchasers may also photocopy the supplemental materials provided with the ASQ:SE-2 questionnaires. Photocopies may only be made from a set of original questionnaires and/or an original User's Guide. See Photocopying Release for certain restrictions.

NUMBER OF ASQ:SE-2 BOXES NEEDED

My organization has many locations throughout the state. How many ASQ:SE-2 boxes do I need to buy?
Each location (i.e., branch office or physical site) that will be using the ASQ:SE-2 system must purchase its own box of original questionnaires with the accompanying CD-ROM; the questionnaire box, CD-ROM, and master forms cannot be shared among sites. Each physical site must also have its own copy of the *ASQ:SE-2 User's Guide.*

I understand that use of ASQ:SE-2 is site specific, but I am not sure how a "site" is defined.
A site is a single physical location, such as an office, clinic, or chid care setting. An organization may have various sites—for example, the downtown office, the East branch, and the North branch. The sites may be located in the same city or town, the same country, the same state, or even different states. For instance, the University of Michigan has three campuses in Michigan: Ann Arbor, Flint, and Dearborn. Each campus is a different site; the main campus in Ann Arbor cannot purchase ASQ:SE-2 and then share copies of it with the two branch campuses

in other cities. Even on one campus, there are different sites; say, if the School of Social Work wanted to use ASQ:SE-2 and the School of Education also wanted to use ASQ:SE-2, each one, as it is a separate department located in a different building, must purchase its own ASQ:SE box. Head Start programs are another example: Even though there are many Head Start programs across the United States, and they are all part of the same organization, the main office of a grantee cannot purchase one ASQ:SE-2 box to share with all of its Head Start programs or sites. Instead, each site must own an original ASQ:SE-2 box and *ASQ:SE-2 User's Guide.* Some ASQ:SE-2 users are pediatricians with more than one office in the same town; each office must own an original ASQ:SE-2 box and *ASQ:SE-2 User's Guide* rather than sharing the ASQ:SE-2 materials between the multiple offices in the same town.

POSTING

Can I post the PDF questionnaires on the CD-ROM on my program's computer network?
The questionnaires, family information sheets, Information Summary sheets, Item Response Sheets, Social-Emotional Development Guides and Activities, Parent Conference Sheet, Child Monitoring Sheet, mailing sheet, What Is ASQ:SE-2?, and ordering guide can be posted on your program's local area network (LAN) or intranet if *only* people in your program at that single physical site have access to the LAN or intranet. Staff can then print and use the questionnaires as needed only from their computers at that single physical site. Remote access from another physical site, including by virtual private network (VPN), file transfer protocol (FTP), tunneling protocols, or other means, is not permitted.

Can I post the ASQ:SE-2 sample questionnaires from www.agesandstages.com on my web site?
No; however, Brookes Publishing encourages and permits linking from your web site to the sample questionnaires at www.agesandstages.com.

Can I post ASQ:SE-2 questionnaires on my web site or my program's web site?
No, posting ASQ:SE-2 questionnaires on any web site, password protected or otherwise, is not permitted.

E-MAILING

Can I e-mail ASQ:SE-2 questionnaires to a colleague or a family?
No, blank questionnaires may not be e-mailed to anyone for any reason. You may, however, share a *completed* questionnaire with a family in the course of your service provision to them.

Can I post online or e-mail the What Is ASQ:SE-2? handout?
Yes, you may post the What Is ASQ:SE-2? handout on your web site or your program's web site. You may e-mail What Is ASQ:SE-2? to a colleague or a family. The sheet may not be altered in any way, however, when posting online or e-mailing, and the copyright protection line at the bottom may not be removed or replaced.

Can I e-mail a Parent Conference Sheet or a Child Monitoring Sheet to a family?
Yes, as long as the sheet is completed, you may e-mail a Parent Conference Sheet or a Child Monitoring Sheet to a family in the course of your service provision to them.

Can I e-mail the letter templates and forms to a family?
Yes, after you've customized the text of the letter templates and forms from the *ASQ:SE-2 User's Guide* to fit your organization's and the family's needs and included the appropriate information, you may e-mail the documents to a family in the course of your service provision to them.

EXTRACTING

Can I use some of the questions from ASQ:SE-2 in a document that I am writing or assessment item or tool that I am creating?
You will need written permission from Brookes Publishing before reformatting, reprinting, reproducing (except as covered by the ASQ:SE-2 Photocopying Release), adapting, or translating the questionnaires, User's Guide, any related materials, or any part thereof in any way. To request permission, please complete a permission request form online at www.brookespublishing.com.

CD-ROM

What can I do with the ASQ:SE-2 CD-ROM?
The CD-ROM can be treated like a more durable version of the paper forms. This means you may print and photocopy the questionnaires and other materials as needed under the terms specified in the Photocopying Release and the End User License Agreement on the CD-ROM.

The questionnaires, family information sheets, Information Summary sheets, Item Response Sheets, Social-Emotional Development Guides and Activities, Parent Conference Sheet, Child Monitoring Sheet, mailing sheet, What Is ASQ:SE-2?, and ordering guide can be posted on your program's local area network (LAN) or intranet if *only* people in your program at that single physical site have access to the LAN or intranet. Staff can print and use the materials as needed only from their computers at that single physical site.

Are the questionnaires on the CD-ROM interactive?
No, the questionnaires on the CD-ROM are not fillable or interactive. The PDF forms on the CD-ROM are essentially a more durable version of the paper forms. You can use the CD-ROM to print the questionnaires and then photocopy them as needed.

ELECTRONIC MEDICAL RECORD/ELECTRONIC HEALTH RECORD

My practice/office uses an electronic medical record/electronic health record (EMR/EHR). Can I incorporate the ASQ:SE-2 questionnaires in our EMR/EHR?
Some uses of ASQ:SE-2 within an EMR/EHR are permitted without explicit permission from Brookes Publishing. These uses also are in compliance with the Photocopying Release and the End User License Agreement. Some EMR/EHR users may want to use ASQ Online to complete the questionnaires and send data to the EMR/EHR. Any use not described in this section requires written permission from Brookes Publishing; go to www.brookespublishing.com to contact your sales representative or request permission from the Subsidiary Rights Department.

For instance, if your practice/office uses a paper questionnaire, asks the parent to complete it, and then enters only the child's score into the EMR/EHR, that would not require any permission from Brookes Publishing. Or if the practice/office's EMR/EHR has fields that identify the ASQ:SE-2 questions by number only (*not* including the text of each question) along with spaces to indicate what the parent has marked for the answers, that would not require any permission from Brookes Publishing. You would not need permission to scan a *completed* ASQ:SE-2 questionnaire (and/or the *completed* Information Summary sheet) into the EMR/EHR, as long as that completed questionnaire is not interactive and not modifiable. This is the equivalent of a practice photocopying completed ASQ:SE-2 questionnaires and placing them in children's paper files or photocopying completed questionnaires for parents to take home and keep for their records.

TRANSLATIONS

I work with a population that does not speak and/or read English. Is ASQ:SE-2 available in other languages?
Yes, ASQ:SE-2 is available in Spanish from Brookes Publishing. Other languages are in development and may be available; please see www.agesandstages.com for the latest information.

I am conducting a research project with a population that does not speak and/or read English, and I would like to use ASQ:SE-2. Can I get permission to translate the questionnaires myself?
Brookes Publishing is pleased to consider requests to translate some or all of the questionnaires. Please contact the Subsidiary Rights Department via Rights & Permissions at www.brookespublishing.com.

MORE INFORMATION

How do I get more information about ASQ:SE-2 usage and rights and permissions?
More information is available in the FAQs at www.agesandstages.com. If your question is not answered by the details provided online, please e-mail your inquiry to Brookes Publishing's Subsidiary Rights Department at rights@brookespublishing.com. E-mails are answered as quickly as possible. Please be advised that it may be approximately 4–6 weeks before you receive a response, however, due to the volume of inquiries received.

I

Overview of ASQ:SE-2

1

Introduction to ASQ:SE-2

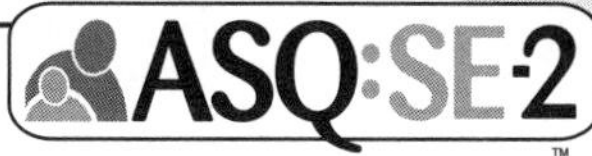

Young children's ability to successfully regulate their emotions and interact with others in positive ways is critical for their well-being and school readiness. Children who appropriately manage their social-emotional behavior are deemed competent, whereas children whose social-emotional behavior is inappropriate and unacceptable to others may be seen as troubled or "disabled." A growing body of evidence suggests that habituated and ingrained social-emotional problems are highly resistant to change and are likely to intensify over time (e.g., Giannoni & Kass, 2012; Walker & Shinn, 2010). As a consequence, the early identification of social-emotional problems in infants, toddlers, and young children is essential to assist them in building their social-emotional competence and reduce the likelihood of their placement in programs designed to address serious behavior or mental health problems.

The need for prevention or early treatment of social-emotional problems in young children is an international concern (Feil et al., 2014; Fernald, Kariger, Engle, & Raikes, 2009). This concern is addressed in the United States through federal legislation such as the Individuals with Disabilities Education Improvement Act (IDEA) of 2004 (PL 108-446) and at regional levels by the creation of state-supported programs. It is important to emphasize, however, that adequate resources are not available at the international, national, and local levels to identify and provide quality services for young children with social-emotional problems (Fernald et al., 2009). This alarming lack of program resources underlines the need for early identification/Child Find through large-scale screening programs to reduce the number of children with serious problems, begin intervention before problems become ingrained, and reduce the need for expensive long-term services.

Assessing infants' and young children's social-emotional development should be completed on a regular basis to identify difficulties as soon as they arise (American Academy of Pediatrics [AAP], 2001, 2006; Halfon et al., 2004; Johnson, Myers, & Council on Children with Disabilities, 2005; Marks & Glascoe, 2010; Marks & LaRosa, 2012; Pizur-Barnekow et al., 2010; Squires & Bricker, 2007; Thomas, Cotton, Pan, & Ratliff-Schaub, 2012). Accurate, affordable strategies to detect social-emotional problems in young children through early screening have been difficult to develop. The challenges include objectively defining target behaviors and how they may vary as a function of settings, measuring the impact of health factors, weighing the influence of family and cultural expectations, and taking the child's developmental status into consideration (Bricker, Macy, Squires, & Marks, 2013; Guralnick, 1997; Squires & Bricker, 2007; Zeanah, 2009). As a consequence, assessment of the social-emotional competence of young children often is not undertaken until problems become serious, thus requiring huge expenditures of intervention resources. Delayed identification is costly to children, families, and communities.

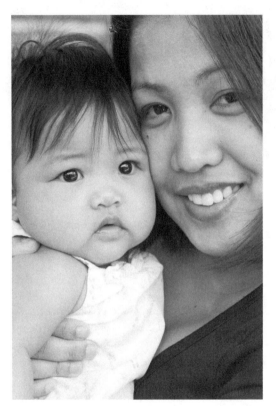

More cost-effective means, such as parent-completed tools, may be better suited for this repeated developmental monitoring (Drotar, Stancin, & Dworkin, 2008; Glascoe & Robertshaw, 2007; Pizur-Barnekow et al., 2010). Professional assessments usually are not performed at regular intervals because they are expensive and time consuming. Parent-completed tools that require less professional time and are more flexible in terms of administration are more easily applied in large-scale screening efforts. The *Ages & Stages Questionnaires®: Social-Emotional, Second Edition (ASQ:SE-2™): A Parent-Completed Child Monitoring System for Social-Emotional Behaviors* was developed to be low cost, effective, and well suited for large-scale implementation.

One purpose of the *ASQ:SE-2™ User's Guide* is to provide potential adopters of ASQ:SE-2 with a clear rationale for examining the social-emotional competence of infants, toddlers, and preschool-age children. The User's Guide also provides a detailed description of the ASQ:SE-2 system, which is designed to offer an accurate and low-cost method of screening young children's social-emotional competence.

WHAT IS ASQ:SE?

The first edition of ASQ:SE became commercially available in 2002 (Squires, Bricker, & Twombly, 2002). ASQ:SE-2 was developed to complement the *Ages & Stages Questionnaires®, Third Edition (ASQ-3™)*—a broad-based, general development screening measure. ASQ-3 is composed of 21 questionnaires designed to identify infants and young children who need more comprehensive developmental assessment of their communication, gross motor, fine motor, problem-solving, and personal-social skills. ASQ:SE-2 focuses exclusively on a child's social-emotional behavior and should be used in conjunction with ASQ-3 or another screening measure that provides more broad-based information about children's developmental status. Information about ASQ-3 can be found at www.agesandstages.com and in the *ASQ-3™ User's Guide* (Squires, Twombly, Bricker, & Potter, 2009).

The authors began the revision of ASQ:SE in 2009. Six objectives guided revisions and required that data be collected from a large sample of children and parents. The first objective was to establish new cutoff scores based on a sample of children that is more representative of the current U.S. population than was available for the first edition. It was necessary to update the normative sample to better reflect 2010 U.S. Census demographics in order to reach this objective. The second objective entailed examining certain psychometric properties of the revised measure, including its validity, reliability, and utility.

The third objective was to improve existing items or add items to address assessment deficiencies. The second edition includes new items that increase the questionnaires' sensitivity to autism and other social-emotional delays (see Table 1.1). These new items target early social-communication, adaptive, and autonomous behaviors. In addition, the authors deleted one item and rewrote items that parents reported were unclear. A fourth objective was to expand the age range of the questionnaire intervals. The age range of ASQ:SE-2 was extended in both directions—to include infants from 1 month to children 72 months (6 years). A new 2 month ASQ:SE-2 interval was developed, tested, and added. It can be used with children from 1 month 0 days through 2 months 30 days.

The fifth objective was to modify the scoring system. The questionnaire format was changed to include new response options (i.e., *often or always, sometimes, rarely or never*), and each questionnaire has a new Information Summary sheet. The sixth and final objective entailed adding a monitoring zone similar to the one used with ASQ-3. This change aids score interpretation and follow-up decision making. See Table 1.2 for a comparison of features between the first and second editions of ASQ:SE. See Chapter 2 for more in-depth information about items and social-emotional areas addressed in the ASQ:SE-2 system.

The ASQ:SE-2 System

ASQ:SE-2 is a comprehensive system designed to permit early identification/Child Find across large groups of children in an economical way. The heart of the system is a series of nine simple-to-complete questionnaires designed to identify infants and young children who need more comprehensive assessment of their social-emotional behavioral repertoire. The questionnaires are completed by parents when a child is 2, 6, 12, 18, 24, 30, 36, 48, and 60 months of age. Throughout the User's Guide and in other ASQ:SE-2 materials, the term *parents* is used to refer to all significant caregivers, such as grandparents, older siblings, and other relatives; foster care parents and guardians; teachers; and others who know the child well and consistently spend 15–20 or more hours per week with the child and are in a position to answer the questions.

When to Administer ASQ:SE-2

Questionnaires can be used individually (e.g., just the 18 month questionnaire) for a one-time screening "snapshot" or in combination (e.g., the 6, 12, 24, and 36 month questionnaires) for monitoring social-emotional development over time, depending on the needs of the child and the program's resources. Children are identified as needing further testing and possible referral to mental health, early intervention, or other community parent support services when their ASQ:SE-2 score is above a designated cutoff point. The ASQ:SE-2 system includes a comprehensive set of implementation procedures, outlined in this User's Guide, that can be adapted for a range of communities with varying goals and resources. The system also includes a wide range of support materials to promote successful implementation of the ASQ:SE-2 screening/monitoring program.

Table 1.1. Additional ASQ:SE-2 items by interval

ASQ:SE-2 interval	Additional scored items
6 month	19. Does your baby make sounds and look at you while playing with you? 20. Does your baby make sounds or use gestures to get your attention? 21. When you smile at your baby, does he smile back at you? 22. When you talk or make sounds to your baby, does she make sounds back?
12 month	22. Does your baby try to show you things? For example, does she hold out a toy and look at you? 23. Does your baby respond to his name when you call him? For example, does he turn his head and look at you? 24. When you point at something, does your baby look in the direction you are pointing? 25. Does your baby make sounds or use gestures to let you know she wants something (for example, by reaching)? 26. When you copy sounds your baby makes, does your baby repeat the same sounds back to you?
18 month	26. Does your child try to show you things by pointing at them and looking back at you? 27. Does your child make sounds or use words or gestures to let you know he wants something (for example, by reaching)? 28. Does your child play with objects by pretending? For example, does your child pretend to talk on the phone, feed a doll, or fly a toy airplane? 29. Does your child wake three or more times during the night? 30. Does your child respond to her name when you call her? For example, does she turn her head and look at you?
24 month	26. Does your child try to show you things by pointing at them and looking back at you? 27. Does your child play with objects by pretending? For example, does your child pretend to talk on the phone, feed a doll, or fly a toy airplane? 28. Does your child wake three or more times during the night? 29. Does your child respond to his name when you call him? For example, does he turn his head and look at you? 30. Is your child too worried or fearful? If "sometimes" or "often or always," please describe:
30 month	28. Does your child try to show you things by pointing at them and looking back at you? 29. Does your child use at least two words to ask for things he wants? For example, does he say "want ball" or "more apple"? 30. Does your child play with objects by pretending? For example, does your child pretend to talk on the phone, feed a doll, or fly a toy airplane? 31. Does your child wake three or more times during the night? 32. Is your child too worried or fearful? If "sometimes" or "often or always," please describe:
36 month	31. Does your child try to show you things by pointing at them and looking back at you? 32. Does your child pretend objects are something else? For example, does he pretend a banana is a phone? 33. Does your child wake three or more times during the night? 34. Is your child too worried or fearful? If "sometimes" or "often or always," please describe:
48 and 60 month	33. Does your child wake three or more times during the night? 34. Is your child too worried or fearful? If "sometimes" or "often or always," please describe: 35. Does your child have simple back-and-forth conversations with you? For example, Parent: "It's raining!" Child: "And cold outside." Parent: "Let's get your coat." Child: "I got it!"

Note: The 2 month questionnaire is new to ASQ:SE-2.

Table 1.2. Comparison of ASQ:SE editions

Feature	First edition	Second edition
Questionnaire age intervals	8 intervals: 6, 12, 18, 24, 30, 36, 48, and 60 months	9 intervals: 2, 6, 12, 18, 24, 30, 36, 48, and 60 months
Screening "window"	3 months to 5.5 years	1 month to 6 years
Items added	Not applicable	New items added to increase sensitivity to autism, social-emotional competence, and early communicative and regulatory behaviors
Correction for prematurity	Optional	Recommended (adjusted age was used in validity and reliability studies)
Number of scored items	Between 19 items (6 months) and 33 (60 months)	Between 16 items (2 months) and 36 items (60 months)
Item response options	Most of the time, sometimes, rarely or never	Often or always, sometimes, rarely or never
Results	Above cutoff, below cutoff	Above cutoff, monitoring zone, below cutoff
Normative sample (*N*)	3,014	14,074 (16,424 questionnaires)
Concurrent validity sample	1,041	2,862
Overall sensitivity; overall specificity	78% (sensitivity) 94% (specificity)	81% (sensitivity) 84% (specificity)
Overall agreement	92%	83%

MATERIALS IN THE ASQ:SE-2 SYSTEM

This section briefly describes materials in the ASQ:SE-2 system, beginning with the *ASQ:SE-2™ Starter Kit,* the User's Guide, and the English and Spanish questionnaires. Then, other key materials in the ASQ:SE-2 system are introduced, including the *ASQ:SE-2™ Quick Start Guide, ASQ:SE-2™ Learning Activities,* and training materials. The section next offers an overview of ASQ Online, which offers data management and online questionnaire completion for the ASQ:SE-2 and ASQ-3. Finally, the section provides information about translations of ASQ:SE-2 available in other languages.

ASQ:SE-2 Starter Kit

The Starter Kit is for program personnel who are considering use of the questionnaires, exploring their potential use, or initiating their use. Each Starter Kit includes

1. Questionnaires box (in English or Spanish)
    - Nine reproducible master questionnaires and Information Summary sheets for scoring
    - CD-ROM with printable PDFs of the questionnaires
    - Social-Emotional Development Guides and Activities
2. User's Guide
3. Quick Start Guide

ASQ:SE-2 User's Guide

This User's Guide provides a comprehensive description of the entire system and can help personnel make appropriate adaptations of the questionnaire system to meet the needs of the populations they serve and their available resources. The User's Guide describes the assessment items, offers strategies for using the ASQ:SE-2 system, and explains how to contend with factors that may affect results (e.g., the time and setting variables in a child's development and health). In addition, the User's Guide contains useful appendixes designed to aid in the screening and monitoring process. More information about chapter contents and appendixes is provided at the end of this chapter.

ASQ:SE-2 Questionnaires

As noted, ASQ:SE-2 questionnaires are the heart of the system. There are nine reproducible master questionnaires and nine reproducible, age-appropriate Information Summary sheets—available in the ASQ:SE-2 box as a paper set and in PDF format on CD-ROM. In addition, the keycode on the ASQ:SE-2 box opens access to questionnaires within an ASQ Online data management subscription (ASQ Pro or ASQ Enterprise) or a questionnaire completion subscription (ASQ Family Access). Program personnel can select the appropriate format option(s) and age interval(s) needed and reproduce only the number of questionnaires necessary. The boxed set of questionnaires (in English or Spanish) also includes a brief Product Overview booklet and reproducible supplemental materials designed to support the use of ASQ:SE-2.

ASQ:SE-2 in Spanish

The ASQ:SE-2 questionnaires are available in Spanish and are supported by other ASQ:SE-2 Spanish materials, including the Quick Start Guide, parent letters and forms (see Appendix D), and Social-Emotional Development Guides and Activities (see Appendix E). The Spanish questionnaires have been field-tested with Spanish-speaking parents in a variety of geographic regions across the United States (e.g., Arizona, Texas, Washington State). Separate cutoff points have not been empirically derived, however. Differential item functioning analyses indicate that English and Spanish items function similarly for young children in both languages, for the most part.

The ASQ:SE-2 Spanish translation was reviewed by a panel of experts with knowledge of different Spanish dialects (e.g., Mexican, Puerto Rican, Chilean, Uruguayan) to ensure the translation is accurate and as widely accessible as possible for the variety of Spanish dialects spoken by families in the United States. These experts offered feedback about appropriate word usage and readability, which was carefully reviewed and incorporated by the translator—a professional with numerous years of experience translating materials for the early care and education field.

ASQ:SE-2 Quick Start Guide

The Quick Start Guide is a brief overview that helps people quickly learn how to use the screening system. The laminated Quick Start Guide provides administration and scoring basics in an easy reference format. It offers an inexpensive way for programs to make sure that all staff using ASQ:SE-2 have key information and guidance to administer and score when they do not have the User's Guide available. The Quick Start Guide is available in packs of five in either English or Spanish.

ASQ:SE-2 Learning Activities

The *ASQ:SE-2™ Learning Activities* are available in English and Spanish and provide information about developmentally appropriate expectations and strategies that programs can offer to parents in areas related to children's social-emotional development. This resource provides simple, fun social-emotional activities as well as information about topics that affect social-emotional development such as positive feeding routines (including breast feeding), typical sleeping patterns for different ages, toilet learning, and positive guidance.

ASQ:SE-2 Training Materials

The *ASQ:SE-2™ in Practice* DVD describes procedures for using and scoring the questionnaires. Programs may use this DVD training tool to introduce ASQ:SE-2 and show staff how to screen, score, and interpret results. The *Ages & Stages Questionnaires® on a Home Visit* DVD and *ASQ-3™ Scoring & Referral* DVD may be useful supplements for staff learning about screening and the ASQ system. The ASQ-3 and ASQ:SE informational web site (www.agesandstages.com) is updated with information about additional training materials for administrators and program staff as they are developed and become available.

Regularly hosted seminars and customized, on-site training seminars are available for ASQ:SE-2 users through Brookes Publishing's professional development program, Brookes On Location. The seminars give an introduction to social-emotional screening, a detailed overview of ASQ:SE-2, an overview of the role of parents in the screening process, and specific information on how to interpret ASQ:SE-2 scores and make referral decisions. Please visit www.brookesonlocation.com for more information.

ASQ Online System

ASQ:SE-2 and ASQ-3 users can manage their screening program within the ASQ Online system. Subscribers use the keycode printed on their ASQ:SE-2 or ASQ-3 box to access the appropriate questionnaires (ASQ:SE-2 in English or Spanish, or ASQ-3 in English or Spanish). ASQ Pro (for single-site programs and practices) or ASQ Enterprise (for multisite programs) include automated scoring, easy report generation, and other features designed to help programs organize their screening program, administer ASQ:SE-2 and ASQ-3, and manage data. ASQ Pro and ASQ Enterprise help personnel

- Create and manage child and program records
- Select the right questionnaire age interval
- Eliminate scoring errors and improve over- and underreferral rates
- Store results and follow-up decisions in child records
- Track when children need to be screened again
- Analyze results with child and program reports
- Access activities parents can try at home to encourage child progress
- Generate aggregate reports that show trends across multiple screening programs (ASQ Enterprise only)

An ASQ Hub account allows states or large organizations to link, aggregate, and review data from programs that use ASQ Pro and ASQ Enterprise in order to monitor ASQ:SE-2 and ASQ-3 screening across multiple programs while keeping child data secure and confidential.

ASQ Family Access permits parents to complete ASQ:SE-2 and ASQ-3 questionnaires for their children online using a secure, private web site. Programs may add ASQ Family Access to a Pro or Enterprise account. They can tailor a welcome page and customize it with their logo and contact information. ASQ Family Access is flexible, user friendly, and cost effective.

Translations

The ASQ:SE-2 questionnaires are available in English and Spanish through Brookes Publishing, and work is underway for translations into other languages. Please visit www.agesandstages.com for information about translations that are available for the previous edition or currently under development for ASQ:SE-2.

OTHER MATERIALS AND INFORMATION SUPPORTING ASQ USERS

Updated information about the ASQ:SE-2 and ASQ-3 family of products can be found at www.agesandstages.com. This robust web site offers news and research updates, user case stories, a searchable resource library with supplemental content and basic training materials, videos, and answers to frequently asked questions. The web site also offers a free calculator for selecting the correct ASQ:SE-2 interval and for adjusting scoring when items are omitted. *ASQ News & Updates* is a free monthly newsletter that includes articles, case studies, and helpful user tips. Users may subscribe at www.brookespublishing.com/newsletters. Users may gain access to ASQ information via social media, including Facebook (https://www.facebook.com/agesandstagesquestionnaires), Twitter (https://twitter.com/BrookesASQ), and Pinterest (https://www.pinterest.com/ASQScreener), for additional news and updates.

THE RELATIONSHIP BETWEEN ASQ:SE-2 AND ASQ-3

Because ASQ:SE-2 specifically focuses on a child's social-emotional behavior, it should be used in conjunction with ASQ-3 or another screening measure that provides information on a child's communicative, motor, problem-solving, and adaptive behaviors. ASQ-3 questionnaires are sold separately and are a series of developmental questionnaires used to identify the need for further developmental evaluation for children from 1 month to 72 months of age. ASQ-3 is available in English, Spanish, and a few additional languages. ASQ-3 addresses five developmental areas: communication, gross motor, fine motor, problem solving, and personal-social. An Overall section asks questions that are indicative of potential developmental problems in young children. The accompanying *ASQ-3™ User's Guide* (Squires et al., 2009) is available to assist professionals using ASQ-3 questionnaires.

USING THE ASQ:SE-2 SYSTEM

The ASQ:SE-2 system is designed for two important purposes. First, it is a comprehensive, first-level screening system for infants and young children. It can be used with large groups of children whose parents complete simple questionnaires on the status of their children's social-emotional competence. Second, the system can be used to longitudinally monitor (i.e., track over time) the behavioral development of children who are at risk for social-emotional disabilities or delays. Children who are at risk for medical or environmental reasons may benefit from monitoring. Risk factors may include prematurity, health problems, poverty, parental substance abuse, or parental depression. Monitoring children's social-emotional status using ASQ:SE-2 provides information about children's development over time and provides opportunities for parents to ask about their children's behavior and have their concerns addressed early.

As noted previously, the questionnaires can be used in a variety of ways. For example, questionnaires can be used at each available interval (e.g., 2, 6, 12, 18, 24, 30, 36, 48, and 60 months), one time only (e.g., 12 months), or at a few selected intervals (e.g., 12, 24, and 36 months). The questionnaires are designed to be completed by a child's parent and can be used by educational, health, or social services programs in a wide variety of ways. Program staff can complete questionnaires with parents at home during home visits; they can send questionnaires home via mail or during contact with families (e.g., distributing them in a child's "mailbox" at preschool, following a meeting or office visit); or they can send parents a link to a secure ASQ Family Access web site to complete questionnaires. Paper and online questionnaires also can be completed in clinics, schools, and child care settings. Chapters 8 and 9 provide detailed information on ASQ:SE-2 administration methods and settings.

Administration and Scoring

Although the questionnaires are designed to be completed by parents, ASQ:SE-2 requires professional involvement. Using an interdisciplinary team of professionals (e.g., health, educational, mental health, and parent support professionals) to determine appropriate follow-up action is recommended because of the complex nature of social-emotional behaviors and potential interventions. One or more professionals are needed to establish the screening and monitoring system, develop the necessary interfaces to community connections and resources, and assist individuals in the use of ASQ:SE-2. Once the screening program is operational, paraprofessionals and support staff can manage much of the system by scoring the questionnaires and providing routine feedback to families of children identified as not requiring further assessment or monitoring. Questionnaires generally can be completed by parents in 10–15 minutes, and scoring by professionals takes less than 5 minutes. Professional staff members must be available to provide feedback to parents and make appropriate referrals when concerns are identified during the screening process.

An ASQ:SE-2 Information Summary sheet for each age interval is included with the questionnaire. This form not only provides space for recording basic information about the child and scoring the questionnaire but also guides the professional in interpreting the results and determining appropriate follow-up. If parents keep the questionnaire for further reference about their child's social-emotional development, then this sheet offers a quick summary of questionnaire results, parent concerns, and follow-up action decisions. The Information Summary sheet may be shared with a child's pediatrician or other professionals with parent permission.

To score a questionnaire, the parent responses (*often or always, sometimes,* and *rarely or never*) to each item are converted to points—0, 5, or 10. In addition, parents may indicate if the behavior addressed in an item is of concern. If the Concern box is checked, then 5 points are added to that item score. Once totaled, a child's score is compared with an empirically derived cutoff point that is shown on the ASQ:SE-2 Information Summary sheet. A score below the cutoff indicates that the child appears to show typical social-emotional development at the time of administration. A child whose score is in the monitoring zone should be considered for referral, especially if the child is a girl. Parent concerns should be addressed, and the child should be re-screened within a few months. If a child's score is above the cutoff, then further diagnostic assessment is required. Regardless of a child's score, if a parent indicates any behaviors of concern, then program staff should follow up, providing support and information and making referrals if deemed appropriate.

ADVANTAGES OF ASQ:SE-2

The ASQ:SE-2 system has several important advantages. First, it is cost effective and accurate. ASQ:SE-2 relies on parents to observe their children and complete simple questionnaires about social-emotional behaviors, which helps reduce screening administration costs and enhances the accuracy of screening assessments by tapping into parents' extensive knowledge of their children (Dieterich, Landry, Smith, Swank, & Hebert, 2006; Fenson et al., 2007; O'Neill, 2007).

A second advantage is that using parent-completed tools such as ASQ:SE-2 promotes family engagement and addresses important requirements for programs such as IDEA 2004 that call for parents to be partners in their children's assessment and intervention activities. Completing the questionnaires helps parents gain valuable information about their children's development in relation to important social-emotional behaviors.

Flexibility is a third advantage of the ASQ:SE-2 system. ASQ:SE-2 can be used in a wide variety of settings, including homes, health care clinics, child care centers, and preschools, and in targeted programs, such as those for teenage parents. How the questionnaires are completed also is flexible. For example, questionnaires can be completed independently by parents; by parents during home visits from nurses, social workers, or paraprofessionals; or by teachers or caregivers who spend at least 15–20 hours per week with a child. Professionals can determine when and how often to conduct screening, ranging from one-time completion to administration at regular intervals for children who are at high risk. ASQ:SE-2's flexibility is further enhanced by providing program personnel with a master set of questionnaires. Screening programs may choose ASQ:SE-2 age intervals to accommodate their programs' goals and resources and the populations they serve. For example, medical practitioners may use the 18 month ASQ:SE-2 interval because it corresponds to the time of well-child visits. Public health home visiting programs may choose the 2 month and 12 month questionnaires because these intervals correspond to home visiting schedules. Head Start programs may use the 36, 48, and 60 month questionnaires to address program guidelines. Finally, the ASQ Family Access online questionnaire completion system offers great flexibility because it allows parents to complete ASQ:SE-2 questionnaires in their homes or wherever they access the Internet. Additional advantages of the ASQ:SE-2 system, such as ease of questionnaire completion and questionnaire scoring, are discussed in Chapter 2.

The advantages of parental involvement, low costs, easy completion, and flexible use all may be belied if the measure is not valid and reliable. The next sections explain why programs need to be concerned about the psychometric data for a screening tool and provide a brief overview of selected psychometric properties of ASQ:SE-2. The measure has been extensively studied, and results offer assurance that the questionnaires accurately evaluate the social-emotional status of young children.

IMPORTANCE OF PSYCHOMETRIC DATA

Users of screening measures should take time to review and understand the psychometric data collected on validity, reliability, and utility. They should make sure that the screening test has been used with a similar population of children and families and that there are studies that provide evidence that the test identifies children accurately. They should exercise caution in using a measure if it lacks psychometric information or data to support its reliability or validity.

A screening measure may miss children who have delays or disabilities if it is not accurate. The measure should correctly identify children as developing typically when in fact they are (i.e., specificity). In addition, children whose behaviors do not match age expectations should be correctly identified as at risk (i.e., sensitivity). Examining test sensitivity and specificity is crucial. No screening measure has perfect sensitivity or specificity because of the brevity of this type of measure. Nonetheless, a measure should be studied thoroughly and the findings should provide assurance of reasonable validity and reliability so that users can trust the results.

OVERVIEW OF ASQ:SE-2 PSYCHOMETRIC DATA

Psychometric data reported on the first edition of ASQ:SE offered reasonable assurance of the measure's reliability and validity as well as its utility (Squires et al., 2002). With development of this second edition also came the requirement of collecting data to ensure psychometric soundness. From 2009 to 2013, data were collected on more than 14,000 children ranging in age from 1 to 72 months. These data were used to establish new cutoff scores for ASQ:SE-2. In addition, subsamples of these data were used to examine selected psychometric properties of the revision.

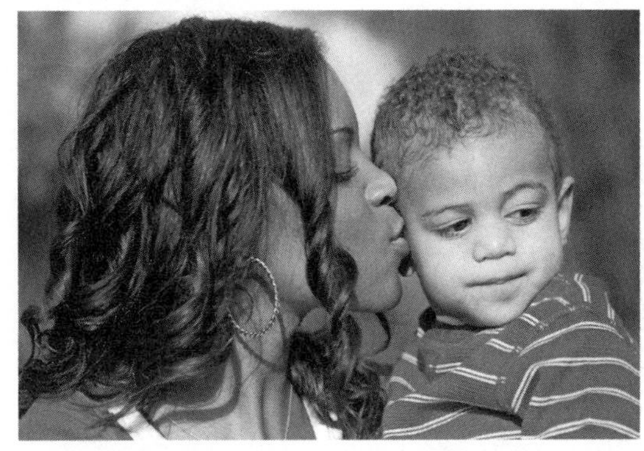

Perhaps the most important psychometric findings address the accuracy of ASQ:SE-2 as determined by its sensitivity and specificity. *Sensitivity,* or the ability of the screening tool to identify those children with social-emotional disabilities, ranges from 77% to 84%, with 81% overall sensitivity. *Specificity,* or the ability of the screening tool to correctly identify those children without social-emotional delays, ranges from 76% to 98%, with 84% overall specificity. In addition, reliability data suggest that scores tended to remain the same over time. Finally, utility data suggest that the questionnaires are easy for parents to complete within an acceptable time frame.

These results support the overall accuracy of ASQ:SE-2 in discriminating between children with social-emotional problems and those who appear to be developing typically in terms of social-emotional behaviors. The ASQ:SE-2 cutoff scores and psychometric studies are described in detail in Appendix C.

HOW THIS GUIDE IS ORGANIZED

This User's Guide is written for professionals who plan to use the ASQ:SE-2 system. The chapters that follow provide information about the need for screening children's social-emotional competency; key guidance about planning, using, and evaluating an ASQ:SE-2 screening/monitoring system; and specific information and examples for implementing ASQ:SE-2.

- Chapter 2 examines the need for screening and monitoring, previous approaches to screening, problems with these approaches, and the inception and development of the ASQ:SE-2 system.

- Chapter 3 provides an overview of the ASQ:SE-2 system, including its components and phases.
- Chapter 4 describes how to plan a screening/monitoring program and the methods for using and scoring ASQ:SE-2.
- Chapter 5 outlines how to organize and manage ASQ:SE-2 within a program.
- Chapter 6 explains the essentials of ASQ:SE-2 administration, scoring, and follow-up.
- Chapter 7 offers information about evaluating the implementation of the system.
- Chapter 8 describes various completion methods for ASQ:SE-2.
- Chapter 9 describes various settings in which ASQ:SE-2 may be used.
- Chapter 10 shares family case studies to illustrate use of ASQ:SE-2 in different settings.

The User's Guide appendixes provide supplemental information to support ASQ:SE-2 users. Appendix A lists recommended readings related to ASQ:SE-2 and developmental screening. Appendix B is a glossary to use when planning and implementing a screening or monitoring program. Appendix C provides a description of the psychometric data collected on ASQ:SE-2 as well as a comparison of the cutoff scores for ASQ:SE and ASQ:SE-2. Appendixes D and E contain reproducible materials to support implementation of ASQ:SE-2, including sample letters and forms and social-emotional guides and parent–child activities to encourage a child's development. Appendix F lists useful resources related to social-emotional development. Appendix G outlines recommended procedures for translating and adapting ASQ:SE-2 to meet the needs of families across cultures.

2

The Need for ASQ:SE-2

ASQ:SE-2™

The quality of life experience during infancy and early childhood has a significant effect on subsequent development (Campbell et al., 2014; Knitzer & Perry, 2009; National Scientific Council on the Developing Child, 2007). Serious medical, biological, and environmental problems demand swift attention and remediation to ensure children's healthy developmental outcomes (AAP, 2006; Durlak, Weissberg, Dymnicki, Taylor, & Shellinger, 2011; Giannoni & Kass, 2012; Squires & Bricker, 2007). Therefore, early identification of children whose developmental or behavioral trajectory is delayed or atypical is essential in order to institute timely action to correct or attenuate problems. Early identification of children with developmental or behavior problems is predicated on the assumption that it is possible to distinguish between children who are developing typically or whose problems are transitory and children who are facing serious and persistent challenges (Bricker, Macy, Squires, & Marks, 2013; Giannoni & Kass, 2012). Acknowledging the importance of early identification/Child Find has led to steady progress toward the timely detection of children with developmental and social-emotional delays since the mid-1980s (Macy, 2012; Pizur-Barnekow et al., 2010; Simard, Luu, & Gosselin, 2012).

NEED FOR SCREENING AND MONITORING

In addition to a general societal consensus that early detection of problems is a worthwhile goal, other important factors have contributed to the growing commitment by local, state, and federally funded agencies to monitor the development of designated groups of infants and young children, including the following:

- A growing population of infants and young children at risk for developmental and social-emotional problems because of environmental conditions, such as poverty, parental drug abuse, neglect, and homelessness
- Increased emphasis on prevention of developmental and social-emotional disabilities and chronic illnesses
- Evidence for the effectiveness of quality early intervention
- Legal and statutory regulations addressing the need for early and effective early identification/Child Find programs

These factors, among others, have led to a growing number of federal- and state-supported programs designed to identify and track the development of infants and young children who are at risk for future problems. The growth in early identification and monitoring of risk groups underlines the need for reliable and cost-effective screening and monitoring approaches. To be effective, screening measures and procedures must accurately discriminate between children who require further, more comprehensive assessment and those who do not. In addition, screening large groups of infants and young children becomes prohibitively expensive unless low-cost strategies are used.

Although early identification/Child Find efforts were initially focused on groups at risk, there is a growing awareness of and need for the screening of all infants and young children for two important reasons. First, in terms of absolute numbers, more children requiring intervention services are initially seen as typically developing as opposed to being assigned to a risk condition. Second, development varies over time, and the ability to predict outcomes by age 6 years remains imperfect. The developers of ASQ-3 and ASQ:SE-2, as well as professional organizations, are now advocating for the universal screening of all children in the United States (Bricker et al., 2013).

The need for accurate and low-cost screening and monitoring of infants and young children was the impetus for the development of the original ASQ and ASQ:SE as well as their subsequent revisions. These measures were created to offer a simple, economical solution to the early identification/Child Find needs of communities throughout the United States. The first step of developing ASQ was to define the target areas of children's development. Likewise, the first step in the development of the ASQ:SE and its revision, ASQ:SE-2, was to define social-emotional competence.

DEFINING SOCIAL-EMOTIONAL COMPETENCE

Raver and Zigler (1997), Squires and Bricker (2007), Zeanah and Zeanah (2009), and others noted a growing need to examine young children's social-emotional competence. Defining and accurately measuring young children's social-emotional abilities and potential difficulties is a complex undertaking, however. Accurate assessment is complex because the parameters of acceptable behavior are influenced by age (e.g., it is acceptable for an infant to cry when hungry, but it is not for an 8-year-old child under most circumstances); by cultural and family values (e.g., some families/cultures encourage children to be active inquisitors, whereas others do not); and by environmental circumstances (e.g., it is generally acceptable to yell and run on the playground, but it is not acceptable to do so in most stores). The complexities inherent in defining appropriate social-emotional behaviors for children at different developmental levels led to significant variability in what individuals, families, and communities identify as acceptable. Behavior occurs on a continuum. It often is not clear to peers, siblings, or adults when a child's behavioral response has crossed the line from an appropriate but immature response (e.g., sucking one's thumb) or temporary misbehavior (e.g., an infrequent temper tantrum) to a repeated behavior (e.g., physically attacking other children) that will cause serious difficulties for the child. Descriptions of young children who have serious social-emotional problems suggest a gradual acceleration in frequency of troubling behavior, severity of the behavioral response, or both, until the child crosses a line that at least some adults or peers deem unacceptable.

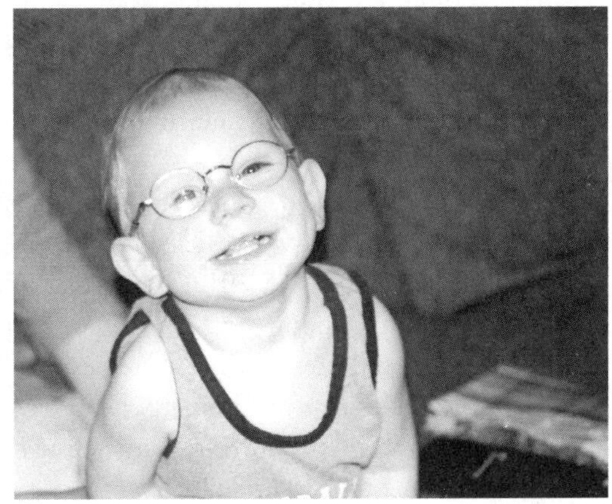

The complexities surrounding the definitions of social competence and emotional competence likely explain, in part, the lag in the timely identification of these problems in comparison with the more accurate and timely identification of cognitive, communication, and motor problems in young children (Feil et al., 2014; Jones & Bouffard, 2012). Our past inability to reliably identify children who require immediate intervention or those who are at significant risk for the development of serious social-emotional problems is particularly troublesome given the broad agreement that early identification of social-emotional problems or potential problems is the most effective prevention/intervention strategy that exists (Campbell et al., 2014; Feil et al., 2014; Yoshikawa et al., 2013).

The conceptual underpinnings for ASQ:SE and ASQ:SE-2 include the social learning model (Bandura, 1997; Patterson, Reid, & Dishion, 1992), which posits that social learning occurs as a function of the child's daily social interactions. In addition, the developmental organizational theory of Cicchetti (1993; Cicchetti, Ackerman, & Izard, 1995) and the marginal deviation model (Dishion, French, & Patterson, 1995; Reid, 1993) provide useful complements to the social learning theory. These theories suggest that deviation from normal developmental trajectories occurs when the important social-emotional, cognitive, and social-cognitive processes are not meaningfully integrated into more advanced levels of complex functioning. For example, if children are not taught to identify and label their emotions as preschoolers, their tantrums and acting-out behaviors may escalate. Disturbances (or inappropriate social learning) at earlier levels likely will cause continuing and more serious disturbances (faulty learning) at subsequent levels (Diamond, Barnett, Thomas, & Munro, 2007; Jones & Bouffard, 2012).

IDEA 2004 requires the use of assessment procedures that address children's social-emotional competence as well as delays and disabilities; however, social and emotional competence and disability are not clearly defined in federal regulations, and many states wait until school entrance to address these disabilities. This deficit likely has been the impetus for a growing literature whose purpose is to understand and appreciate social-emotional development and what constitutes competence and disability.

Social competence and emotional competence are clearly connected; however, we, and others, believe that the constructs of social competence and emotional competence represent distinct though overlapping developmental areas and behavioral processes. Grappling with definitional problems associated with social-emotional behavior has concerned a number of important contributors to developmental psychology (e.g., Emde, Korfmacher, & Kubicek, 2000; Jones & Bouffard, 2012; Landy, 2009; Raver & Zigler, 1997; Waters & Sroufe, 1983). Two important working assumptions can be gleaned from these authors' writings. First, the constructs of the behavioral domains of social competence and emotional competence can be usefully separated into two areas, with the understanding that there is also overlap, in order to have a comprehensive and detailed understanding of young children's behavior. Second, the definitions of these constructs need to address setting/time and children's development, children's health, and family/cultural variables in order to be useful. That is, definitions composed of specific behaviors (e.g., child shares toys with peers) cannot adequately account for wide variations in social-emotional competence. Rather, definitions need to address general processes that transcend setting; time; and developmental, health, and family/cultural variables and accommodate wide variation in specific behavioral indices. The definitions of social competence and emotional competence and their relationship are shown in Figure 2.1.

Social competence can be defined as an array of behaviors that permits one to develop and engage in positive interactions with peers, siblings, parents, and other adults (see Figure 2.1) (Jones & Bouffard, 2012; Raver & Zigler, 1997). For example, 4-year-old José, who typically engages his siblings and peers in appropriate play, elicits helpful assistance from teachers and parents, and uses positive strategies to solve problems, will likely be seen as a socially competent child. Four-year-old Linda, who typically fights over toys, is noncompliant, and attempts to solve problems by hitting, may not be seen as socially competent or at least may be seen as less socially competent than José.

Determining if children similar to José are socially competent often is more straightforward than identifying those children who are lacking such competence, such as Linda. For example, when 3-year-old Tommy yells and snatches a toy, this social behavior may be deemed appropriate if the toy was originally taken from Tommy, or it may be deemed inappropriate if Tommy instigated the aggression. When children exhibit prosocial behavior, the analysis is generally simple and straightforward; however, when children behave negatively, aggressively, or inappropriately, one cannot automatically conclude that the response indicates an issue with social competence.

Using a definition that transcends specific behaviors, *emotional competence* can be defined as the ability to effectively regulate emotions to accomplish one's goals (Campos et al., 1994). Emotional reactions can occur alone or overlay other responses, such as verbal responses. For example, if a toy is taken from Yolinda, she can cry or she can cry while delivering the verbal message, "Give it back." The 3-year-old who calms easily after a frightening experience, who controls his or her anger when disciplined, and who smiles and laughs at funny stories likely is seen as emotionally competent. The 3-year-old who cries uncontrollably at an unfamiliar sight, who screams frequently, and who is unresponsive for extended periods may be seen as having emotional problems. As with social behavior, however, the appropriateness of an emotional response is affected by setting/time and the child's development, his or her health, and

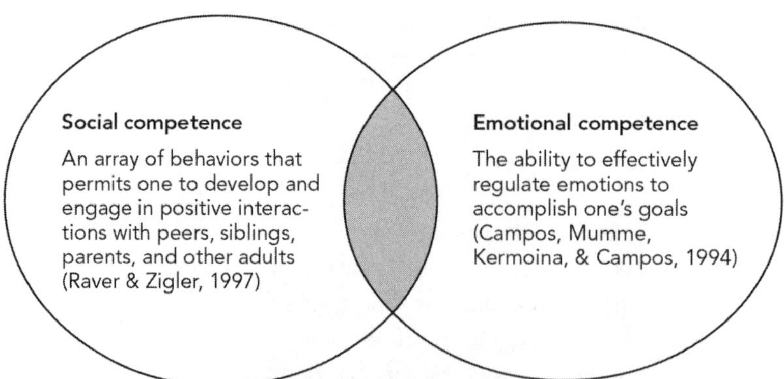
Social competence
An array of behaviors that permits one to develop and engage in positive interactions with peers, siblings, parents, and other adults (Raver & Zigler, 1997)
Emotional competence
The ability to effectively regulate emotions to accomplish one's goals (Campos, Mumme, Kermoina, & Campos, 1994)

Figure 2.1. Relationship between the behavioral domains of social competence and emotional competence.

family/cultural variables. As with defining social competence, it is generally easier to decide if a child is emotionally competent than to decide if a child has emotional problems and needs intervention.

NEED FOR THE ASQ:SE-2 SYSTEM

A significant need exists for a psychometrically sound, low-cost screening instrument that can accurately reflect the social-emotional competence of infants, toddlers, and preschool-age children. Many of the available social-emotional tools are not designed for large-scale screening of children and therefore do not meet the criteria for low-cost screening. Some instruments take considerable time to complete, involve complex scoring, and require highly trained professionals to interpret results. In addition, many tools have limited data available on their reliability, validity, and utility. Finally, some instruments do not include parents in a meaningful capacity.

ASQ:SE and its revision, ASQ:SE-2, were specifically designed to be low-cost screening instruments with established validity and reliability. Using ASQ:SE-2 is economical because it relies on parents to complete simple, easy-to-read questions about their children at designated age intervals—from 1 month to 72 months. This approach ensures meaningful participation by parents. Parents report that the questionnaires take little time to complete (i.e., 10–15 minutes). Scoring the questionnaires is simple and can be done by a variety of practitioners, such as teachers and child care professionals. Interpreting the results is straightforward because children's scores can be compared with empirically derived cutoffs that indicate if children's development appears to be on track at the time of administration, if children should be monitored, or if they should receive further evaluation. The ASQ:SE-2 normative group closely approximates the demographics of the 2010 U.S. Census data (Bureau of the Census, 2011) for income, level of education, race, and ethnicity, and it includes a sizeable, representative number of children at each age interval. In addition, reliability (e.g., test–retest, internal consistency) and validity (e.g., concurrent) of ASQ:SE-2 have been studied with large groups of children. Both underreferral (i.e., children who should be identified are missed) and overreferral (i.e., children are identified who should not be) rates for ASQ:SE-2 are acceptable, indicating that, in most cases, the measure accurately identifies children who need further evaluation (i.e., sensitivity) and those who do not (i.e., specificity) (Briggs et al., 2012; Heo & Squires, 2012; Squires, Bricker, Heo, & Twombly, 2001; Squires, Bricker, & Twombly, 2004). See Appendix C for more details about the psychometric properties of ASQ:SE-2.

The most effective use of any screening instrument is within larger, coordinated early identification/Child Find systems and not as an isolated activity (Bricker et al., 2013); therefore, procedures for developing a comprehensive community-based screening program are included later in this User's Guide. Other screening and monitoring procedures are reviewed next to provide a context for the ASQ:SE-2 approach.

SCREENING AND MONITORING APPROACHES

Screening and monitoring of infants and young children have primarily been conducted by means of periodic follow-up with designated groups considered to be at risk for developmental disabilities. The major exceptions to this basic approach have been the general screening procedures conducted by the public schools with children entering kindergarten or programs such as Head Start that have mandated universal screening of enrolled children. Expanded efforts are underway to universally screen children from birth onward (Bricker et al., 2013) because of mounting evidence regarding the importance of early identification and effectiveness of early intervention for children with disabilities such as autism (Boyd, Odom, Humphreys, & Sam, 2010; Kim et al., 2011; Wallace & Rogers, 2010). Screening approaches can be classified as follows: the professionally based multidisciplinary team approach, the well-child checkup approach, the community-based evaluation roundup approach, the parent monitoring approach, and the universal screening approach.

Multidisciplinary Team Approach

The multidisciplinary team approach began in the 1970s and assesses designated groups of infants and young children at risk for developmental disabilities. Screening groups of premature infants with low birth weights who meet specific criteria (e.g., Casey, Whiteside-Mansell, Barrett, Bradley, & Gargus, 2006; Serenius et al., 2013) at designated intervals is an example of this type of approach. Much of the screening conducted by multidisciplinary teams is designed to determine the frequency of problems in specific populations of infants and/or locate variables that predict potential problems. Infants are brought to evaluation centers at established intervals and assessed with one or more standardized measures by highly trained professionals representing a range of disciplines. The children often are given medical or neurological examinations.

Well-Child Checkup Approach

A second approach to screening and monitoring is identifying infants and young children who are at risk for developmental delays at well-child checkups in physicians' offices or in public health facilities. The AAP (2014) recommends developmental surveillance at every well-child visit and emphasizes the importance of using formal, validated tools at 9, 18, and 24 or 30 months of age as well as screening for autism at 18 and 24 months (Johnson, Myers, & Council on Children with Disabilities, 2007). This method is a universal approach in that the goal is to screen all children who participate in well-child checkups at these ages—not only children who appear to have significant delays or whose parents express concern. National studies indicated that pediatricians are making progress toward this goal, with 48% reporting that they are screening children younger than 36 months using a standardized screening test, a 25% increase since 2002 (Radecki, Sand-Loud, O'Connor, Sharp, & Olson, 2011). Tests such as ASQ-3, Denver II (Frankenburg et al., 1996), and the Pediatric Symptom Checklist (Jellinek et al., 1999) are used by professionals or paraprofessionals to assess a child's developmental status. The tests used in this approach generally are quick to administer and can be used with young children at any age. Although this approach is often called universal, it is not because many children do not participate in well-child checkups.

Community-Based Evaluation Roundup Approach

Community-based evaluation roundup is a third approach to screening and monitoring. Roundups permit parents to bring their infants or young children to an evaluation center for screening. Roundups typically are scheduled one to four times per year and are staffed by professionals and volunteers. Measures are easy to administer and are appropriate for large groups of children. Frequently used measures include the Developmental Indicators for the Assessment of Learning–Fourth Edition (Mardell, & Goldenberg, 2011) and the Early Screening Inventory–Revised (Meisels, Marsden, Wiske, & Henderson, 2008).

Parent Monitoring Approach

Having parents monitor their children's development is a fourth approach to screening (Bricker et al., 2013; Heo, Squires, Yovanoff, & Lee, 2006; Squires et al., 2014; Squires, Bricker, & Potter, 1997; Squires, Nickel, & Bricker, 1990; Squires, Nickel, & Eisert, 1996). Measures suitable for a parent monitoring approach require minimal professional input and can be used at any age. One tool used is the Denver Prescreening Developmental Questionnaire II (Frankenburg & Bresnick, 1998), which is designed to be completed by parents in a physician's office. Knobloch and her associates (Knobloch, Stevens, Malone, Ellison, & Risemburg, 1979) developed the Revised Parent Developmental Questionnaire for the same purpose. Parents' Evaluation of Developmental Status (PEDS; Glascoe & Robertshaw, 2007) is a third example of a parent-completed screening questionnaire. PEDS asks parents about their general concerns in 10 developmental areas and is easily completed in pediatric and other settings. ASQ-3 is a final example that uses a parent monitoring approach. Although ASQ-3 shares similarities with each of the tests previously discussed, it differs in important ways that are discussed later in this chapter.

Universal Screening Approach

Some states are working toward a universal screening approach that will provide the opportunity for all children to have access to developmental and social-emotional screening at regular intervals. Universal screening approaches require large-scale coordination and collaboration between agencies that provide services to children and families—including but not limited to early intervention (IDEA Part C), early childhood special education (IDEA Part B, Section 619), Early Head Start, Head Start, child care, home visiting, primary health care, newborn hearing screening (Early Hearing Detection and Intervention), family support, parenting programs, and the child welfare system. To effectively track children, states are working to coordinate key health, educational, and social services data systems and are using unique child identifiers to share data between these systems. Several states are beginning to pilot electronic systems for screening, referral, and the exchange of data related to the referral and evaluation process. In turn, efforts are underway to create unified state early childhood comprehensive systems that include early education programs, Head Start grantees, early learning advisory councils, Child Care and Development Fund (CCDF) agencies, and quality rating and improvement systems (QRIS), all of which can serve as partners in the coordination of statewide screening efforts. Although there is much work to be done to make universal screening of children a reality, these efforts are heartening first steps.

CHALLENGES TO SCREENING/MONITORING PROGRAMS

Screening and monitoring young children's social-emotional development presents several challenges, including variability in children's social-emotional development, parent involvement, and cost. Each challenge is discussed next.

Children's Social-Emotional Development

As mentioned previously, the dynamic and complex nature of social-emotional development is perhaps the first and most important challenge for the timely identification of problems in infants and young children. Social-emotional development in most children, however, proceeds at a predictable rate and in a predictable fashion (Cicchetti et al., 1995; Freeman, 2014; Martoccio, Brophy-Herb, & Onaga, 2014). The child's early experiences within his or her family can either promote or interfere with learning to successfully regulate emotions and learning to develop and maintain positive social relationships. Families who provide safe, supportive, and enriching environments do much to foster healthy and appropriate social-emotional behavior. Living in families in which child abuse, neglect, or domestic violence are present, however, can lead to problems in social-emotional development and subsequent poor mental health outcomes as demonstrated by the Adverse Childhood Experiences (ACES) study (Centers for Disease Control and Prevention, 2014). In addition, children with physiologically based behavior problems (e.g., autism) are at high risk for a host of negative developmental and behavioral outcomes.

For a variety of reasons, children who do not follow a typical trajectory of social-emotional development may or may not be identified in a timely manner. Some behavior variations do not cause parental concern (e.g., a child who is withdrawn or anxious may be considered an "easy" child), whereas other behavior variations are quickly seen as problems (e.g., a child who has tantrums frequently, a child who is aggressive with peers). Social-emotional variations also do not occur at specified times—children may develop difficulties at any point. For example, a feeding problem during infancy may have a brief or a lasting effect on the child's subsequent social-emotional development.

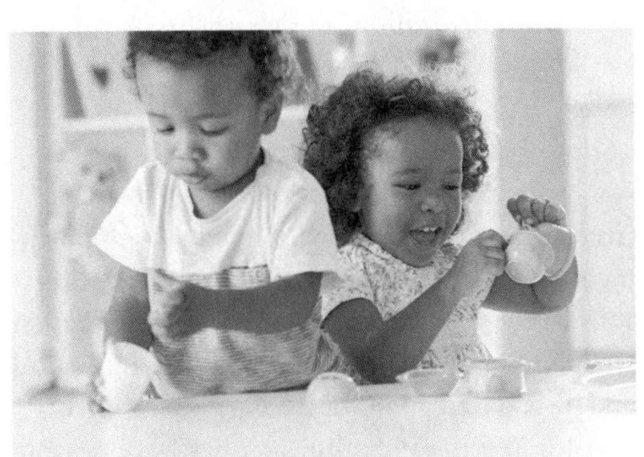

The transactional theory of development (Sameroff & Chandler, 1975) posits that caregiver–child interactions influence how children will develop. Physiological or environmental conditions confronting individual children can change and thus cannot be reliably predicted over time. One should not assume that because a child's social-emotional trajectory is on target at 9 months, it will remain on target as the child ages. In addition, one should not assume that an infant who has behaviors that are of concern at 4 months will continue to develop poorly. As a consequence, the dynamic nature of social-emotional development makes it prudent to repeatedly screen children over time and quickly address behaviors of concern. Screening programs that assess children at one point in time may overlook children whose problems occur after the assessment interval. In addition, if initial screening occurs when children are age 4 or 5 years old, then timely identification of problems and subsequent interventions may literally have been delayed by years. Programs that repeatedly screen children but at infrequent intervals also run the risk of untimely detection of social-emotional problems in children. All children should be screened at frequent intervals—that is, universal periodic screening of all children—to ensure the timely identification of children with suspect development.

Parent Involvement

Including parents and caregivers in assessing their children's developmental status is a second challenge for screening and monitoring programs. Families may be concerned about screening, or they may not want to participate for a variety of reasons. These reasons can range from reservations about "testing" their child, to fear of intrusive "systems," to annoyance with paperwork, to frustration with finding time. Some parents may be challenging to involve due to instability in their lives or cognitive or mental health challenges. Screening and monitoring measures that are completed by professionals with minimal parental input, however, do not reflect the intent of U.S. federal law or recommended practices, nor can they present a full picture of a child's developmental status.

Federal legislation has made it increasingly clear that parents have the right and responsibility to be involved in their child's assessment, intervention, and evaluation efforts, beginning with the Education of the Handicapped Act Amendments of 1983 (PL 98-199), followed by the Education of the Handicapped Act Amendments of 1986 (PL 99-457), and finally with the Individuals with Disabilities Education Act Amendments (IDEA) of 1997 (PL 105-17) and IDEA 2004. Using screening systems that do not include parents in meaningful and useful ways disregards this important mandate.

In addition, recommended practice dictates involving parents and other caregivers to ensure that their rich, extensive reservoir of information about the child is accessed (Sandall, Hemmeter, Smith, & McLean, 2005). Failure to gather and use parental information for determining the child's social-emotional status results in, at best, an incomplete assessment picture. Most parents know what their children can do and how they behave in familiar and unfamiliar environments. An assessment that takes place outside the home in a relatively short period of time may be inaccurate because children behave differently in different settings, at different times of day, and with different caregivers.

Engaging families and other caregivers in child assessment activities is also a recommended practice because this involvement has the potential to help parents acquire critical information concerning their child as well as learn more appropriate behavioral expectations for their child. Participation in a simple, straightforward assessment may alert parents to developmental skills important for their child to acquire and may alert parents to future developmental goals for their child. Participation in screening also may present parents with opportunities to ask questions about their child's behavior and seek information on the type of activities that may promote development in specific areas.

It is important to note that not all parents are equipped to accurately assess their child's behavior. In particular, parents with serious mental health problems, substance abuse issues, and other social-emotional disorders may not be capable of viewing their child objectively. In such cases, other screening strategies may be necessary as alternatives or for corroboration if a parent-completed measure is used.

Cost

Cost is a third challenge for screening and monitoring programs. Screening and monitoring large groups of children can be expensive. Yearly cost can be determined by calculating cost in two ways. First, cost can be calculated by multiplying the cost per child by the total number of children screened. For example, if it costs $10 per child and 100 children are screened, then the total cost is $1,000. A second way to determine cost is by number of children identified. This method may be particularly relevant for developmental screening because large numbers of children require screening in order to detect the few that need further assessment. Depending on risk factors associated with groups of children, only 15%–30% will be identified during the screening process (Bricker, Squires, Kaminski, & Mounts, 1988; Centers for Disease Control and Prevention, 2007; Hack et al., 2005; Serenius et al., 2013). Thus, if 100 children are screened at $10 per child and 30 children are detected, then the cost per detected child becomes much higher. These figures emphasize the importance of keeping cost per child low if communities are to conduct periodic screening for all their young children. The cost of frequent screening may become prohibitive when highly skilled professionals conduct screenings with designated target populations. For example, if a group of 100 children is screened by a skilled professional once per year for 6 years at the rate of $50 per screening, then the total cost of screening the children is $30,000, or $300 per child. On the contrary, first-level screening approaches that employ parents to complete developmental questionnaires can significantly reduce the cost of screening and monitoring large groups of children. For example, cost can be controlled by having paraprofessionals or office staff distribute the measures, score the results, and provide feedback to families of children who are typically developing. Professional expertise can be reserved to help families of children who require further assessment.

ASQ:SE-2 SYSTEM

The ASQ:SE-2 system was specifically developed to address the challenges described in the previous section. The ASQ:SE-2 system addresses the dynamic nature of social-emotional development by offering multiple assessment intervals. Parental participation is ensured by having parents evaluate their child's social-emotional status through answering simple, straightforward items about their child's behavior. Finally, having parents complete the questionnaires instead of professional test administration helps ensure that the system is cost effective.

Chapter 3 provides an overview of the ASQ:SE-2 system, which has three components: 1) questionnaires, 2) procedures for their use, and 3) support materials for adapting the system. In addition, the system has four phases: 1) planning the screening/monitoring program; 2) preparing, organizing, and managing the screening/monitoring system; 3) administering and scoring the questionnaires and conducting follow-up; and 4) evaluating the screening/monitoring program. Each of these phases is discussed in detail in Section II (Chapters 4–7).

Advantages of the ASQ:SE-2 System

ASQ:SE-2 has several key advantages, including parental involvement, ease of scoring and completion, flexibility, and cost effectiveness. Supported by extensive research, ASQ-SE-2 can be used in a wide range of settings and can meet the needs of a variety of programs, communities, and individuals.

Parent Engagement

Parental participation in assessing children's social-emotional development is the primary advantage of using ASQ:SE-2. Creating a screening/monitoring system that requires parental participation and encourages parent engagement addresses three important goals. First, ASQ:SE-2 meets federal and state guidelines that mandate the meaningful inclusion of parents in their child's assessment process. Second, using ASQ:SE-2 helps educate parents about social-emotional development and about whether their child's behavior is similar to that of same-age peers. Completing questionnaires may aid parents in understanding their child's strengths or areas that may benefit from attention. Third, including parents makes using ASQ:SE-2 one of the least costly screening strategies currently available.

Extensive Research Base

Developers of ASQ:SE-2 have collected extensive data on selected parameters of its utility, reliability, and validity. In addition, normative data from more than 14,000 children have been assembled and used to derive cutoff scores for each ASQ:SE-2 age interval. Users report that the questionnaires address important social-emotional behaviors and that they are easy to complete within a reasonable time frame. Validity findings support the accuracy of ASQ:SE-2 in identifying children whose social-emotional status requires further assessment, with excellent sensitivity (.81) and specificity (.84). Test–retest reliability findings suggest that there is high stability of scores over time. Details on cutoff norms and psychometric findings are provided in Appendix C.

Ease of Questionnaire Completion

ASQ:SE-2 questionnaires are intentionally short and contain differing numbers of items, depending on the age of the child and complexity of behaviors being evaluated. The number of items ranges from 19 (on the 2 month interval) to 39 (on the 60 month interval). The reading level is at a fourth- to sixth-grade level to ensure that the questionnaires are understandable to most parents without any training or professional input. Although a few parents will need assistance (e.g., those who cannot read), most parents can successfully complete a questionnaire whether it is mailed to them, they access it on the Internet, or they are offered a print copy to complete in person. Parents are required to read each item, check a score box, and indicate if the behavior in the item is of concern. Parents generally report a completion time of 10–15 minutes. This small time investment is acceptable to most parents, although there are those with significant challenges in their lives (e.g., mental health problems, substance abuse, mental disability) for whom independent completion of the questionnaires is not possible.

Ease of Questionnaire Scoring

Scoring a completed ASQ:SE-2 questionnaire is simple and can be done in approximately 3–5 minutes. Scoring requires summing the checked responses and concerns for each item. Item scores are added and then a total is compared with a cutoff score for each age interval. The age interval cutoff score is provided on the Information Summary sheet for each questionnaire. Children's scores dictate subsequent actions. Children with results below the cutoff score are considered to be typically functioning at the time of administration. Children with results close to the cutoff are in the monitoring zone; they are considered to be at risk and require monitoring, with possible follow-up action needed. Children with scores above the cutoff should be referred for further assessment.

Questionnaire scoring is automated for programs using the ASQ Online system. For programs with an ASQ Family Access subscription for questionnaire completion, results are transferred to their ASQ Pro or Enterprise account for scoring and professional evaluation.

Flexibility of Screening Administration

The ASQ:SE-2 system can be adapted to meet the specific needs of communities and programs that may have widely varying goals, populations served, and available resources. Programs may decide to mail questionnaires to families' homes, ask parents to complete questionnaires online on a secure web site, or provide questionnaires for parents to complete during home visits. Other choices may entail completion during a parent and child visit to an evaluation center, a well-child checkup, or a visit to a physician's office, or completion during a telephone interview with the parents. Some communities and programs may choose to combine strategies so that most parents receive questionnaires through the mail or online, while a few parents (e.g., those who cannot read) complete questionnaires through telephone interviews. Some communities may develop a system in which all physicians and clinical staff ask parents to complete questionnaires prior to every well-child visit.

Cost Effectiveness of ASQ:SE-2

ASQ:SE-2 is a low-cost option for developmental-behavioral screening and monitoring for two reasons. First, parents complete the questionnaires rather than skilled professionals. Second, each program site need only make a one-time purchase of the ASQ:SE-2 box of questionnaires. The questionnaires can be reproduced and used for all participating families over time. The boxed set of masters contains nine questionnaires appropriate for screening children from 1 month to 72 months of age, included in reproducible formats—users can photocopy the paper masters or print questionnaires from the CD-ROM. ASQ Family Access, the online questionnaire completion system, is even more cost effective because it eliminates paper and postage costs. Because ASQ:SE-2 is a first-level screener, results from completed questionnaires clearly indicate whether a referral is needed, eliminating time and cost associated with second-level screening.

Challenges for the ASQ:SE-2 System

As with all screening/monitoring systems, ASQ:SE-2 has limitations and may present implementation challenges for program personnel.

Organizational Requirements

Using ASQ:SE-2 requires an organizational structure that ensures parents are receiving and returning questionnaires as directed by the program. Processes need to be in place and monitored to confirm that 1) questionnaires are mailed or given to parents; 2) information is collected at specified intervals; 3) questionnaires are returned and appropriately scored; and 4) parents are given the necessary feedback. It is also essential to confirm that support is provided and referrals are made as indicated by screening results. When screening large groups of children, procedures should be in place to ensure that the approach is implemented as planned. ASQ Online users can access technical assistance and ongoing updates to enhance their use of the ASQ:SE-2 system.

Need for Parent Cooperation

ASQ:SE-2 may not be appropriate for use with all families. Some parents may be unwilling or find it intrusive to complete questionnaires. In addition, some families may experience significant chaos in their lives, rendering them unable to complete a questionnaire. Parents who have cognitive or emotional impairments may be unable to understand the questionnaires, or their answers to questions may be more reflective of their own emotional state than the social-emotional development of their child. Alternatives may be necessary for these parents and families.

Cultural and Language Modifications

It may be necessary to make cultural and/or linguistic modifications to the questionnaires for some families because there is no screening tool that is appropriate for all families in all settings. Items that are not compatible with a family's cultural norms (e.g., making eye contact) may need to be omitted (Heo & Squires, 2012; Lyman, Njoroge, & Willis, 2007). Language and other modifications to items or questionnaires also may be required. Although ASQ:SE has been translated into numerous languages (e.g., Spanish, French, Vietnamese, Chinese, Norwegian, Thai, Hmong, Somali), there will be families who speak languages and dialects for which a translation is not available. Experienced community members with knowledge of the culture and community support programs will need to assist program personnel in effectively using ASQ:SE-2 with families who speak different languages and who are from different cultural backgrounds. Chapter 10 presents examples that illustrate how to use ASQ:SE-2 with families from diverse backgrounds. Appendix G provides detailed information on considerations and procedures for translating and adapting ASQ:SE-2 for use with families of different linguistic and/or cultural backgrounds. Cultural guidelines on translating ASQ:SE-2 and ASQ-3 can be found at www.agesandstages.com.

Accuracy of Screeners

By definition, screening instruments are brief and easy to complete and score. They are not always accurate in their assessment of children's developmental status, however, because of their brevity. All screening measures misclassify some children; thus, it is important for users to examine the specificity and sensitivity of measures to ensure that they are using a tool that correctly classifies the majority of children. Although ASQ:SE-2 has excellent psychometric properties and will correctly identify the majority of children, it will occasionally overidentify or underidentify children. This is why it is especially important to review parent concerns and discuss when screening results may not reflect what adults have previously observed about the child's development.

CONCLUSION

Involving parents or caregivers is at the heart of ASQ:SE-2. The pivotal role of parents in the ASQ:SE-2 system addresses mandates for meaningful family involvement while keeping screening costs relatively low. In addition, flexibility in completing and scoring questionnaires and implementing the ASQ:SE-2 system provide a strong rationale for using this parent-completed questionnaire as a first-level screening approach. An overview of components and phases of the ASQ:SE-2 system is presented in Chapter 3.

3

The ASQ:SE-2 System

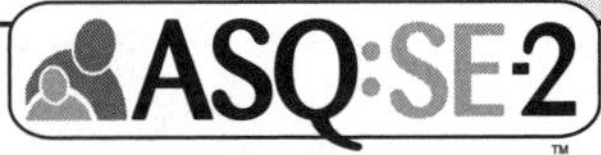

Assessing social-emotional competence and development in young children can be challenging because it is critical to evaluate children's responses through four important lenses—setting/time, development, health, and family/culture (see Chapter 2). Table 3.1 summarizes these four classes of variables, which are discussed next; it also lists examples of questions to consider when addressing each variable.

ASSESSING SOCIAL-EMOTIONAL COMPETENCE

Setting and time variables can affect the interpretation of children's behavior because a child's responses may vary across environments (e.g., home, school). These differences may occur for a variety of reasons, including the child's familiarity with a setting or situation-specific feedback. For example, a parent who responds to a tantrum at home by giving the child attention may be reinforcing that behavior and causing tantrums to occur more frequently and with increasing intensity. The same behavior, ignored at school, may quickly disappear.

Table 3.1. Variables and associated questions to consider when assessing social and emotional competence in young children

Variable	Questions to consider
Setting/time	Where, when, and under what environmental conditions does the behavior occur?
Development	What is the child's developmental level?
Health	What is the child's health status?
Family/cultural	What family/cultural factors are potentially associated with the behavior?

The social-emotional competence of children also needs to be viewed through a developmental lens. That is, the developmental level of children has a significant bearing on how acceptable or unacceptable people find specific behaviors. For example, a toddler who cries when confronted by a stranger may be seen as normal by most adults, who understand that the child is passing through a developmental stage. Most adults do not find it troubling when a 6-month-old pulls hair but will likely object to the same behavior exhibited by a 3-year-old. It is unacceptable to most adults for an 8-year-old to snatch a toy from a peer, whereas adults may tolerate such behavior from a 2-year-old.

Behaviors may also vary across gender. For example, girls' verbal skills typically develop at a faster pace than boys', and boys typically show more physical aggression in preschool classrooms than girls (Ostrov & Keating, 2004). Differing supports for social-emotional behaviors may be needed for families and classrooms based on these developmental differences.

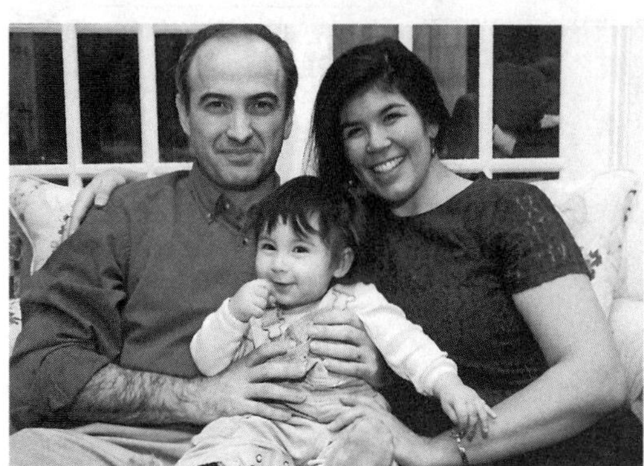

Photo by Terry Joseph Sam.

Evaluation of children's social-emotional behaviors also may require examining them through a health or physical fitness lens. Factors such as whether a child has a chronic illness (e.g., asthma, otitis media) or is tired, hungry, or reacting to a medication likely will affect how the child responds to daily events. A fussy infant who is difficult to soothe may be ill. A child who comes to school tired and hungry may display inappropriate social-emotional behaviors that likely would not occur if the child had adequate sleep and nourishment.

Finally, a child's social-emotional responses need to be considered through the lens of family and cultural values. The interactions among family members, especially a child's relationship to his or her parents, play an important part in the development of social-emotional competence. Family and cultural variables, including family dynamics, cultural norms, and the primary language spoken by family members, may have a significant effect on children's social-emotional behavior. Some families/cultures place great importance on children being quiet and unobtrusive, whereas other families/cultures encourage verbal interactions. As a consequence, a quiet or verbally outspoken child may be behaving in ways consistent with family values. For example, Japanese mothers often use more nonverbal responses with their infants, rocking them and using soothing sounds, whereas American mothers are often more verbal and encourage their infants to respond (Owens, 2010). Finally, young children who experience stress or trauma show signs through their behavior, including changes in sleeping and feeding behaviors.

ASQ:SE and its revision, ASQ:SE-2, were created with an appreciation for settings and times, children's development, children's health, and families' cultural values. Questionnaire items and guidance for interpreting results were written with an eye toward these important evaluative lenses. In addition, the developers adopted a conceptual framework that guided the creation of questionnaire items. This conceptual framework is described next.

CONCEPTUAL BASIS FOR ASQ:SE-2 CONTENT

The questionnaires' item content addresses seven behavioral constructs—self-regulation, compliance, adaptive functioning, autonomy, affect, social-communication, and interaction with people. Table 3.2 presents the seven behavioral constructs and their definitions. The separation into seven areas as well as the area names (e.g., self-regulation) are somewhat arbitrary but may help professionals understand the organization of ASQ:SE-2 and the intent of the individual questions.

Table 3.2. Seven behavioral areas of ASQ:SE-2 and associated definitions

Behavioral area	Associated definition
Self-regulation	Items address the child's ability or willingness to calm or settle down or adjust to physiological or environmental conditions or stimulation.
Compliance	Items address the child's ability or willingness to conform to the direction of others and follow rules.
Adaptive functioning	Items address the child's success or ability to cope with physiological needs (e.g., sleeping, eating, elimination, safety).
Autonomy	Items address the child's ability or willingness to self-initiate or respond without guidance (i.e., moving to independence).
Affect	Items address the child's ability or willingness to demonstrate his or her own feelings and empathy for others.
Social-communication	Items address the child's ability or willingness to interact with others by responding to or initiating verbal or nonverbal signals to indicate interests or needs, feelings, and affective or internal states.
Interaction	Items address the child's ability or willingness to respond to or initiate social responses to parents, other adults, and peers.

With the conceptual framework for questionnaire content in place, the developers examined the content of norm-referenced, standardized tests and other resources and gathered input from a multidisciplinary team of experts. Content that matched a specific age interval (e.g., 2, 6, 12 months) was used as the basis to develop specific items. The developers formulated items to assess competence and detect problem behaviors. Examples of competence-related items include the following: "Is your baby able to calm herself down (for example, by sucking her hand or pacifier)?" "Does your baby like to be picked up and held?" and "Does your baby let you know when she is hungry, tired, or uncomfortable? For example, does she fuss or cry?" Examples of items related to problem behaviors include the following: "Does your child have eating problems? For example, does he stuff food, vomit, eat things that are not food, or ___?" and "Does your child hurt himself on purpose?"

After content was selected for each age interval, the developers wrote the questionnaire items to ensure content met the following criteria:

- The item addresses important social-emotional milestones or problem behaviors that are indicative of social-emotional difficulties.
- The behavior the item addresses is easy for parents to observe and evaluate.
- The item text was written at or below a sixth-grade reading level.

Small illustrations are included to increase readability. Figure 3.1 shows an item from the 24 month questionnaire.

24. Does your child like to be around other children? For example, does she move close to or look at other children?

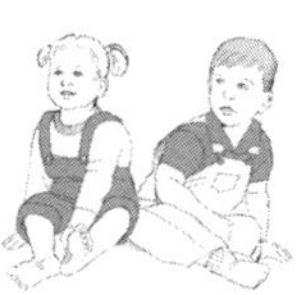

Figure 3.1. ASQ:SE-2 item example. Each ASQ:SE-2 questionnaire includes 19–39 simply worded questions, like the one above. Some items are accompanied by illustrations to assist parents in answering the questions about their child's behavior.

Table 3.3 presents the seven behavioral areas, their associated general content, and the specific ASQ:SE-2 items by age interval. ASQ:SE-2 items are not evenly distributed across the seven behavioral areas. The number and content of items varies across age intervals to reflect changes in child development.

The primary purpose of ASQ:SE-2 is to assist parents, educators, social services staff, and health/medical personnel in the timely identification of children with responses or patterns of responses that indicate the possibility of the development of future social-emotional difficulties. In other words, ASQ:SE-2 is designed to identify children whose social-emotional competence differs in some way from expectations associated with their chronological age. ASQ:SE-2 is not a diagnostic tool for identifying children with serious social-emotional disorders; rather, it should be seen as an aid in identifying young children who may benefit from more in-depth evaluation and/or preventive interventions designed to improve their social-emotional competence.

The next section describes the three components of the ASQ:SE-2 system—the questionnaires, the procedures for using and scoring the questionnaires, and the support materials. The remainder of the chapter discusses the four phases for using the ASQ:SE-2 system: 1) planning the screening/monitoring program; 2) preparing, organizing, and managing the screening/monitoring program; 3) administering and scoring ASQ:SE-2 and following up; and 4) evaluating the screening/monitoring program.

COMPONENTS OF THE SYSTEM

As noted, ASQ:SE-2 is a system composed of separate but linked and coordinated parts or components, each of which is described next.

Component 1: Questionnaires

ASQ:SE-2 is composed of nine questionnaires designed to be completed by parents to assess the social-emotional competence of their children. ASQ:SE-2 questionnaires can be used with all children from 1 month to 72 months of age. The nine age intervals are at 2, 6, 12, 18, 24, 30, 36, 48, and 60 months. The 2 month questionnaire has the shortest range and can be used with infants 1 month 0 days through 2 months 30 days, whereas the 6 through 30 month questionnaires each span 6-month age intervals, and the 36 through 60 month questionnaires each span longer age intervals of more than 6 months. For example, the 6 month questionnaire is used with infants from 3 months to 8 months, and the 12 month questionnaire is for infants from 9 months to 14 months. The 48 month questionnaire can be used with children from 42 months to 53 months, and the 60 month questionnaire is used with children from 54 months to 72 months. It is important to note that there are no gaps between age intervals, so the questionnaires are appropriate for use with any child from 1 month 0 days through 72 months 0 days.

The format for each questionnaire interval is the same. The first page is a family information sheet that asks for identifying information about the child and the person completing the questionnaire. The pages that follow contain the ASQ:SE-2 items—these are simple questions about a child's social-emotional behaviors. In addition to responding to each item, parents may indicate if any behavior targeted in an item is of concern to them. The last questions are open-ended and are designed to elicit overall parental concerns (e.g., "Do you have any concerns about your child's eating or sleeping behaviors? If yes, please explain"). The final page of each age interval is the Information Summary sheet, which serves as the scoring sheet and as a guide

Table 3.3. Behavioral areas, associated content, and specific items by ASQ:SE-2 age interval

		ASQ:SE-2 items by age interval								
Behavioral area	Associated content	2m	6m	12m	18m	24m	30m	36m	48m	60m
Self-regulation	Can calm self?	7	8	10						
	Body relaxed?	9	10	8	5	4				
	Trouble falling asleep at naptime or night?		16	15	13	16				
	Calms within half hour when upset? Calms within 15 minutes?	1	1	5	7	8	14	5	4	5
	Cries for long periods of time? Cries, screams, or has tantrums for long periods?	8	9	9	9	11	9	19	8	9
	Tries to hurt others (children, adults, animals)?			21	25	25	27	29	31	30
	Does things over and over and gets upset when stopped?				11	21	10	21	22	22
	Seems more active than other children?							12	16	16
	Settles after exciting activities?						8	7	7	7
	Stays with activities for at least [3, 5, 10, or 15] minutes?						11	13	18	13
	Moves easily from one activity to another?						22	8	20	20
	Destroys or damages things on purpose?						24	24	25	25
Total number of self-regulation items		**4**	**5**	**6**	**6**	**6**	**8**	**9**	**9**	**9**
Compliance	Follows [simple or routine] directions? Follows rules at home or child care?				19	18	20	18	24	24
	Does what you ask?						12	11	13	15
Total number of compliance items		**0**	**0**	**0**	**1**	**1**	**2**	**2**	**2**	**2**
Adaptive functioning	Trouble sucking from breast or bottle?	10	11							
	Stays awake for hour or more at one time during the day?	14	15							
	Feeding takes longer than 30 minutes?	11	12	12						
	Gets constipated or has diarrhea?		18	18	17	17				
	Eating problems [stuffing food, vomiting, eating nonfood]?	13	14	14	12	13	15	15	11	12
	Sleeps at least [8 or 10] hours in a 24-hour period?	15	17	17	15	14	18	16	15	17
	Hurts self on purpose?				23	23	25	22	23	23
	Stays away from dangerous things?						23	23	26	26
	Unusual interest in or knowledge of sexual language and activity?							30	32	32
	Stays dry during the day? Goes to bathroom by self?								10	11
	*Wakes 3 or more times at night?				29	28	31	33	33	33
Total number of adaptive functioning items		**5**	**6**	**4**	**5**	**5**	**5**	**6**	**7**	**7**

(continued)

Table 3.3. *(continued)*

		ASQ:SE-2 items by age interval								
Behavioral area	Associated content	2m	6m	12m	18m	24m	30m	36m	48m	60m
Autonomy	Checks that you are near when exploring? Explores new places?				21	20	21	20	21	21
	*Too worried or fearful?					30	32	34	34	34
	Clings more than you expect?						3	4	2	2
Total number of autonomy items		**0**	**0**	**0**	**1**	**2**	**3**	**3**	**3**	**3**
Affect	Likes to be picked up and held? Likes to be hugged or cuddled?	2	3	4	6	7	2	2	5	3
	Stiffens and arches back when picked up?	3	4	6	8	9				
	Interested in things (people, toys, and foods)?			11	10	10	13	10	9	10
	Seems happy?						5	9	14	8
	Shows concern for other people's feelings?								28	27
Total number of affect items		**2**	**2**	**3**	**3**	**3**	**3**	**3**	**4**	**4**
Social-communication	*Makes sounds and looks at you while playing with you?		19							
	*Makes sounds or gestures to get attention?		20							
	*Smiles back at you?		21							
	*Makes sounds back when you talk?		22							
	Looks at you and seems to listen when you talk? Turns head, looks, or smiles when you talk? Looks at you when you talk to him?	4	5	20	1	1	1	1	1	1
	Makes babbling sounds?			16						
	Lets you know when [hungry, tired, uncomfortable, sick, hurt]? Lets you know feelings with gestures or words? Uses words for wants or needs?	5	6	19	18	19	19	17	17	18
	Uses words to describe own and others' feelings?							25	19	19
	*Looks in the direction you point?			24	16	15	17			
	*Tries to show you things?			22						
	*Responds to name?			23	30	29				
	*Uses sounds or gestures to communicate wants? Uses sounds, words, or gestures to let you know wants?			25	27					
	*When you copy sounds baby makes, repeats same sounds back?			26						
	*Shows you things by pointing and looking back at you?				26	26	28	31		
	*Plays with objects by pretending?				28	27	30			
	*Uses 2 words to ask for wants?						29			
	*Pretends objects are something else?							32		
	*Has simple back-and-forth conversations with you?								35	35
Total number of social-communication items		**2**	**6**	**8**	**7**	**6**	**6**	**5**	**4**	**4**

Behavioral area	Associated content	ASQ:SE-2 items by age interval								
		2m	6m	12m	18m	24m	30m	36m	48m	60m
Interaction *Parents and other adults*	Smiles at you and family members? Laughs or smiles [with you and family members, when playing with you]?		2	1	3	3				
	Seems to enjoy watching or listening to people? Likes to play games such as Peekaboo? Likes hearing stories [and, or] singing songs?	6	7	7	22	22	6			
	Stays upset more than an hour when you leave?				2	5				
	Enjoy [feeding times, mealtimes] together?	12	13	13	14	12	16	14	12	14
	Likes to play near or be with family and friends? Greets familiar adults? Talks or plays with familiar adults?			3	20	6	4	3	3	4
	Looks for you when stranger comes near? Friendly with strangers?			2	4	2	7	6	6	6
Peers	Likes to be around other children? Plays next to other children?				24	24	26			
	Can name a friend? Takes turns and shares during play with children?							26	27	31
	Other children like to play with child?							27	29	28
	Likes to play with other children?							28	30	29
Total number of interaction items		**2**	**3**	**5**	**7**	**7**	**5**	**6**	**6**	**6**
General concerns and Overall comments	Anyone shared concerns about behaviors?	16	23	27	31	31	33	35	36	36
	Parent concerns about [eating, sleeping, or toileting behavior/habits]?	17	24	28	32	32	34	36	37	37
	Parent worries about [baby, child]?	18	25	29	33	33	35	37	38	38
	What parent enjoys about [baby, child]?	19	26	30	34	34	36	38	39	39
Total number of general concerns and Overall items		**4**	**4**	**4**	**4**	**4**	**4**	**4**	**4**	**4**
Total number of ASQ:SE-2 items per interval		**19**	**26**	**30**	**34**	**34**	**36**	**38**	**39**	**39**

Note: Numbers next to abbreviated items indicate item number on the specific ASQ:SE-2 questionnaire.
*Indicates the item is new in ASQ:SE-2.

to interpreting the child's results. This sheet provides space for the professional to summarize the child's total score and compare it with the cutoff, record parent concerns, and indicate follow-up decisions made.

Most parents can complete a questionnaire in 10–15 minutes, depending on the length of the specific questionnaire and the time it takes for the individual parent to read and mark appropriate responses. The text is at a fourth- to sixth-grade reading level. As with any parent-completed assessment tool, not all parents will be able to read, understand, and accurately complete ASQ:SE-2 without support. The questionnaires can be used as an interview tool for parents who do not read English or Spanish at a fourth- to sixth-grade level. The questionnaires also can be used as an interview tool for parents with cognitive and/or emotional disabilities; however, it may be helpful to gather information from other caregivers or to use a professionally administered tool. Each questionnaire consists of three parts, as follows:

1. *Family information sheet:* This page indicates the questionnaire age range and interval at the top. It asks for identifying information about the child and the person completing the questionnaire. It also provides space to enter program information.
2. *Item pages*: These pages start with brief instructions to the parent completing the questionnaire and include space for the program to indicate a date for return and contact information if there are questions. ASQ:SE-2 items appropriate for each age interval follow. Table 3.4 shows the number of scored questions per age interval. Questionnaires vary in length from three to five pages. Items use simple, straightforward language at a fourth- to sixth-grade reading level. Each questionnaire also includes three general questions to elicit parental concerns and a final question that asks, "What do you enjoy about your baby/child?" For scored items, parents choose from three response options: *often or always, sometimes,* or *rarely or never.* Parents indicate their response by checking the box that best describes their child's behavior. In the last column, parents may check the circle to indicate if that behavior is of concern to them. Items are coded *Z, V,* or *X* to permit quick scoring by the professional. Next to each item, the professional can translate parent responses into point values of 0, 5, or 10, respectively, adding 5 points to any item if the parent indicates that the behavior is of concern (both the item response score and the concern score inform the child's total score). Total points per page can be recorded at the bottom of each page. These page totals are combined on the Information Summary sheet to calculate the child's total score.
3. *Information Summary sheet:* This final page has two purposes: 1) to assist with scoring and follow-up and 2) to provide a summary of the child's performance on the questionnaire. This sheet is for professional use, and program staff can choose to use the entire Information Summary or only the scoring section. Each Information Summary includes a scoring chart section to calculate the child's total score and record the score next to the established cutoff, and a score interpretation section with a graphic that displays whether the child's total score indicates no or low risk, monitoring, or further assessment. A high total score indicates potential problems, whereas a low score suggests that the child's social-emotional development is consistent with age expectations. Children whose total scores exceed the established cutoff should be referred for a diagnostic evaluation, whereas children whose scores are in the monitoring zone should be screened again in 2–4 months. Children whose scores are in the monitoring zone may need referral, especially if the children are girls and if parents have concerns. The Information Summary also includes an area to record parent concerns and responses to Overall items. Each sheet guides the professional through follow-up and referral considerations and offers a section to note follow-up decisions and actions. The Information Summary sheet can be retained by program staff as a record of the child's performance so that the questionnaire itself can be returned to parents (or service providers) for future reference. If the program needs a record of all item responses for a questionnaire, then these can be recorded, along with any parent notes, on the optional Item Response Sheet.

Table 3.4. Number of scored ASQ:SE-2 items by age interval

	ASQ:SE-2 age interval								
	2	6	12	18	24	30	36	48	60
Number of items	16	23	27	31	31	33	35	36	36

Component 2: Procedures for Using and Scoring Questionnaires

ASQ:SE-2 can be used in a variety of ways. Frequently used options include mailing questionnaires to families' homes, supporting parents to complete questionnaires during home visits, asking parents to electronically complete questionnaires on a secure web site, and having parents or service providers complete questionnaires on site at a clinic or child care center. Programs also may use a combination of these options (e.g., giving parents a questionnaire during a home visit, asking them to bring the completed questionnaire to the next well-child visit, having them share their questionnaire responses electronically on site via kiosk or tablet). Each of these options is discussed in detail in Chapter 8.

Several factors will influence the option choice. First, available resources likely will have much to do with selecting completion methods. If personnel are available to conduct home visits, then this may be the best option for some families. This option, however, may not be feasible for some programs, may not fit program goals, or may be more intensive and costly than other available options. Second, the characteristics of the families involved may influence the option choice. Many families will be ready, comfortable, and able to independently complete a questionnaire. Other families may benefit from support to complete a questionnaire. In a study conducted by Lyman et al. (2007) on using ASQ:SE with diverse families, the authors highly recommended having a provider present when parents complete ASQ:SE to reframe questions and support the omission of items that may be inappropriate for a given culture. Parents with cognitive, physical, or emotional difficulties may require support to complete questionnaires. Home visits or on-site completion may need to be considered in these cases. Third, family preference may be a factor in choosing which option to use. Some families may want to complete a questionnaire when both parents or other family members are available, according to cultural practice or preferences, and then return the questionnaire by mail or by dropping it off at the pediatrician's office or preschool. Other families may prefer completing the questionnaires with a home visitor during the day. The completion methods for some families may change as life circumstances change.

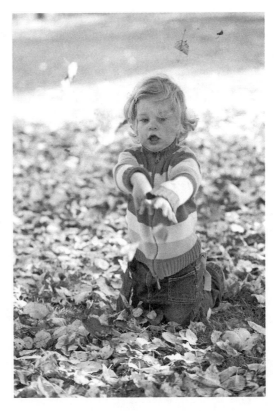

Component 3: Support Materials

The ASQ:SE-2 system has numerous support materials available to facilitate successful use. Some materials are included in this User's Guide, and some are available with the questionnaires box. Some materials are available at www.agesandstages.com, whereas others are separate products available for purchase. Materials included in this User's Guide are as follows:

- Referral guidelines in Chapter 6 (pp. 98–103)
- Suggested readings about screening and ASQ in Appendix A
- A glossary of relevant screening terms in Appendix B
- The complete ASQ:SE-2 technical report, which summarizes psychometric data on the questionnaires, in Appendix C
- Sample forms and letters for parents, professionals, and program use (in English and in Spanish) in Appendix D
- Handouts about social-emotional development milestones and parent–child activities for each age interval in Appendix E
- Information about recommended social-emotional resources in Appendix F
- Guidelines for cultural and linguistic adaptation in Appendix G

In addition to the resources in the User's Guide, other commercially available materials can help assist programs using ASQ:SE-2. These materials include

- *ASQ:SE-2 Quick Start Guide* (in English and Spanish): This is a handy reference for professionals that outlines administration and scoring basics.
- *ASQ:SE-2 in Practice:* This training DVD shows ASQ:SE-2 administration with a family, from the initial introduction of the tool to considerations for interpreting ASQ:SE-2 results.
- *ASQ Pro and ASQ Enterprise:* These online management subscriptions allow programs to track and manage ASQ-3 and ASQ:SE-2 data.
- *ASQ Family Access:* This subscription allows parents to complete ASQ:SE-2 and ASQ-3 questionnaires via a secure, customizable web site.

More information about these products and other products associated with ASQ-3 is found at www.agesandstages.com. In addition, users may gain access to numerous free resources available to support implementation. The agesandstages.com web site offers news and research updates, user stories, a searchable resource library, videos, answers to frequently asked questions, and a free calculator for determining a child's age and adjusting scoring when items are omitted. A free monthly newsletter includes articles, case studies, and helpful user tips. Additional ASQ news and updates are available via social media, including Facebook, Twitter, and Pinterest.

PHASES OF THE SYSTEM

The ASQ:SE-2 system is composed of four phases, each of which is outlined briefly next and more extensively in Section II of this User's Guide. Figure 3.2 provides an overview of the phases and their relationship.

Phase I: Planning the Screening/Monitoring Program

The first phase of the ASQ:SE-2 system involves screening program planning so that key information is gathered and decisions are made prior to implementation. Planning the screening/monitoring program involves the following nine steps:

1. Communicate with community partners.
2. Include parent perspectives.
3. Involve health and mental health care providers.
4. Determine target population.
5. Finalize goals and objectives.
6. Determine program resources.
7. Determine administration methods and settings.
8. Determine depth and breadth of program.
9. Select referral criteria.

These steps, discussed in detail in Chapter 4, are suggested areas to consider before initiating the screening program. Some agencies, centers, or offices may not need to devote planning time to all of the steps because existing policies may already address them. For example, program goals and objectives may already be delineated, and administration methods may already be defined by state guidelines. Completing the planning phase helps ensure that the screening/monitoring program will run smoothly and efficiently.

Phase II: Preparing, Organizing, and Managing the Screening/Monitoring Program

The second phase of the ASQ:SE-2 system focuses on *organization and operations management*—paper or electronic tickler (to-do) programs, record keeping, forms, policies, and procedures for determining follow-up for children who are identified as needing further assessment—and staff training. This phase, which contains the details for organizing the daily operation of the screening/monitoring program, includes the following steps:

10. Create a management system.
11. Prepare questionnaires.
12. Develop forms, letters, and a referral guide.
13. Articulate screening policies and procedures.
14. Provide staff training and support.

Chapter 5 outlines each of these steps and includes suggestions for maintaining child and family records and establishing management systems. This chapter also includes brief information

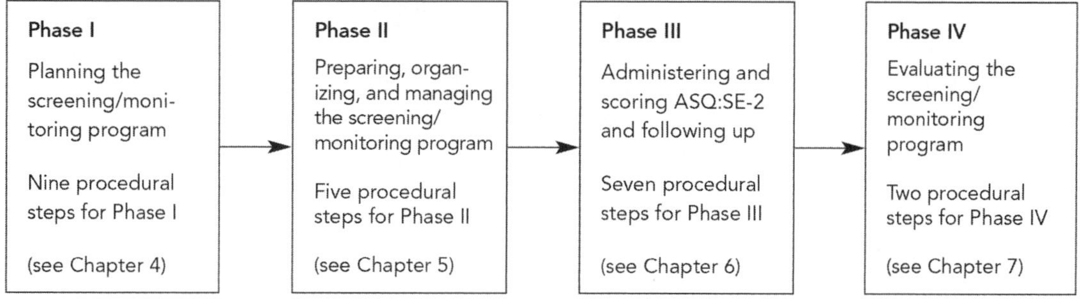

Figure 3.2. An overview of the four interrelated phases of the ASQ:SE-2 system. Each phase includes a number of steps to be performed before the phase is completed.

about managing the ASQ:SE-2 screening process online through ASQ Pro and ASQ Enterprise. Suggestions for developing forms, letters, and samples are given (blank samples or templates appear in Appendix D). Staff training and ongoing support, an essential element of an effective screening/monitoring program, are also discussed in Chapter 5.

Phase III: Administering and Scoring ASQ:SE-2 and Following Up

The third phase of the ASQ:SE-2 system includes steps needed for *administering and scoring* questionnaires and establishing referral guidelines for families. Chapter 6 includes step-by-step directions for this phase. The steps for the third phase are as follows:

15. Select the appropriate ASQ:SE-2 age interval.
16. Support parent completion of ASQ:SE-2.
17. Score ASQ:SE-2.
18. Review written comments on scored and unscored sections of ASQ:SE-2.
19. Interpret ASQ:SE-2 scores.
20. Communicate results with families.
21. Determine appropriate follow-up.

Chapter 6 discusses these seven steps, illustrating in detail how to administer, score, and interpret ASQ:SE-2 results. The chapter provides guidelines for follow-up action, including how to communicate with families. Chapter 6 explains the nuts and bolts of administration, from how to select an ASQ:SE-2 questionnaire based on a child's age or adjusted age and how to prepare ASQ:SE-2 materials prior to the screening, to how to support parent completion of questionnaires and how to determine the type of follow-up a child may need.

Phase IV: Evaluating the Screening/Monitoring Program

The final phase of the ASQ:SE-2 system focuses on ongoing *evaluation* of the screening/monitoring program implementation to determine progress and effectiveness. This fourth phase has two steps:

22. Assess progress in establishing and maintaining the screening/monitoring program.
23. Evaluate the program's effectiveness.

Chapter 7 describes this final phase and includes a worksheet to guide evaluation of progress. Information helpful in measuring effectiveness is given, including how to calculate over- and underidentification rates and how to survey parents for feedback. Completing evaluation activities on an ongoing basis helps ensure that program procedures are efficient and that the screening/monitoring system is effective—that is, that children in need of further diagnostic assessment are being identified.

ASQ:SE-2 IN PRACTICE

Section III of the User's Guide provides practical information on the various ways in which ASQ:SE-2 can be implemented. Chapter 8 illustrates options for administering ASQ:SE-2, and Chapter 9 describes how ASQ:SE-2 can be used across a variety of settings. Chapter 10 presents case studies about using ASQ:SE-2 with families.

CONCLUSION

This chapter provides an overview of the ASQ:SE-2 system components—the questionnaires, the procedures for using and scoring the questionnaires, and support materials. The heart of the ASQ:SE-2 system are the nine questionnaires that cover the age range 1 month to 72 months (6 years) of age. Explicit procedures for planning, organizing, administering, and evaluating the screening/monitoring program support successful implementation of ASQ:SE-2. A broad range of support materials assist with starting and maintaining the ASQ:SE-2 system.

II

Implementation of ASQ:SE-2

4

Phase I
Planning the Screening/Monitoring Program Using ASQ:SE-2

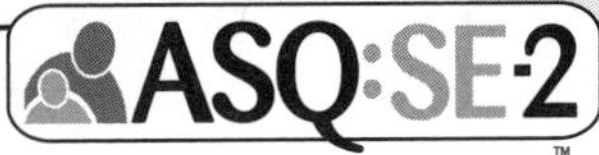

A number of critical factors should be considered when initiating a screening/monitoring program such as the ASQ:SE-2 system. This chapter describes each of the steps involved in the planning phase.

IMPORTANCE OF THE PLANNING PHASE

The planning phase includes important steps toward establishing a successful screening/monitoring program. Unless careful thought is given to each step of the planning phase, serious difficulties may arise later when the system is in operation. This chapter presents detailed information on how to plan and develop a program designed to screen and monitor the social-emotional development of young children ages 1 month to 72 months (6 years) using ASQ:SE-2. Planning the program and collaborating with relevant community agencies prior to implementation are essential to the success of any relatively large-scale screening program that requires input and coordination across a variety of agencies and personnel. This chapter describes nine steps, beginning with initial planning and moving to implementation of a program designed to assist communities in the early identification of young children with potential social-emotional problems.

The purpose of screening and monitoring programs is twofold. One goal is to accurately identify children who should receive follow-up attention to determine if a problem exists. A second goal is to conduct the program in a manner that permits the assessment of large groups of children at a low cost per child. Effective screening programs are able to acquire reliable targeted information on large groups of individuals in economical ways. Screening programs fail if the outcomes are in error (i.e., the information is inaccurate or unreliable) and if per-individual costs are high (i.e., the cost of conducting the screening exceeds the usefulness of the outcome). As a consequence, effective screening of children for social-emotional problems requires a tool or procedure that is low in cost to use and yields accurate outcomes (e.g., acceptable over- and underidentification rates).

Screening generally refers to a one-time administration of a tool or procedure. For example, kindergarten roundups are generally conducted as a one-time observation and testing of children before they enter first grade. Monitoring implies ongoing surveillance of the target population over time. For example, infants discharged from a neonatal intensive care unit (NICU) might be tested at 2, 6, 12, 24, and 36 months. ASQ:SE-2 can be used as a one-time screener, or, preferably, it can be used to monitor children over time by using the questionnaires at designated intervals. The program described in this User's Guide is generally referred to as both a screening and monitoring program, although the terms are used separately. See Chapters 8 and 9 for more detailed information about administering ASQ:SE-2 with varying options for methods and settings.

STEPS IN THE PLANNING PHASE

Figure 4.1 provides a schematic of the steps necessary to begin screening and monitoring a designated population of children using the ASQ:SE-2 system. Although the figure shows a linear, one-step-at-a-time approach to planning, it is possible to work on more than one step simultaneously or to rearrange the order of the steps as needed.

1. Communicate with Community Partners

Collaboration, or establishing connections between systems that historically have not interacted with one another, is one of the most important features of successful community mental health screening and intervention programs for young children (Bricker et al., 2013; Guralnick, 2011; Knitzer, 2000). Pooling knowledge and resources is particularly important when dealing with the complex issues surrounding young children's mental health. Because the roots of problems may or may not be organically based, issues such as the quality of parent–child interactions, parental drug and alcohol abuse, maternal depression, poverty, domestic violence, and child abuse should be dealt with concurrently for interventions to have lasting effects. In addition, given the general lack of resources available to young children and their families, it is

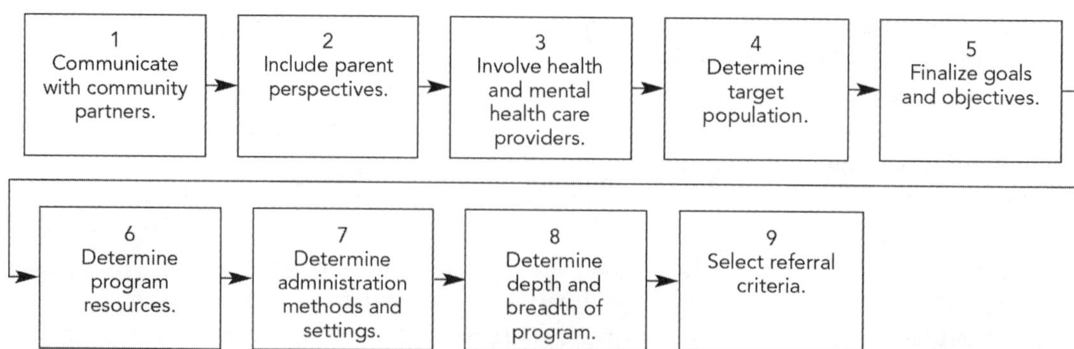

Figure 4.1. The nine important steps of the ASQ:SE-2 system planning phase. These steps can be performed one at a time, or some may be undertaken simultaneously. Sometimes program staff will choose to complete the steps in a different order from the one shown here.

important to use available resources efficiently and avoid duplicating services. Making agreements regarding which agencies will screen children, how information will be shared between service providers, and who is available in the community to provide needed follow-up is an important step in using limited resources wisely.

Many community agencies that provide services to young children and their families include social-emotional screening as part of their services. Some programs, such as Early Head Start and Head Start, are mandated in their performance standards to screen all children within a certain period of time after children's entry into the program. Other agencies, such as child welfare agencies, operate under federal mandates that require personnel to refer children for developmental screening. For example, children younger than 3 years old with documented abuse or neglect must be referred for developmental screening under the Keeping Children and Families Safe Act of 2003 (PL 108-36), which amends the Child Abuse Prevention and Treatment Act (CAPTA) of 1974 (PL 93-247), as well as under the Individuals with Disabilities Education Improvement Act (IDEA) of 2004 (PL 108-446).

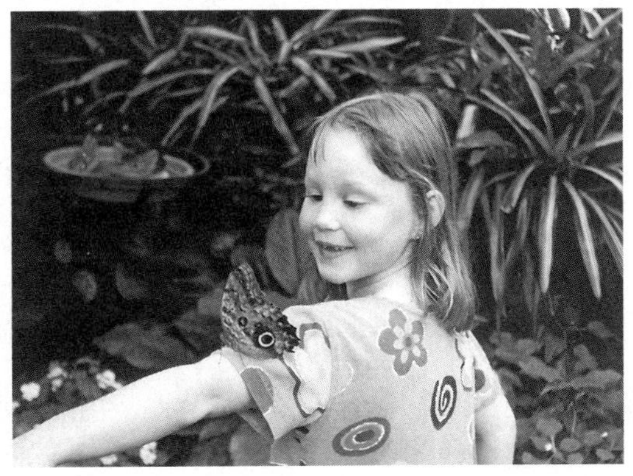

A useful place to begin is to arrange regular meetings or conversations with the Local Early Intervention Interagency Coordinating Council (LICC). The LICC is an interagency group that operates in most communities to coordinate services under IDEA. In addition, community and statewide efforts are underway to create unified early childhood comprehensive systems that include Head Start, Early Head Start, Early Learning Advisory Councils, Child Care and Development Fund agencies, and quality rating and improvement systems (QRIS), all of which can serve as partners in coordinating screening efforts. Creating work groups or establishing an ongoing dialogue among community agencies that provide services for young children with social-emotional problems is essential to determining what services currently are available and where gaps exist. A single coordinated system with cross-agency policies, procedures, and data management is the most effective approach for screening and monitoring systems and will avoid unnecessary and costly duplication of resources (Bricker et al., 2013; Guralnick, 2013).

Part C of IDEA 2004 establishes a program for providing intervention services to infants and toddlers and specifies the developmental services to be provided in the areas of physical, cognitive, communication, social-emotional, and adaptive development. Services included under Part C include family counseling, psychological services, social work services, occupational and physical therapy, speech-language therapy, and early identification through screening and assessment. These types of services should be available in every community for even the youngest child meeting state eligibility requirements. If services are not available and the need is present, then this service gap should be addressed by the LICC.

Part C eligibility under IDEA 2004 is determined by each state's definition of developmental delay and includes children with "diagnosed physical or mental condition that has a high probability of resulting in developmental delay" (§ 632[5][A][iii]). Children with these "established conditions" are eligible for services under Part C of IDEA by virtue of their diagnosis, regardless of whether a measurable delay is present. These infants and toddlers do not need to undergo the same eligibility evaluation procedures required by children who are referred with a suspected delay. States may also choose to include children *at risk* for disabilities in the eligible group. The intention of Part C services for children at risk or children with an established condition is to ameliorate or prevent secondary delays. See your state Part C eligibility definitions to determine which conditions make a child automatically eligible for Part C services. Review these criteria to ensure compatibility between the screening/monitoring program and evaluation procedures used to determine eligibility for services. For example, if your state is one that includes drug-exposed infants in the category of established conditions, your procedures should clarify that these infants can be referred directly from the hospital to early intervention with documentation of their substance exposure. These babies do not need to undergo further screening or evaluation to determine eligibility but can move directly to the development of an individualized family service plan (IFSP) and receive services.

Part B of IDEA 2004 mandates special education and related services for children ages 3 years through 21 years. Section 619 of Part B pertains to children ages 3 years through 5 years. Services included under Section 619 are education, occupational and physical therapy, speech-language therapy, and services for children with learning disabilities and with serious emotional disturbance. Section 619 services are provided by local school districts in most states.

The screening program can contact school districts and the lead agency for Part C service provision (which varies by state) to begin establishing links between Part B and Part C services. Meetings can be arranged between these representatives and the screening program.

In conclusion, to reduce duplication and increase effectiveness of screening and referral for families of young children, a wide range of state and local agencies should coordinate screening and monitoring efforts, including but not limited to the following: Part C and Part B Section 619; Early Head Start; child care; home visiting; physical (Children's Health Insurance Program [CHIP], Special Supplemental Nutrition Program for Woman, Infants, and Children [WIC]) and mental health care providers and systems; newborn hearing screening (Early Hearing Detection and Intervention); family support networks; foster care; and parenting groups. A broad range of personnel from these systems should convene to discuss community screening efforts and establish one unified, cross-agency system. Community representatives should consider the following:

- What screening/monitoring efforts currently are underway in the community? Does the medical community provide social-emotional screening services? What other community agencies (e.g., school district, Head Start, child welfare, public health agencies) provide screening?
- What populations are being screened/monitored, and are there gaps? Do certain geographic regions of the community have better identification rates than other regions? What different cultural groups are there in the community? Do these groups have access to social-emotional screening? Can diverse members of the community be reached in culturally appropriate ways?
- How can duplication of screening/monitoring efforts be reduced? Can agreements be reached regarding which agency will take the primary role in screening and then share screening information among agencies? Should using a common child identification number to share information be considered? How can data be shared across agencies, protecting child and family privacy?
- Are there mechanisms in place for immediately referring children to community services without gaining access to screening services? For example, are there children with established risk factors, such as children in foster care who were removed from their home environment due to parental abuse/neglect, who should be immediately referred for early intervention/early childhood special education (EI/ECSE) services?

- What types of screening tests are being used, and are these tests valid and reliable? Can community agencies agree on the use of common screening tests? Are tests being used to screen social-emotional development or for early autism detection?
- What types of resources are available in the community, and how can these resources be maximized? Do agencies need to prioritize which children are most vulnerable for social-emotional delays? Are physicians aware of reimbursements for social-emotional/behavioral health screening? Are current methods of screening costly?
- Is a comprehensive inventory of community resources available? What types of community resources are available for referral (e.g., EI/ECSE, parenting education programs, mental health services, parent–child interactive therapies, respite, family support services)? Are community agencies ready to receive referrals?

States that receive funds under CAPTA are mandated to develop and implement provisions and procedures for referring infants and toddlers with substantiated cases of abuse or neglect to Part C early intervention services. To comply with this mandate, a consortium of infant mental health and child therapists in a region of the Northwest has been identified to provide social-emotional screening and assessment of this very vulnerable population. The therapists have established relationships and referral procedures with other agencies that provide critical services that may be indicated following screening with ASQ:SE-2, including EI/ECSE providers, county mental health providers, community Head Start and Early Head Start programs, the Child Care Resource and Referral agency, local women's and men's alcohol and drug treatment programs, three homeless shelters, the Sacred Mary Hospital Newborn Intensive Care Unit, Centro-Latino, and a number of community pediatricians. Representatives from these agencies, as well as several parent representatives, serve on an advisory board that provides ongoing advice and direction for the screening/monitoring program. One decision the advisory board made was to screen and assess not only the infants and toddlers mandated under CAPTA but also any child younger than school age with a substantiated case of abuse or neglect.

---

2. Include Parent Perspectives

Involving families in planning and developing the screening/monitoring program is a second important step in the planning phase. Families' suggestions regarding procedures and agencies to include in the process provide an important and useful perspective. How to successfully provide screening/monitoring services to families is critical to consider during the planning process. Family members can advise agencies on how to involve families with young children and can communicate what types of follow-up services are needed in communities. It is important to provide services in a culturally appropriate and respectful manner because most communities are home to a variety of families with different backgrounds, experiences, and cultural values. Inviting family members with diverse backgrounds, including those who can serve as "cultural guides," to participate in a planning group can help others understand a variety of parental perspectives on screening and monitoring. Family members who represent different groups can help review proposed screening protocols as well as provide feedback regarding the cultural appropriateness of the proposed screening tools. Items on forms and assessments may need to be adapted or reinterpreted to become more meaningful to families. For example, a large community of ethnic Hmong families in Minnesota created the impetus for an audio version of ASQ:SE. This was a key change because the Hmong culture has a strong oral tradition, and parents are less comfortable with written information. Although ASQ:SE-2 is available in languages other than English (see www.agesandstages.com for more information), parent and other caregiver input may be essential to devising plans that best accommodate families with cultural experiences that may differ significantly in terms of practice and values. A discussion of factors to consider when translating/adapting ASQ:SE-2 appears in Appendix G.

3. Involve Health and Mental Health Care Providers

Primary health and mental health care providers in most communities wish to be informed about their young patients' participation in screening/monitoring programs. Staff implementing a screening/monitoring program should involve primary health and mental health care providers of participating children for four important reasons. First, health care providers have valuable health information about their patients and young children that serves to enhance screening, referral, and follow-up decisions. Second, collaboration among professionals and program personnel will produce the greatest benefits for young children and their families. Third, primary health care providers have the ability to make referrals and access services for young children through health systems that are not available through EI/ECSE systems. Fourth, providers need to be aware of services being provided to their patients so that services are not duplicated.

The AAP issued policy statements that make clear the importance of developmental and social-emotional screening and the critical role pediatricians should play in the early identification of children at risk for developmental delays, including autism. The AAP (2006) policy statement on screening recommended that pediatricians and other primary care providers screen all infants and young children for developmental and social-emotional/behavioral delays during preventive care visits and refer families to community-based resources based on results. Recommendations on screening for autism suggested that pediatricians and other primary care providers should screen for autism and related disorders at 18 months and 24 months (Johnson et al., 2007). At the very least, physicians should be informed when their young patients are participating in screening/monitoring programs (after written consent to share results has been obtained from parents). In some cases, health care providers and their offices will be the ones conducting the ASQ:SE-2 screening. See Chapter 9 for additional information on different screening providers and locations.

It is important to determine what medically sponsored and/or operated screening activities are in place (e.g., well-child checkups at specific age intervals) during the planning phase and support these screening efforts by augmenting or complementing these services rather than trying to replace them. In addition, screening/monitoring programs should develop strategies to communicate screening results to the physicians of children being screened. Figure 4.2 shows a sample letter designed to explain a family's participation in the screening/monitoring program to health care providers when another office is conducting the screening. Figure 4.3 contains a sample letter designed to assist health care providers in understanding ASQ:SE-2 screening results of their young patients. (Blank letter templates appear in Appendix D.)

4. Determine Target Population

Many states and communities have begun to plan universal screening efforts that create opportunities for children to thrive by fostering the early and timely identification of problems or

Dear Dr. Goldenberg:

The parents or guardians of your patient, Sophia Martinez, have agreed to complete the Ages & Stages Questionnaires: Social-Emotional, Second Edition (ASQ:SE-2), as part of our screening/monitoring program. The purpose of this program is to monitor children's social-emotional development, refer as indicated by results, and provide support to caregivers when social-emotional/behavioral concerns are identified.

ASQ:SE-2—a series of nine parent-completed questionnaires for children from 1 month to 72 months (6 years) of age—screens children's social-emotional development and identifies potential social-emotional issues. ASQ:SE-2 is a companion tool to the Ages & Stages Questionnaires, Third Edition (ASQ-3), which is designed to screen children's developmental skills/milestones periodically over time.

Parents or guardians are asked at repeated intervals to respond to questions about their child's social-emotional behaviors. If the child obtains a score above an established cutoff point on a questionnaire, the parents/guardians and you will be notified so that further behavioral evaluation can be scheduled. More information on use of ASQ:SE-2 in a medical setting can be found at www.agesandstages.com.

Please contact Jennifer Davis at 541-555-0112 if you would like more information about this program.

Sincerely,

Katherine Kephart
Steps-Ahead

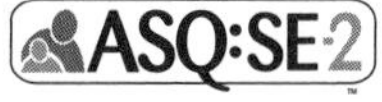

Figure 4.2. A sample Physician Information Letter to health care providers. Appendix D contains a blank, photocopiable version of this letter.

conditions that may affect child development. Universal screening efforts may include a goal such as screening every child in a given community at a minimum of every 12 months using valid and reliable screening tools. In recent years, states have expanded publically funded pre-K programs and developed QRIS that work closely with child care providers to improve the quality of caregiving environments. Some of these "universal" initiatives include developmental screening as a provided service or a quality indicator. AAP recommends universal developmental screening of young children by primary care providers at 9-month, 18-month, and 24- or 30-month well-child visits. Many community programs will need to prioritize and develop objective criteria for selecting whom to screen and monitor, however, because of limited resources. During the planning phase, advisory groups or program personnel may want to consider targeting groups with specific risk factors (or multiple risk factors), certain geographical regions that are underserved, specific minority groups that may be at high risk, or an age range that may maximize screening efforts (e.g., 36 months). Screening advisory groups can help determine where gaps exist in community services.

Dear Dr. Williams:

Ages & Stages Questionnaires: Social-Emotional, Second Edition (ASQ:SE-2), is a series of nine parent-completed questionnaires developed for screening children from 1 month to 72 months (6 years). ASQ:SE-2 helps monitor children's social-emotional development and identify potential social-emotional/behavioral issues. ASQ:SE-2 is a companion tool to the Ages & Stages Questionnaires, Third Edition (ASQ-3), which is designed to screen children's developmental skills/milestones. More information on use of ASQ:SE-2 in a medical setting can be found at www.agesandstages.com.

An ASQ:SE-2 questionnaire was recently completed by Lindy Savage for your patient, Aiden Savage, date of birth 5/16/2009. A copy of the ASQ:SE-2 Information Summary sheet is provided for your records.

The checked box below provides a brief summary of the results of that questionnaire:

- ☐ The child's ASQ:SE-2 score is **below the established cutoff,** indicating social-emotional development appears to be on schedule at this time.
- ☒ The child's ASQ:SE-2 score is **close to the established cutoff** (within the monitoring zone). We have provided information to the family and will monitor the child's development.
- ☐ The child's ASQ:SE-2 score is **above the established cutoff,** indicating a need for further social-emotional/behavioral evaluation. We have discussed referral options with the family.

The checked box below indicates the needed follow-up action:

- ☐ **No follow-up action needed.**
- ☒ **Follow-up action needed.** Attached is the completed ASQ:SE-2 with specific behavioral concerns highlighted. We hope you can discuss these concerns with the caregiver during the child's upcoming appointment to help the family determine the most effective next steps.

Please contact me if you have any questions.

Sincerely,

Cynthia Stewart
Steps-Ahead

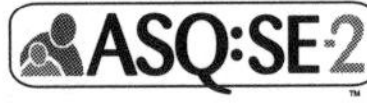

Figure 4.3. A sample Physician Results Letter explaining ASQ:SE-2 screening results to the child's medical provider. Appendix D contains a blank, photocopiable version of this letter.

Several studies found that although biological factors play a major role in predicting severe cognitive delays, these factors play only a minor role in predicting mild delays. A wide variety of risk factors affect individual children (Cicchetti & Toth, 2000; Duncan & Brooks-Gunn, 2000; Garbarino & Ganzel, 2000; Guralnick, 2013). These factors can potentially act as barriers to healthy social-emotional development. Studies that have monitored the development of at-risk populations over time report that the most reliable outcome predictors are not individual variables such as prematurity, teen parenthood, or poverty but rather the number of risk factors to which a child is exposed (Garbarino & Ganzel, 2000; Sameroff, 2009, 2010; Sameroff & Fiese, 2000). Children who experience two to three risk factors are far more likely to develop problems than children who are exposed to one risk factor. The likelihood of poor developmental and social-emotional outcomes is significantly increased for children exposed to four or more risk factors. Such results strongly suggest that programs should use the number of risk factors as their primary criterion rather than selecting specific risk factors. Table 4.1 shows the number of risk factors and priority recommendations for screening and monitoring. It should be recognized, however, that there are a few risk factors—such as parental psychopathology—that often occur in conjunction with other risk factors, such as substance abuse and child maltreatment. These constitute severe dysfunction in parenting that can lead to serious child maladjustment and behavior problems (Guralnick, 2013; Wade, Moore, Astington, Frampton, & Jenkins, 2015; Osofsky & Thompson, 2000). For example, maternal depression is known to contribute to maladaptive parenting and to emotional problems in infants and children (Knitzer, Theberge, & Johnson, 2008; Sontag-Padilla et al., 2013). Instances of parental psychopathology warrant careful monitoring of the child's social-emotional development.

Program resources and goals must be consistent with the risk factors chosen by the screening program personnel. Programs with limited resources may wish to target only children with multiple risk factors because these children are more likely to experience developmental delays. If program resources are sparse, then targeting these children may be an especially compelling recommendation. Once the criteria are selected to determine the target population, they should be clearly written so that they are understood by personnel in different community agencies who may refer or identify potentially eligible children/families. The selection criteria should also be formulated to be respectful of families to the greatest extent possible. "Multiple risk factors" can be used as a category rather than "troubled families," for example.

In addition, when identifying risk factors for a screening/monitoring program, it is important to review federal and state mandates, as well as examine selection criteria used by existing programs that may be serving the same community.

Federal and State Guidelines for Determining Eligibility for Part C Services

As discussed previously, IDEA Part C eligibility is determined by each state's definition of developmental delay and includes children with "established physical or mental conditions with a high probability of resulting in developmental delay" (IDEA 2004, § 303.21). States also may choose to include children at risk for disabilities in the eligible group. Review your state's eligibility criteria carefully to determine which children may be automatically eligible for services by virtue of an established condition or risk factor.

Table 4.1. Recommended screening and monitoring priority for numbers of co-occurring risk factors

Number of co-occurring risk factors and screening and monitoring priority	Examples of risk factors
Four or more *Mandatory*: must be screened and monitored **Three** *High*: should be screened and monitored if at all possible **Two** *Moderate*: should be screened and monitored if resources allow **One** *Low*: screen and monitor if possible	Poverty Low birth weight Substance abuse Teen parent Premature birth Parent has no high school education Chromosomal abnormality *Abuse/neglect *Parent mental illness or psychopathology

*Always warrants careful monitoring of child's social-emotional development.

Amendments to Child Abuse Prevention and Treatment Act

The Keeping Children and Families Safe Act of 2003, also called the CAPTA amendment of 2003, requires that each state develop "provisions and procedures for referral of a child under the age of 3 who is involved in a substantiated case of child abuse or neglect to early intervention services funded under Part C of the Individuals with Disabilities Education Act" (42 U.S.C. §5106a). Most of these children have experienced a range of risk conditions and likely should be screened periodically, thus requiring the inclusion of abuse/neglect as a risk factor.

Risk Factors Used by Other National, State, and Local Programs

Reviewing the populations served by other programs available in the community can help ensure effective use of resources in targeting population needs. These programs might include those established to serve homeless children under the McKinney-Vento Homeless Assistance Act of 1987 (PL 100-77), as well as local Early Head Start, Head Start, Healthy Start, Healthy Families America, Nurse-Family Partnership, and Parents as Teachers programs. Reviewing the risk factors addressed by these existing state or local screening/monitoring programs may permit the legitimate elimination of those factors from a new community program. For example, if a state medical program is providing follow-up monitoring of low birth weight infants, then low birth weight can be eliminated as a risk factor for a new screening/monitoring program.

The Steps-Ahead staff acknowledged limited resources by modifying their original goal of screening and monitoring all children from birth to 5 years of age who were identified as having at least one risk factor. After consulting with the advisory board, Steps-Ahead staff decided they would need to reduce the number of children to be screened. To do this, the selection factors for participation in the program were changed. Instead of one risk factor, three risk factors were required to qualify an infant or young child for participation. Given the change in risk criteria, staff recognized that fewer families in the community would be served. Steps-Ahead staff prepared to refer families they were unable to serve to other community resources and programs.

---

5. Finalize Goals and Objectives

Careful delineation of the screening/monitoring program's goals and objectives by the major stakeholders (i.e., parents, program staff, community agency staff) during the planning phase will help ensure that the program operates and uses resources efficiently and effectively. Several meetings of individuals from participating or receiving agencies may be required to develop a set of reasonable and generally acceptable goals. Time spent during this step is likely to result in a screening/monitoring program that better meets child, family, community, regional, and state needs. The success of any monitoring program, no matter what its resources are, is dependent on matching its goals to available resources. For many programs, establishing goals and determining program resources are activities best done simultaneously. If these phases are conducted separately, then it may be necessary to revise program goals once resources are analyzed and allocated. The following goals are offered as examples for screening/monitoring programs designed to identify children with social-emotional problems:

- Increase understanding among families, care providers, and communities about the importance of nurturing young children's healthy social-emotional development.
- Conduct community-based screening of infants' and young children's social-emotional development at designated intervals.
- Identify early and accurately those infants and young children who require further evaluation in the area of social-emotional competence.
- Increase involvement of parents in the assessment of their children's social-emotional health.
- Refer children for social-emotional evaluations and services when necessary and in a timely manner.
- Identify professionals qualified to undertake comprehensive evaluation of young children's social-emotional development.
- Increase access to mental health services for infants, young children, and their families.

Program staff should modify these suggested goals to fit the needs of their community and screening/monitoring program. After developing program goals, the next phase is to determine the resources available to operate the program and to allocate them appropriately.

6. Determine Program Resources

The success of any screening/monitoring program, no matter how economical, is dependent on matching its goals to available resources. The flexibility of the ASQ:SE-2 system may provide additional opportunities for communities to efficiently utilize resources and expand screening efforts. All screening/monitoring programs require resources to operate and support families when concerns arise; however, having parents observing and gathering information on their child's development may permit the use of limited resources for other purposes.

The ASQ:SE-2 system was designed to be used by parents or other caregivers with minimal support from program personnel. Completing a questionnaire independently requires reading skills at a fourth- to sixth-grade reading level. Independent completion requires that parents are able to read, observe, and report on their children's behaviors without assistance.

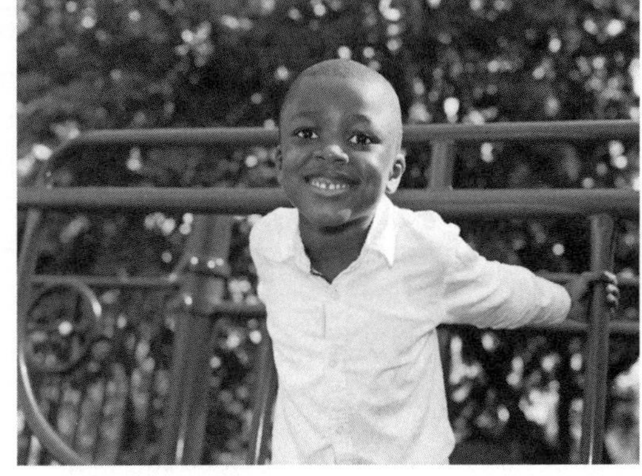

Clearly, not all parents will be able to complete questionnaires independently for a variety of reasons (e.g., cognitive disability, substance abuse, limited reading skills). Thus, families may require support from program staff to successfully complete a questionnaire. Some parents may need minimal assistance, such as item clarification or assistance reading some items. Other parents may need more in-depth assistance. For example, a parent with a cognitive disability may require someone to read and explain the intent of items. Also, a parent who speaks a language or dialect unfamiliar to program personnel may require an interpreter. Finally, a parent may need assistance with siblings in order to focus on the target child and complete the questionnaire. Even if parents initially require assistance, over time (and given the opportunity) they may become more independent and confident about their ability to report on their child's social-emotional behaviors.

Determining resources may require some modification of the chosen goals and objectives in at least three ways. First, limited resources may require changes in program goals and objectives. For example, a program may have set a goal to monitor all infants discharged from the local hospital NICU for a period of 3 years. An examination of resources may indicate that the necessary personnel and funds are not available to conduct such a large project; however, support may be available to monitor a smaller subgroup of infants who have two or more risk factors, thus requiring a modification in the program goal.

Second, limited resources may require changes in the means by which a goal is accomplished. Monitoring a group of infants may not be possible through home visits to every family, but it may be possible to monitor some children by mailing their parents an ASQ:SE-2 questionnaire to complete, freeing up resources for home visits to families with children who have more intensive needs.

Third, modifying goals may be necessary when a specific resource is unavailable. Education-related resources may not be available for infants and toddlers because of the narrow definition of eligibility under a state's definition of Part C. Although the mental health field is making great strides in their understanding and provision of services to children younger than 3 years, these services are still not readily understood or available in many communities (Bricker et al., 2013). Therefore, referral sources may be scarce, and planning groups will need to scan their local communities for appropriate and available follow-up referral sources prior to implementing a large-scale social-emotional screening/monitoring program.

As soon as goals are selected and necessary resources are identified to meet those goals, agency personnel can begin to address the specific settings and methods needed to start a screening/monitoring program using ASQ:SE-2.

During a planning meeting for the development of a social-emotional monitoring program at the Green Water Child Protective Services, personnel identified logistics and time constraints as potential barriers to screening and monitoring children in their foster care program. During the discussion, however, several participants were able to identify existing systems in the agency that could support screening and monitoring of children in foster care. For example, prior to every 6-month review of active cases, caseworkers send a request for updated information to foster care providers. It was suggested that ASQ:SE-2 could be enclosed with this mailing for the foster parents to complete.

---

7. Determine Administration Methods and Settings

The ASQ:SE-2 system is flexible in that it can be used in different settings with a range of administration methods and differing levels of support to caregivers who are completing questionnaires. Most programs use a combination of settings or administration methods, depending on the varying needs of families. (See Chapter 8 for a more detailed discussion of methods for using ASQ:SE-2.) Specific issues should be considered in each setting, however, prior to implementing a screening/monitoring program. Careful planning will ensure that the administration method chosen will provide accurate screening results as well as continue to maintain the underlying principle of ASQ—the meaningful inclusion of parents in their child's screening.

Methods of administration, settings, procedures, considerations, and potential uses for the ASQ:SE-2 system are described in Tables 4.2 and 4.3. Families may receive and complete a

Table 4.2. Completion methods for ASQ:SE-2

Completion method	Procedure	Considerations	Potential agencies, settings, or uses
Mail-out	Staff mail questionnaires to parents. Parents complete questionnaires independently and return for scoring and feedback. Staff score questionnaires. Staff send replies (e.g., letters) to parents whose children are not identified as at risk. Staff contact parents who indicate concerns or whose children are identified as at risk (i.e., personalized response: telephone call, face-to-face contact with parent).	This is a cost-effective strategy for screening large numbers of children. Return rates for questionnaires can be increased with a variety of strategies. Computer systems are not needed to support this method.	Statewide and universal screening initiatives Community-based programs with limited resources Child welfare screening under Child Abuse Prevention and Treatment Act (CAPTA) of 1974 (PL 93-247)
Online	Staff invite parents to complete questionnaires online at secure ASQ Family Access URL. Parents independently complete questionnaires online. Online management system (ASQ Pro, ASQ Enterprise) scores and generates reports for staff review. Staff generate replies (e.g., letters) through the online management system (ASQ Pro, ASQ Enterprise) for parents whose children are not identified as at risk. Staff contact parents who indicate concerns or whose children are identified as at risk (i.e., personalized response: telephone call, face-to-face contact with parent).	This is the most cost-effective strategy for screening large numbers of children, although initial costs may be higher. This strategy may not work well for families with limited literacy or no access to computers.	Statewide and universal screening initiatives Primary health care screening
Interview	Staff give questionnaires to parents. Staff make follow-up telephone calls to support questionnaire completion. Parents read items and ask questions, or parents have help from staff to read and understand items. Staff score questionnaires and discuss results with parents.	This is an effective strategy when parents do not return questionnaires, omit responses, or may have limited English, Spanish, or literacy skills. This is also an effective strategy for families who may need questions reframed or omitted to make sense given their cultural context.	Early intervention and early childhood special education (EI/ECSE) assessment and eligibility Child welfare screening under CAPTA and its amendments
Face to face	Staff provide questionnaires in advance for parents to review and complete independently and follow up with a home visit; *or* Staff provide questionnaires and the support necessary for parents to complete the questionnaires. Staff score questionnaires and discuss results with parents.	This is an effective strategy for families at high risk. Staff should provide the minimum support parents need to complete questionnaires. Staff should not offer opinions about a child's behavior while parents are answering questions. Staff should plan adequate time to debrief results with families and address concerns or follow up at the next visit.	Public health Caregiving or educational settings (e.g., Early Head Start) Parent education Child abuse prevention home visiting programs Child welfare screening under CAPTA and its amendments

Table 4.3. Completion settings for ASQ:SE-2

Completion setting	Procedure	Considerations	Potential agencies, settings, or uses
Screening clinics	Staff have parents complete questionnaires on paper or using a computer kiosk/tablet connected to an online system. Staff score and interpret results, review with parents, and discuss referral options.	Staff should provide the minimal support parents need to complete questionnaires.	Early intervention/early childhood special education (EI/ECSE) eligibility screening Child Find Health fair Children's museum Public library outreach
Education and child care settings	Staff give parents questionnaires to complete and return. Staff score and interpret results, review with parents, and discuss referral options.	Parents should complete questionnaires independently. If there are concerns, then teachers may complete questionnaires based on their classroom observations of children.	Head Start program Preschool Child care center Family child care home
Primary health care offices	Staff mail or direct parents to online questionnaires prior to visit. Parents bring completed questionnaires to visit; *or* Parents complete questionnaires at the office on paper or using a computer kiosk/tablet connected to an online system. Staff score the questionnaires; *or* Online system scores the questionnaires Staff interpret results, review with parents, and discuss referral options.	Staff can monitor children by screening at regular intervals that correspond with well-child visits. Staff should provide the minimal support parents need to complete questionnaires.	Pediatric office Family care practice Public health clinic

questionnaire through a mail-out system, online, or with the help of a professional or other staff member over the telephone or in the family's home. Settings for questionnaire administration can include screening clinics, education and child care facilities, and health care provider offices or clinics. Support can be provided for any of these administration methods and settings (e.g., support can be provided in a mail-out system by calling parents and helping them complete ASQ:SE-2 over the telephone). An important consideration is to only provide as much assistance as is needed by each individual. Chapters 8 and 9 describe administration methods and settings in greater detail. The following four factors may affect the distribution method and settings chosen:

1. Type of program (e.g., early intervention or special education, child care, child welfare, primary health care)
2. Available resources (e.g., financial resources, personnel and clerical support, computer and online access)
3. Characteristics of parents (e.g., languages and cultures, literacy levels)
4. Program goals (e.g., identifying eligible children for special education services, increasing parental knowledge of child social-emotional development, preventing child abuse)

Four Corners Head Start staff were interested in implementing a system to screen and monitor the social-emotional behaviors of the children in their Early Head Start program. The staff were concerned, however, about their ability to take on this task and follow up with families of children who were identified as needing further evaluation. At the time, there was only one half-time child mental health specialist for an organization that served 500 families. The staff developed a two-level system in which ASQ:SE-2 questionnaires were distributed by the teacher or home visitor to all families in the fall. The mental health specialist then limited her follow-up to families who did not return questionnaires and to children whose scores on ASQ:SE-2 indicated a need for follow-up or were in the monitoring zone near the cutoff. She contacted each of the 106 families who did not return questionnaires, by telephone or in person, and assisted them, when appropriate, in completing ASQ:SE-2. She met individually with families with behavioral concerns or whose child's ASQ:SE-2 score indicated potential problems. Together with families, she determined appropriate follow-up and assisted the families with gaining access to community resources and supports.

8. Determine Depth and Breadth of Program

Advisory groups and program personnel need to make decisions about the comprehensiveness of the screening/monitoring program during the planning phase. These decisions will be influenced by the goals and objectives of the program, available resources, and recommendations from the field regarding best practice. In particular, three elements should be considered—frequency of screening, breadth of screening, and type of screening measure.

Frequency of ASQ:SE-2 Screening

ASQ:SE-2 can be used to screen a child's social-emotional development at one point in time or may be used to repeatedly monitor the child using more than one ASQ:SE-2 age interval. It is ideal to screen children at regular intervals, from 1 month to 6 years, if possible. Using each of ASQ:SE-2 age intervals (i.e., 2, 6, 12, 18, 24, 30, 36, 48, and 60 months) is a reasonable monitoring schedule. Programs with fewer resources may choose specific intervals for their monitoring efforts. It is advisable to monitor children over time, considering the rapid social-emotional changes that occur in children between birth and 6 years of age. Parents also have different needs at different stages of a child's development. For example, some parents are very comfortable and at ease about parenting infants but begin to feel challenged when their child becomes a toddler and moves away from them in a strive for independence. In addition, any change in children's homes, schools, or health status may greatly affect their social-emotional development. For all of these reasons, monitoring is recommended.

Although the ASQ:SE-2 system was developed to monitor children over time, the questionnaires can be also used for one-time screening. Some programs may not be able to mount a full-time monitoring program but be able to screen children once. Programs that work with families in transition may encounter situations in which only a one-time screening is possible. Programs that choose this approach should be prepared to respond immediately to concerns that parents note or make a referral if appropriate. For example, programs should have information on hand about a variety of topics (e.g., toileting, feeding) or should have staff members who can discuss these concerns with the parents. Professionals should be prepared to refer children for follow-up when it is indicated by screening results and conversations with the parents.

Children who are referred and found eligible for EI/ECSE services or mental health services based on social delays or behavioral concerns should not receive further screening with ASQ:SE-2. Children who score above the cutoffs and are referred for a more comprehensive assessment but do not qualify for services should continue to be screened regularly. These children have a higher likelihood of exhibiting a social-emotional problem later on (Glascoe, 2001; Guralnick, 2013).

Breadth of Screening

Recommended practice suggests that children's social-emotional development should be screened at least annually. If parents or others have concerns about a child's behavior or if the child has experienced risk factors—such as neglect and extreme poverty—then social-emotional screening should be conducted more frequently, preferably every 6 months. In addition, programs should ensure that developmental screening is addressed in the major areas of development (i.e., motor, communication, cognitive, personal-social).

Type of Screening Measure

The AAP (2006, 2007) recommends using a standardized developmental screening tool such as ASQ-3 for children who appear to be at low risk for developmental problems at 9, 18, and 24 and/or 30 months. Children with suspected developmental problems should be screened with standardized tests more frequently. Screening for social-emotional delays, including autism, is recommended to begin at 18 months using formal standardized measures (AAP, 2014; Johnson & Myers 2007). Screening specifically for autism spectrum disorder is recommended at 18 months and 24 months (AAP, 2014). In addition to using formal screening measures, AAP recommends that health care professionals perform developmental surveillance (informal assessments) at every well-child preventive visit, including asking for parent concerns, obtaining a developmental history, and identifying risk and protective factors. ASQ:SE-2 has been revised to be more sensitive to screening for autism spectrum disorder and early regulatory disorders, with a number of items added that are early red flags for autism.

9. Select Referral Criteria

The final step of the planning phase focuses on discussing and selecting the criteria that program personnel will use to refer children for more extensive assessment. Examining children's performances on ASQ:SE-2 offers a straightforward way to determine those children who should be referred, those who should be carefully monitored, and those whose social-emotional development appears to be proceeding without problem. ASQ:SE-2 generally identifies children who require further assessment and may be eligible for services and generally does not identify children who are not eligible for services. When scoring the questionnaires, users can identify those children who need further assessment and those who do not by comparing a child's score with the ASQ:SE-2 cutoff score. Each interval's cutoff score provides the marker that separates children who require referral and assessment or monitoring from those who do not. (Chapter 6 provides detailed guidelines on scoring ASQ:SE-2.)

The cutoff score for each questionnaire is included in Table 4.4. These cutoff scores were empirically derived using a large number of completed questionnaires, and the empirically derived cutoff points were chosen to minimize under- and overidentification; however, it should

Table 4.4. ASQ:SE-2 monitoring areas, cutoff points, and 90th percentiles as illustrated on ASQ:SE-2 Information Summary sheets

ASQ:SE-2 interval	Monitoring zone[a, b]	Referral above cutoff[c]	90th percentile[d]
2	25–35	35	55
6	30–45	45	55
12	40–50	50	75
18	50–65	65	105
24	50–65	65	110
30	65–85	85	135
36	75–105	105	155
48	70–85	85	150
60	70–95	95	155

[a]Scores below monitoring zone indicate typical development.

[b]Scores in monitoring zone may need further investigation.

[c]Scores above referral cutoff indicate a possible delay in social-emotional development (further evaluation with a professional is recommended).

[d]At this point, a child's score is higher than 90% of scores gathered in the normative sample.

be emphasized that all screening measures make errors. Program personnel may decide to adjust referral criteria or cutoff points during the planning stage so children who are identified as having problems do, in fact, require further assessment.

ASQ:SE-2 Cutoff Scores

Cutoff scores for social-emotional development are available for each questionnaire age interval and have been statistically determined. Total scores, means, and score distributions were determined using data from more than 16,000 questionnaires. Using nearly 3,000 ASQ:SE-2 questionnaires and paired convergent validity outcomes, cutoff points were derived to maximize identification of those children with potential social-emotional delays. A detailed discussion of how cutoff points were determined is contained in Appendix C. Using the ASQ:SE-2 cutoff scores, the following referral criteria are recommended:

- *Refer* a child whose score is above the established cutoff for further assessment.
- *Monitor* a child whose score is in the monitoring zone. Some programs may choose to provide information and resources to parents and then rescreen in a short period of time. Scores in the monitoring zone may also result in a referral to a community agency, as indicated by the results and conversations with the parent.
- *Follow up* on a child whose score is below the cutoff score but whose parent has indicated a concern on any of the items or Overall questions on ASQ:SE-2. Concerns may trigger a potential referral to any number of community agencies, from primary health care to parenting support groups.

The monitoring zone was added to ASQ:SE-2 to help practitioners and families identify those children who may need additional resources and supports. Children with scores in the monitoring zone have an increased number of behaviors that may be of concern to parents and teachers. Parents can decide which follow-up activities will be most helpful, and children can be rescreened more frequently. Girls' scores on ASQ:SE-2 were significantly lower than boys' from 12 months on (see Appendix C). Therefore, girls whose scores are in the monitoring zone need special consideration and possible referral.

Steps-Ahead decided to use the referral criteria as recommended in the *ASQ:SE-2 User's Guide*. Children whose scores are above the cutoffs on ASQ:SE-2 are referred to the early intervention program of Lane County for a developmental assessment. If these children do not qualify for the early intervention program, then Steps-Ahead continues to monitor them using the ASQ:SE-2 system. When Miguel's score was in the monitoring zone, his parents were referred to other community agencies or providers (e.g., the child's pediatrician, parenting support group) and were given parenting information as indicated by ASQ:SE-2 results. Miguel was rescreened in 5 months. When the questionnaire indicated parent concerns, the social worker contacted Miguel's parents and discussed the concerns. Based on the discussion, Miguel continued to be monitored by Steps-Ahead and the family was linked with other needed services.

CONCLUSION

As previously noted, time devoted to the planning steps described in this chapter likely will be well spent in terms of ensuring the long-term success of a screening/monitoring program. The steps in Phase I provide a foundation on which the day-to-day activities of using the ASQ:SE-2 system with young children and their families can be built. The next chapter describes preparing, organizing, and managing your screening/monitoring system, including systems for managing data, preparing questionnaires, and developing strategies to train and support staff. Forms to assist with organizing and maintaining the ASQ:SE-2 screening/monitoring system are included.

5

Phase II
Preparing, Organizing, and Managing the ASQ:SE-2 Screening/Monitoring Program

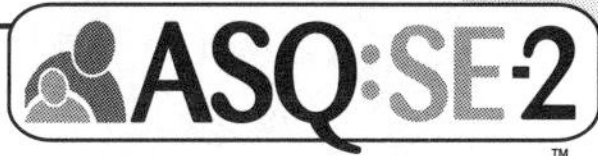

Once the planning phase is complete, program personnel need to allocate sufficient time to prepare, organize, and develop strategies for managing all aspects of the screening/monitoring program.

STEPS IN THE PREPARING, ORGANIZING, AND MANAGING PHASE

This chapter discusses the five steps shown in Figure 5.1 that compose Phase II, including creating a management system; preparing questionnaires; developing forms, letters, and a referral guide; articulating screening policies and procedures; and providing staff training and support.

10. Create a Management System

This first step describes a series of strategies that permits the efficient operation of a screening/monitoring program, beginning with managing paperwork and ending with developing systems to manage the timely sending and retrieving of questionnaires. A program may be enhanced through use of the ASQ Online management system (ASQ Pro and ASQ Enterprise), which supports programs in effectively organizing and managing child and family data for both ASQ-3 and ASQ:SE-2.

Assemble Paper or Electronic Files

Developing a process for assembling individual paper or electronic files for each child ensures that all questionnaires and forms concerning the child and family will be kept in a single

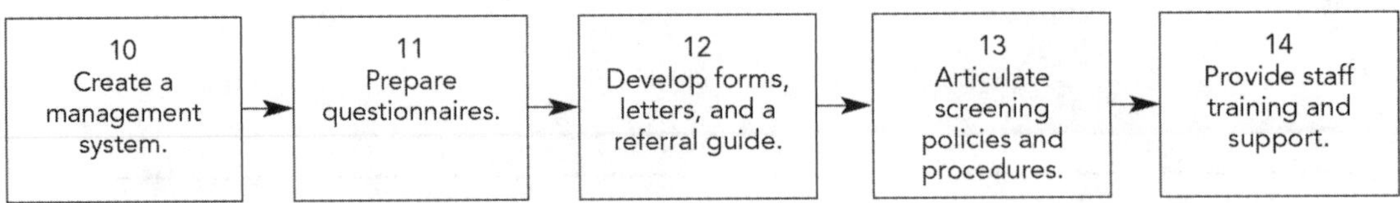

Figure 5.1. Phase II of ASQ:SE-2 implementation and associated steps.

location. All of the information in the paper or electronic files should be periodically updated. Developing paper or electronic files entails the following important steps:

1. Assign the child an identification (ID) number—the first child to join the program might be assigned the number 001, the second 002, and so forth. ID numbers should be assigned for two reasons. First, children with the same or similar last names are less likely to be confused if ID numbers are assigned. Second, the use of ID numbers can help ensure confidentiality when necessary. The ASQ Online management system generates a unique ID number for each child and also allows previously assigned numbers to be recorded if desired by the user or program.
2. Place the Demographic Information Sheet in the child's paper or electronic file for easy access. The Demographic Information Sheet is discussed in detail later in this chapter and shown as Figure 5.8. Appendix D contains sample forms that programs may use.
3. Label the paper file with the child's name or other information that program staff may find essential in order to locate the child's file, or input basic information into the electronic file in order to create a child's profile.

Create a Master List

Having a master list of participating children and associated activities, such as ASQ intervals to be sent, is essential to the smooth and efficient operation of a screening/monitoring program. The master list helps program personnel ensure that necessary information is collected and questionnaires are completed for each child participating in a screening/monitoring program in a given agency. Figure 5.2 shows a master list format that can be used effectively for tracking on paper (a full-size photocopiable version appears in Appendix D). The ASQ Online management system has various features that show listings of participating children.

Create a System to Manage ASQ:SE-2 Implementation

When developing a screening/monitoring system, it is essential to adopt accurate and efficient procedures to permit timely distribution and completion of questionnaires. The integrity of the ASQ:SE-2 system is dependent on reasonable adherence to a preset schedule. The schedule ensures that parents, caregivers, and/or service providers receive and complete questionnaires in a timely manner, within the target age range indicated for the ASQ:SE-2 questionnaire interval—within 1 month of the youngest age interval (i.e., the 2 month ASQ:SE-2), within 3 months of the younger age intervals (i.e., the 6, 12, 18, 24, and 30 month intervals), and within 6 months of the older age intervals (i.e., the 36, 48, and 60 month intervals). Table 5.1 provides guidelines for which interval is appropriate for a child's age, and the age range is clearly indicated on each questionnaire.

Correct for Prematurity

The authors recommend that programs create a screening/monitoring schedule with ASQ:SE-2 that adjusts for prematurity if a child was born 3 or more weeks before his or her due date and is chronologically younger than 2 years of age. This adjustment ensures that the correct age interval questionnaires are used with children born prematurely. The ASQ system uses two methods for adjusting age for prematurity:

- *Adjusted age:* The first method for adjusting age for prematurity is calculating *adjusted age.* The adjusted age is calculated by subtracting the number of weeks of prematurity from the child's chronological age. The resulting adjusted age is used to determine the appropriate ASQ:SE-2 interval to administer on any given day.
- *Corrected date of birth:* The second method for adjusting age for prematurity is termed *corrected date of birth* (CDOB). The CDOB is calculated by adding the number of weeks the infant was born premature to the child's date of birth (the CDOB is essentially the same date as the child's original due date). The target date for administering ASQ:SE-2 is then determined by adding the desired number of months (e.g., 16 months for the 16 month ASQ:SE-2) to the child's CDOB.

After determining the child's CDOB or adjusted age, Table 5.1 should be used to determine the correct ASQ:SE-2 age interval. The ASQ age calculator found at www.agesandstages.com or

ASQ:SE-2 Master List

Program name/site: ______

Child's name	Child ID #	Parent consent on file	Demographic Information Sheet	Physician Information Letter	2 month ASQ:SE-2	6 month ASQ:SE-2	12 month ASQ:SE-2	18 month ASQ:SE-2	24 month ASQ:SE-2	30 month ASQ:SE-2	36 month ASQ:SE-2	48 month ASQ:SE-2	60 month ASQ:SE-2

Instructions: After filling in the program name and site, program staff should be diligent in keeping the ASQ:SE-2 Master List up-to-date. Every child who is participating in the program should be listed by name and ID number on this form or on one like it. In the spaces provided next to the child's name, record the date(s) any item in the top row was completed. For the questionnaires, program staff may also want to note an *S* after the date for a Spanish questionnaire or *IC* for a questionnaire that was returned incomplete and therefore could not be scored. Programs that use the ASQ Online management system (ASQ Pro, ASQ Enterprise) do not need to maintain an ASQ:SE-2 Master List on paper (the information is stored in the online system instead).

ASQ:SE-2

Figure 5.2. ASQ:SE-2 Master List. Appendix D contains a blank, photocopiable version.

Table 5.1. ASQ:SE-2 age administration chart

Child's age	Use this ASQ:SE-2
1 month 0 days *through* 2 months 30 days	2 month
3 months 0 days *through* 8 months 30 days	6 month
9 months 0 days *through* 14 months 30 days	12 month
15 months 0 days *through* 20 months 30 days	18 month
21 months 0 days *through* 26 months 30 days	24 month
27 months 0 days *through* 32 months 30 days	30 month
33 months 0 days *through* 41 months 30 days	36 month
42 months 0 days *through* 53 months 30 days	48 month
54 months 0 days *through* 72 months 0 days	60 month

the apps for mobile devices and tablets in the App Store and Google Play can be used to assist professionals with this adjustment.

If a program does not correct for prematurity, then scores above the cutoff need to be interpreted with caution. Premature infants often have difficulties with regulatory behaviors (e.g., feeding difficulties) that will elevate ASQ:SE-2 scores. In these cases, ensuring that caregivers are receiving appropriate support services is critical, whereas a referral for a mental health evaluation may be less appropriate.

Select a Questionnaire Distribution System

The method of use selected by the program or agency (e.g., mail-out, online, home visit) will affect the way in which questionnaires are distributed and completed; however, some guidelines generally apply. Questionnaire distribution and receipt can be overseen through use of a variety of systems, including 1) computer-based systems to notify agency staff that a questionnaire should be distributed to a child at designated age intervals, 2) less technical strategies such as a card file tickler system that are adaptable to a mail-back system, or 3) other systems, such as personal calendars (paper or electronic) to keep track of when children should be screened. The following sections provide general information on computer-based systems, the card file tickler system, and other ASQ:SE-2 tracking systems.

Computer-Based System Agencies that have access to technical expertise in computer-based management systems may decide to create their own system for managing ASQ:SE-2 administration, provided that they do not infringe on copyright and other intellectual property rights of the ASQ:SE-2 product line. (Programs with questions may contact rights@brookespublishing.com.) Or agencies may prefer to subscribe to the ASQ Online management system for ASQ available through Paul H. Brookes Publishing Co. ASQ Pro is designed for single-site programs, and ASQ Enterprise is designed for multisite programs. Subscribers can manage demographic and questionnaire data—for both ASQ:SE-2 and ASQ-3—and organize their screening/monitoring programs. They can create user records for all staff and profiles for the children they serve, generate questionnaire mailings and other communications at targeted intervals, and record completed screening/monitoring tasks/activities as well as plan follow-up. (See www.agesandstages.com for detailed information.)

Tickler System Using a card file tickler system that is adaptable to a mail-out method and other uses is a second method of questionnaire distribution and receipt. The tickler system uses index cards to keep track of the steps involved in mailing ASQ:SE-2 (although the tickler could be adapted for use with other methods of ASQ:SE-2 administration). A file box is sorted by weeks or months in a year, and as cards get pulled and refiled, they alert agency staff as to when certain activities need to occur. Detailed instructions for how to create a card file tickler system can be found in Appendix 8A at the end of Chapter 8. The instructions for the tickler system also include critical information about completing questionnaires within the age administration windows and reminding parents to complete ASQ:SE-2 before the due date if they have not returned it in a timely manner.

Other Systems Developing a system that helps keep track of tasks related to ASQ:SE-2 is a third method of distributing questionnaires. For example, a home visitor could take the birth dates of children on his or her caseload and project when ASQ:SE-2 would need to be administered in the upcoming year. He or she could use a day planner to make note of these dates. Agencies could post a master calendar with all children's projected ASQ:SE-2 monitoring dates. Any number of systems can work to keep track of ASQ:SE-2 activities, the important point being that a system is created.

11. Prepare Questionnaires

ASQ:SE-2 questionnaires are designed to be reproduced from paper or PDF masters as needed by program staff (please see the conditions of the Photocopying Release on p. xx and the End User License Agreement on the CD-ROM). Each questionnaire is clearly labeled at the top with the age interval and age administration range for ease of use by the staff in charge of photocopying, printing, and/or distributing the questionnaires. ASQ Pro and ASQ Enterprise users may assemble and print individual or group questionnaire mailings with the system's communications feature. This enables users to select the appropriate questionnaire(s), customize parent letters or forms, and put the materials together for efficient mailing preparation. ASQ Family Access users may organize their system so that parents complete ASQ:SE-2 questionnaires online.

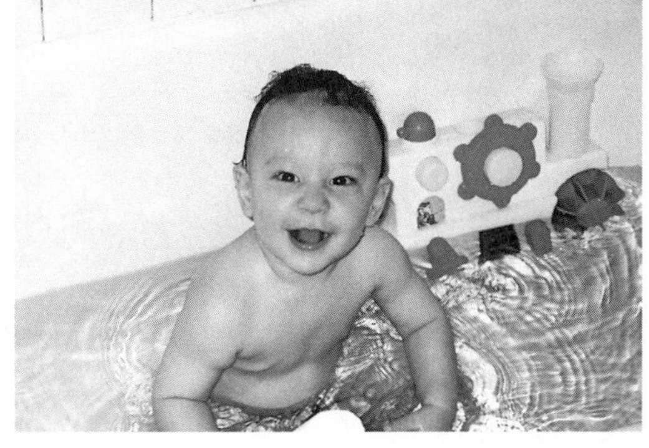

Family Information Sheet

The family information sheet for each questionnaire asks for identifying information about the child and family (see Figure 5.3). The answers to these questions aid staff by indicating who filled out the questionnaire, whether the correct interval has been completed (by comparing the date the questionnaire is completed with the child's date of birth or adjusted age), and whether any assistance was required in completing the questionnaire. The family information sheet is designed to be clear and accessible to parents who may be uncomfortable filling out forms or wary of being part of a "system."

The family information sheet provides space to insert, stamp, type, or write essential identifying information for the program (see Figure 5.3). The program may place its program logo

2 Month Questionnaire

1 month 0 days through 2 months 30 days

ASQ:SE-2 Ages & Stages Questionnaires® Social-Emotional SECOND EDITION

Date ASQ:SE-2 completed: 5/21/16

Baby's information

Baby's first name: Maria Baby's middle initial: V. Baby's last name: Gomez

Baby's date of birth: 4/3/16 If baby was born 3 or more weeks premature, please enter the number of weeks:

Baby's gender: ○ Male ● Female

Person filling out questionnaire

First name: Francesca Middle initial: P. Last name: Gomez

Street address: 300 Dove Road, Apt. 5

City: Baltimore State/province: MD ZIP/postal code: 21227

Country: USA Home telephone number: 202-555-0198 Other telephone number:

E-mail address:

Relationship to baby: ● Parent ○ Guardian ○ Teacher ○ Other: ○ Grandparent/other relative ○ Foster parent ○ Child care provider

People assisting in questionnaire completion:

Program information (For program use only.)

Baby's ID #: Age at administration in months and days:

Program ID #: If premature, adjusted age in months and days:

Program name:

P201020000

Figure 5.3. A sample family information sheet. The sheet is designed to be clear and accessible to parents.

or contact information, if desired, in the space at the top left where the illustration of mother and child is located. Once the screening/monitoring program is operational, staff may wish to enter this information on all of the master family information sheets; the information can be updated if any of the program's identifying information changes over time. Identifying information is vital when mail-out procedures are used. The name and telephone number of a contact person may be indicated on this sheet so that parents know who can answer their questions or address their concerns. ASQ Online management system users can upload a logo and update other program information as needed. The bottom of the family information sheet has a section for information important to the program, which includes the child and program identification numbers as well as the child's age at administration and adjusted age as appropriate.

Questionnaire

The first page of each questionnaire contains brief instructions and important points to remember. It also provides space to provide staff contact information and indicate when the

2 Month Questionnaire *1 month 0 days through 2 months 30 days*

ASQ:SE-2

Questions about behaviors babies may have are listed on the following pages. Please read each question carefully and check the box ☑ that best describes your baby's behavior. Also, check the circle ✓ if the behavior is a concern.

Important Points to Remember:

- ❑ Answer questions based on what you know about your baby's behavior.
- ❑ Answer questions based on your baby's *usual* behavior, not behavior when your baby is sick, very tired, or hungry.
- ❑ Caregivers who know the baby well and spend more than 15–20 hours per week with the baby should complete ASQ:SE-2.
- ❑ Please return this questionnaire by: 6/11/16
- ❑ If you have any questions or concerns about your baby or about this questionnaire, contact: Jenny Smith
- ❑ Thank you and please look forward to filling out another ASQ:SE-2 in 3 months.

	OFTEN OR ALWAYS	SOME-TIMES	RARELY OR NEVER	CHECK IF THIS IS A CONCERN	
1. When upset, can your baby calm down within a half hour?	☒ z	☐ v	☐ x	○ v	___
2. Does your baby like to be picked up and held?	☒ z	☐ v	☐ x	○ v	___
3. Does your baby stiffen and arch her back when picked up?	☐ x	☐ v	☒ z	○ v	___
4. When you talk to your baby, does he look at you and seem to listen?	☒ z	☐ v	☐ x	○ v	___
5. Does your baby let you know when she is hungry, tired, or uncomfortable? For example, does she fuss or cry?	☒ z	☐ v	☐ x	○ v	___
6. When awake, does your baby seem to enjoy watching or listening to people? For example, does he turn his head to look at someone talking?	☒ z	☐ v	☐ x	○ v	___
7. Is your baby able to calm herself down (for example, by sucking her hand or pacifier)?	☒ z	☐ v	☐ x	○ v	___
8. Does your baby cry for long periods of time?	☐ x	☒ v	☐ z	○ v	___

TOTAL POINTS ON PAGE ___

P201020100

Ages & Stages Questionnaires®: Social-Emotional, Second Edition (ASQ:SE-2™), Squires, Bricker, & Twombly.

page 1 of 3

Figure 5.4. A sample first page of an ASQ:SE-2 questionnaire showing important points to remember and questions with responses.

questionnaire should be returned (see Figure 5.4). The questionnaire items immediately follow. Each item is answered by marking the appropriate response option, and a few items have space for the parent to write comments. The last column has a circle the parent can use to indicate if that item is a concern.

ASQ:SE-2 Information Summary Sheet

The ASQ:SE-2 Information Summary sheet provides a summary of the questionnaire results (see Figure 5.5). The top of the sheet indicates the age interval and has space to include brief identifying information about the child. The sheet has space to calculate and record the child's total score and a scoring graphic that shows where a score falls in relation to the cutoff for referral. There is a guide to score interpretation, an area to record parent concerns, a section that outlines important considerations to discuss with families prior to making decisions about referral or follow-up, and a place to record decisions about follow-up action. If programs plan to have families keep the completed questionnaire, then parent answers can be recorded on the optional Item Response Sheet.

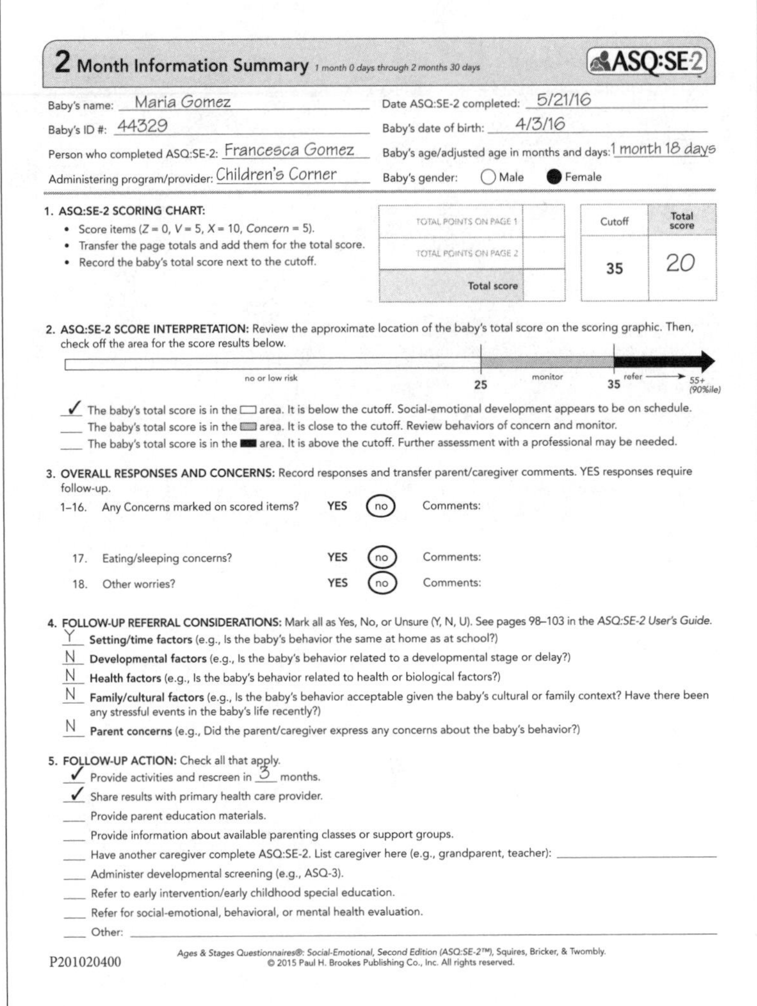

2 Month Information Summary *1 month 0 days through 2 months 30 days* ASQ:SE-2

Baby's name: Maria Gomez
Date ASQ:SE-2 completed: 5/21/16
Baby's ID #: 44329
Baby's date of birth: 4/3/16
Person who completed ASQ:SE-2: Francesca Gomez
Baby's age/adjusted age in months and days: 1 month 18 days
Administering program/provider: Children's Corner
Baby's gender: ○ Male ● Female

1. ASQ:SE-2 SCORING CHART:
- Score items (*Z* = 0, *V* = 5, *X* = 10, *Concern* = 5).
- Transfer the page totals and add them for the total score.
- Record the baby's total score next to the cutoff.

TOTAL POINTS ON PAGE 1	
TOTAL POINTS ON PAGE 2	
Total score	

Cutoff	Total score
35	20

2. ASQ:SE-2 SCORE INTERPRETATION: Review the approximate location of the baby's total score on the scoring graphic. Then, check off the area for the score results below.

no or low risk 25 monitor 35 refer → 55+ (90%ile)

✓ The baby's total score is in the ☐ area. It is below the cutoff. Social-emotional development appears to be on schedule.
___ The baby's total score is in the ▒ area. It is close to the cutoff. Review behaviors of concern and monitor.
___ The baby's total score is in the ■ area. It is above the cutoff. Further assessment with a professional may be needed.

3. OVERALL RESPONSES AND CONCERNS: Record responses and transfer parent/caregiver comments. YES responses require follow-up.

1–16. Any Concerns marked on scored items? YES (no) Comments:

17. Eating/sleeping concerns? YES (no) Comments:
18. Other worries? YES (no) Comments:

4. FOLLOW-UP REFERRAL CONSIDERATIONS: Mark all as Yes, No, or Unsure (Y, N, U). See pages 98–103 in the *ASQ:SE-2 User's Guide*.
Y **Setting/time factors** (e.g., Is the baby's behavior the same at home as at school?)
N **Developmental factors** (e.g., Is the baby's behavior related to a developmental stage or delay?)
N **Health factors** (e.g., Is the baby's behavior related to health or biological factors?)
N **Family/cultural factors** (e.g., Is the baby's behavior acceptable given the baby's cultural or family context? Have there been any stressful events in the baby's life recently?)
N **Parent concerns** (e.g., Did the parent/caregiver express any concerns about the baby's behavior?)

5. FOLLOW-UP ACTION: Check all that apply.
✓ Provide activities and rescreen in 3 months.
✓ Share results with primary health care provider.
___ Provide parent education materials.
___ Provide information about available parenting classes or support groups.
___ Have another caregiver complete ASQ:SE-2. List caregiver here (e.g., grandparent, teacher): ______
___ Administer developmental screening (e.g., ASQ-3).
___ Refer to early intervention/early childhood special education.
___ Refer for social-emotional, behavioral, or mental health evaluation.
___ Other: ______

P201020400

Figure 5.5. A sample ASQ:SE-2 Information Summary sheet. (Blank masters of the ASQ:SE-2 Information Summary sheets appear as hard copies in the ASQ:SE-2 questionnaires box and in PDF format on the CD-ROM included with the ASQ:SE-2 box.)

If agencies have an established agreement to share information about clients, and parents have provided written consent authorizing sharing their child's screening results with outside parties such as medical providers or preschool teachers, then sending the ASQ:SE-2 Information Summary sheet will provide a complete summary of a child's ASQ:SE-2 screening results. The receiving agencies, however, need to understand ASQ:SE-2 and how cutoff scores were derived in order to accurately interpret children's results. Professionals complete the Information Summary sheet rather than parents. (See Chapter 6 for details on completing the Information Summary sheet and interpreting results.)

Cultural and Family Adjustments

Although items on ASQ:SE-2 were carefully selected so that most parents would find the questionnaires easy to understand and use, there may be items that are not appropriate for a given family, culture, or geographic area. Families, especially across different cultures, have different expectations related to attachment and children's self-regulation, feeding, and toileting behaviors. For example, parents may continue to feed their children during the preschool years, or they may encourage self-feeding. Intentional floor time (i.e., "tummy time") is not encouraged in some cultures because the floor is considered unhealthy due to dirt and germs (Lyman et al., 2007). When preparing copies of ASQ:SE-2 to distribute, instructions in a second language such as Arabic could be added. Questions that may be culturally inappropriate can be masked or crossed out. Staff need be trained on culturally sensitive screening and assessment procedures. Professionals can understand expectations, work together on family concerns, and interpret results appropriately by learning more about parent expectations (e.g., "What do you consider a long time to calm down from a tantrum?") or parenting practices (e.g., "How and when do you put your child down to sleep?"). Together, providers and caregivers can discuss follow-up actions that are appropriate for the family's cultural context. Programs ideally should try to employ "community health workers," or providers with experience with a family's specific culture, to assist in the administration and interpretation of ASQ:SE-2 results. Deciding how to handle differences and adjustments can be an important part of organizing the screening/monitoring program. See Appendix G for a detailed discussion about adapting or translating ASQ:SE-2 for use with families from diverse backgrounds.

Several families who recently immigrated to the United States have been referred to the Steps-Ahead program. These families share many common values concerning child development and behavior. For some families, however, there are items on ASQ:SE-2 that do not reflect their parenting practices or do not make sense to them. For example, the question, "When you leave, does your child remain upset and cry for more than an hour?" was confusing for a parent who had never left her child in someone else's care. The Steps-Ahead program provides training to staff on how to administer ASQ:SE-2 with diverse families. When staff introduce ASQ:SE-2, they encourage parents to ask questions and let them know if any ASQ:SE-2 questions do not make sense or seem inappropriate. The previous ASQ:SE-2 item was omitted because it was determined to be inappropriate for the family's parenting practice or values. Steps-Ahead was still able to get a valid ASQ:SE-2 score because it is okay for three or fewer scored items to be omitted on a single questionnaire.

---

12. Develop Forms, Letters, and a Referral Guide

This step covers a range of information associated with developing forms and letters essential for the smooth and efficient operation of a screening/monitoring program. The forms and letters described in this step of Phase II are offered as models or templates and likely will need to be modified by program personnel who choose to use them. Appendix D includes blank samples of forms and letters along with Spanish translations. The ASQ Online management system contains customizable letter templates for use in a screening/monitoring program.

Information and Agreement Letter

Figure 5.6 presents an example of a welcome letter that could be sent to a parent or other caregiver. It contains a brief description of the importance of early development and of the screening/monitoring program. The letter also explains the parent participation expected and the activities of the program personnel. (A blank letter template appears in Appendix D.)

Dear parent/caregiver:

Welcome to our social-emotional screening and monitoring program! The first 5 years of your child's life are very important. Social-emotional development within the first few years of life prepares your child to be confident, trusting, curious, and able to develop positive relationships with others. Your child's positive social-emotional development forms a foundation for learning throughout life.

As part of this service, we provide the Ages & Stages Questionnaires: Social-Emotional, Second Edition (ASQ:SE-2), to help you keep track of your child's social-emotional development. ASQ:SE-2 asks questions about your child's behaviors and social-emotional growth.

If the questionnaire shows that your child is developing without concerns, we will share some activities that you can do at home to encourage your child's social-emotional development. Then, we will give you a questionnaire every 6 months until your child is 3 years old, and then again at 4 and 5 years old.

If completing this questionnaire brings up any questions or concerns, we can talk about information and resources that can help. Information will be shared with other professionals or agencies only with your written consent.

We look forward to your participation in our program. Please call or e-mail me at any time if you have any questions or would like to discuss any concerns about your child's development.

Sincerely,

Violet Jones
Steps-Ahead

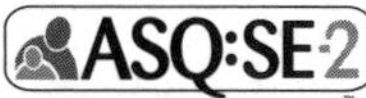

Figure 5.6. A sample Parent Welcome Letter for parents or guardians. Appendix D contains blank, photocopiable versions of this letter in English and Spanish.

Obtaining consent or agreement from a child's parent or guardian is an important prerequisite for participation in a screening/monitoring program. Personnel have four options for obtaining agreement to participate in the program: 1) call the parent or guardian to obtain initial consent, then include a written consent form with the first questionnaire and ask parents to complete and return both; 2) send a letter to the parent or guardian soliciting written consent; 3) obtain consent online; or 4) obtain written consent in person. How parents or guardians are initially approached depends on the program's goals and resources. It is important to provide parents with as much information as possible about the screening/monitoring program when obtaining their consent to participate.

Most programs ask parents to complete a consent form before beginning the screening process. Figure 5.7 offers an example of a form to be completed and signed by parents or guardians indicating their willingness to participate in the screening and monitoring program. (A blank version appears in Appendix D.) The form also gives parents and guardians the option of refusing to participate. Like the letter contained in Figure 5.6, this form should be modified as necessary to meet the specific needs of the program.

Consent Form

The first 5 years of life are very important. Social-emotional development within the first few years of life prepares your child to be confident, trusting, curious, and able to develop positive relationships with others. Your child's positive social-emotional development forms a foundation for learning throughout life.

Please read the text below and mark the desired space to indicate whether you will participate in the screening/monitoring program.

● I have read the information provided about the Ages & Stages Questionnaires: Social-Emotional, Second Edition (ASQ:SE-2), and I wish to have my child participate in the screening/monitoring program. I will fill out questionnaires about my child's social-emotional development and will promptly return the completed questionnaires.

○ I do not wish to participate in the screening/monitoring program. I have read the provided information about the Ages & Stages Questionnaires: Social-Emotional, Second Edition (ASQ:SE-2), and understand the purpose of this program.

Amita Gupta
Parent's or guardian's signature

July 10, 2016
Date

Child's name: Subir Gupta

Child's date of birth: July 1, 2013

If child was born 3 or more weeks premature, # of weeks premature: ____________

Child's primary physician: Dr. Scott

ASQ:SE-2

Figure 5.7. A sample Consent Form to be signed by a child's parent or guardian regarding participation in a screening/monitoring program. Appendix D contains blank, photocopiable versions of this form in English and Spanish.

Demographic Information Sheet

After parents or guardians have signed forms indicating their wish to participate in the screening/monitoring program, a staff member should describe the procedures that will be used in more detail. At this time, parents should be asked to provide demographic information about their child and family. This information may help programs interpret screening results. For example, children who were born with low birth weight may have more regulatory concerns, especially when they are infants, which may affect referral considerations. This information is ideally obtained in person, but it also can be gathered over the telephone or through the mail. Figure 5.8 shows an example of a Demographic Information Sheet. (A full-size photocopiable version appears in Appendix D.) Programs may use this sheet to gather demographic information on the children/families they will serve. The Demographic Information Sheet can be used to update demographic information annually or at shorter or longer intervals, depending on the program's needs. The program can indicate to parents which items to fill out and which sections will be completed by program staff (e.g., the Program Information section).

Demographic Information Sheet

Today's date: 7/30/16
Child's name (first/middle/last): Sarah Ann Rose
Child's date of birth (MM/DD/YYYY): 07 / 18 / 2012
If child was born premature, # of weeks premature:
Child's gender: ○ Male ● Female
Child's race/ethnicity: Mixed
Child's birth weight (pounds/ounces): 6/4
Parent/primary caregiver's name (first/middle/last): Margaret Shiner
Relationship to child: Grandmother
Street address: 84 West Charles Street
City: Topeka
State/province: KS ZIP/postal code: 66629
Home telephone: 202-555-0156 Work telephone: 202-555-0114
Cell/other telephone: none
E-mail address: none
Child's primary language: English
Language(s) spoken in the home: English
Child's primary care physician: Dr. Johnson
Clinic/location/practice name: Topeka, KS
Clinic/practice mailing address: Box 3590
City: Topeka
State/province: KS ZIP/postal code: 66629
Telephone: 202-555-0191 Fax: 202-555-0150
E-mail address:
Please list any medical conditions that your child has: asthma

Please list any other agencies that are involved with your child/family:

Program information
Child ID #: 00592
Date of admission to program: 7/1/16
Child's adjusted age in months and days (if applicable):
Program ID #:
Program name: St. Mary Child Development Center

ASQ:SE-2

Figure 5.8. A sample Demographic Information Sheet. Appendix D contains blank, photocopiable versions of this sheet in English and Spanish.

Before using any demographic form, staff should carefully review it to ensure it meets the program's specific information needs and any confidentiality and information-sharing guidelines that may affect the program. For programs using or planning to use the ASQ Online management system (ASQ Pro and ASQ Enterprise), staff should be sure to gather the demographic data required to create child profiles in the online system. Information needed for the ASQ Online management system includes the child's name, date of birth, number of weeks premature (if applicable), gender, and address, as well as the parent or caregiver's name, relationship to the child, telephone number, address, and primary and secondary home languages.

Program Description Letters

Once parents have indicated their willingness to participate in the screening/monitoring program, staff should provide parents with an expanded verbal or written description of the program. It is important that parent questions and concerns be addressed early. It is equally important to ensure that parents understand the program and the options available to them.

Parents' willingness to be (and remain) involved in the program may hinge on understanding their involvement and role in the screening process. A description letter may accompany the first questionnaire (ideally, the 2 month age interval). A sample program description letter is contained in Figure 5.9. If another option is being used (e.g., home visits, one-time screening, primary health care provider monitoring), then the letter may accompany an appointment card. In any case, the letter should indicate that the parent or guardian may speak to a staff member to ask specific questions.

In addition, the reproducible handout called What Is ASQ:SE-2™? (see Figure 5.10) can be shared with parents at this point if desired. This handout, which appears in Appendix D and in paper as well as PDF format on CD-ROM with the ASQ:SE-2 questionnaires box, offers a simple introduction to developmental screening and ASQ:SE-2. It is designed to facilitate family participation in the screening/monitoring program. It does not describe how to complete the questionnaire.

Once parents have a general understanding of the program, the next step is to familiarize them with the questionnaires and the specific procedures used to complete them.

The Steps-Ahead staff decided that their initial contact with parents would be within 1 month of the infant's birth. Based on information on birth certificates completed in the hospital, the social worker determined whether each family met the required risk criteria. The social worker then sent the What Is ASQ:SE-2? handout along with a letter explaining the program to the parents. She called the parents within 1 week to answer any questions they might have and schedule a home visit. The Steps-Ahead social worker obtained the parents' consent to participate, enrolled the family, and described how to complete the questionnaire during the home visit. The social worker also had parents choose whether they wanted to receive questionnaires during home visits, while at the program site, by mail, or through a telephone interview.

Letter to Primary Health Care Providers

If not conducting the screening themselves, primary health care providers in most communities will appreciate receiving information about their young patients' participation in screening/monitoring programs. Refer to Figure 4.2 in Chapter 4 for a sample letter to a health care provider explaining the family's participation in a screening/monitoring program. Figure 4.3 in Chapter 4 shows a sample letter briefly describing ASQ:SE-2 and how to interpret the cutoff scores. This brief note can be attached when sending ASQ:SE-2 results to primary health care providers. (Blank templates of the physician letters appear in Appendix D.) Health care providers who are administering ASQ:SE-2 to a child may find it helpful to ask the child's family if they are receiving any community services. If so, the health care provider may want to contact this agency (with the parent written consent); this agency will appreciate receiving information about the child's screening/monitoring results.

Steps-Ahead involved physicians both as participants on the advisory board and with individual families when needed. The two physicians serving on the advisory board wrote letters to other physicians in the community describing the Steps-Ahead program. To ensure physician participation, Steps-Ahead staff notified physicians when families who were their patients enrolled in the program. (Parents indicated their child's physician on the ASQ:SE-2 Demographic Information Sheet.) Steps-Ahead staff also shared ASQ:SE-2 results with the child's health care provider after parents had given their written consent.

Dear Mr. and Mrs. Feldman:

Thank you for participating in our child screening/monitoring program. Enclosed is a questionnaire from the Ages & Stages Questionnaires: Social-Emotional, Second Edition (ASQ:SE-2), which is a screening tool that will provide a quick check of your daughter Lily's social-emotional development. This questionnaire asks questions about your child's behaviors and social-emotional growth. The information you supply will help reveal your child's strengths, uncover any areas of concern, and determine if there are community resources or services that may be useful for your child or your family. If completing this questionnaire brings up any questions or concerns, we can talk about information and resources that can help.

We'd like to ask you first to fill out the enclosed family information sheet, which helps us be sure we have the most up-to-date information possible. Please keep these tips and directions in mind while completing ASQ:SE-2.

Tips for completing ASQ:SE-2:

✓ Caregivers who know the child well and spend more than 15–20 hours per week with the child should complete ASQ:SE-2.
✓ Answer based on what you know about your child's behavior.
✓ Answer questions based on your child's *usual* behavior, not behavior when your child is sick, very tired, or hungry.

Directions for completing ASQ:SE-2:

1. Please read each question carefully and check the response that best describes your child's behavior:
   - **Often or always:** My child performs this behavior often or always.
   - **Sometimes:** My child sometimes performs this behavior (not consistently).
   - **Rarely or never:** My child rarely performs this behavior or has never performed the behavior.
2. **Concerns:** Check the circle to the right of a question if the behavior is a concern.
3. Some questions have blank spaces for you to provide examples of your child's behavior. Please be sure to explain your response(s).
4. The Overall section at the end of the questionnaire asks open-ended questions about your child's behaviors. Answer questions by marking ***yes*** or ***no*** and provide an explanation for your responses.

Please be sure to send back the questionnaire within 2 weeks. Please contact me if you have any questions or concerns.

Sincerely,

Violet Jones
Steps-Ahead

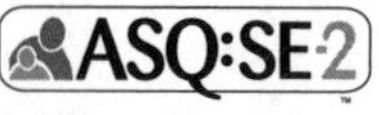

Figure 5.9. A sample ASQ:SE-2 Questionnaire Parent Cover Letter. Appendix D contains blank, photocopiable versions of this letter in English and Spanish.

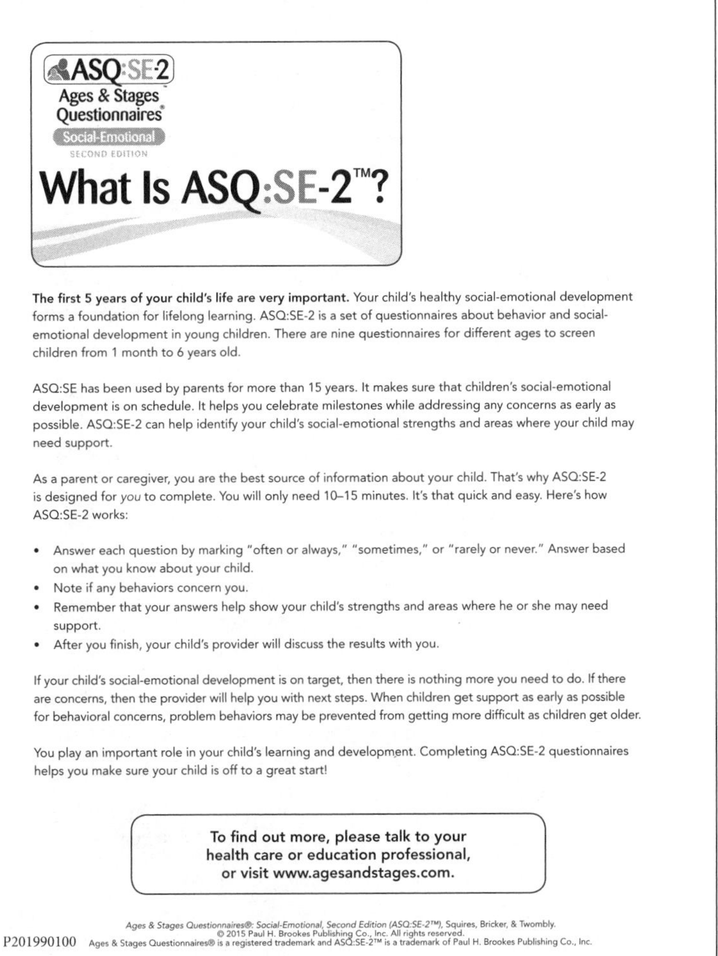

ASQ:SE-2
Ages & Stages Questionnaires®
Social-Emotional
SECOND EDITION

What Is ASQ:SE-2™?

The first 5 years of your child's life are very important. Your child's healthy social-emotional development forms a foundation for lifelong learning. ASQ:SE-2 is a set of questionnaires about behavior and social-emotional development in young children. There are nine questionnaires for different ages to screen children from 1 month to 6 years old.

ASQ:SE has been used by parents for more than 15 years. It makes sure that children's social-emotional development is on schedule. It helps you celebrate milestones while addressing any concerns as early as possible. ASQ:SE-2 can help identify your child's social-emotional strengths and areas where your child may need support.

As a parent or caregiver, you are the best source of information about your child. That's why ASQ:SE-2 is designed for *you* to complete. You will only need 10–15 minutes. It's that quick and easy. Here's how ASQ:SE-2 works:

- Answer each question by marking "often or always," "sometimes," or "rarely or never." Answer based on what you know about your child.
- Note if any behaviors concern you.
- Remember that your answers help show your child's strengths and areas where he or she may need support.
- After you finish, your child's provider will discuss the results with you.

If your child's social-emotional development is on target, then there is nothing more you need to do. If there are concerns, then the provider will help you with next steps. When children get support as early as possible for behavioral concerns, problem behaviors may be prevented from getting more difficult as children get older.

You play an important role in your child's learning and development. Completing ASQ:SE-2 questionnaires helps you make sure your child is off to a great start!

To find out more, please talk to your health care or education professional, or visit www.agesandstages.com.

Figure 5.10. What Is ASQ:SE-2™? parent handout. Appendix D contains blank, photocopiable versions of this handout in English and Spanish. It is also included with the ASQ:SE-2 questionnaire box.

Feedback Letters

Once completed questionnaires are returned, program personnel will want to consider offering at least two types of feedback letters based on results for children who 1) score well below the cutoffs or 2) score near the cutoffs (i.e., in the monitoring zone) and/or whose parents indicate a concern.

When Scores Are Well Below Cutoffs Most children for whom a questionnaire is completed will score well below the established cutoff score. For these children, a letter can be sent to parents explaining that their child's social-emotional development appears to be on schedule and also indicating when the next questionnaire will need to be completed. Figure 5.11 shows a sample feedback letter for parents of children whose scores indicate that their social-emotional development is currently on track.

When Scores Are in the Monitoring Zone For questionnaires on which a child's total score is close to the cutoffs (i.e., in the monitoring zone), a letter may be sent to parents explaining that their child appears to be developing on schedule but might benefit from some additional support in the social-emotional area. The program may choose to provide the social-emotional guides and parent–child activity sheets (in Appendix E at the end of this book and also on the CD-ROM in the ASQ:SE-2 questionnaires box). Parents also can be informed when the next questionnaire should be completed. Figure 5.12 contains a sample feedback letter for parents of children whose scores are in the monitoring zone and who may benefit from additional supports and/or referrals to community agencies.

When Scores Are Above the Cutoffs or Parents Indicate Concerns Parents should be contacted directly if they raise a concern on a questionnaire or if the child's score is above the cutoff. The score or concern should be discussed, and if appropriate, further assessment options should be reviewed. (See Chapter 6 for guidance on how to discuss results with families.) In addition, the child's health care provider should receive a letter indicating further assessment is recommended (see Figure 5.13).

Dear Mrs. Torini:

Thank you for completing the recent questionnaire from the Ages & Stages Questionnaires: Social-Emotional, Second Edition (ASQ:SE-2), for your child. Your responses on the questionnaire show that your child's social-emotional development is on schedule at this time.

Enclosed is some general information about social-emotional development specific to your child's age and activities that you can do together with your child to promote his social-emotional development.

You'll receive another questionnaire in 4 months. Please remember that is very important to complete all items and return it as soon as you finish it.

Please call or e-mail us at any time if you have any questions or concerns about your child's behaviors or development. There is a lot of excellent information we can share with you, and resources are available in our community to support you on your parenting journey.

Sincerely,

Douglas Maahs
Steps-Ahead

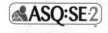

Figure 5.11. A sample Parent Feedback Letter: Typical for parents or guardians whose child's questionnaire score is well below the cutoff. Appendix D contains blank, photocopiable versions of this letter in English and Spanish.

Dear Mr. and Mrs. Singh:

Thank you for completing the recent questionnaire from the Ages & Stages Questionnaires: Social-Emotional, Second Edition (ASQ:SE-2), for your child. Your responses on the questionnaire show that your child's social-emotional development should be monitored for a period of time.

We are enclosing some general information about the social-emotional development of children specific to your child's age and age-appropriate activities that you can do together with your child to promote her social-emotional development. Also included is specific information about some of the behaviors for which you have concerns.

We also suggest that you complete another ASQ:SE-2 questionnaire in 6 months. We will contact you with a reminder and send you an ASQ:SE-2 questionnaire at that time.

I will be e-mailing or calling you in the next week to follow up about the concerns you mentioned in the questionnaire. There is a lot of excellent information we can share with you, and resources are available in our community to support you on your parenting journey.

I'm looking forward to talking to you soon.

Sincerely,

Frances Frye
Steps-Ahead

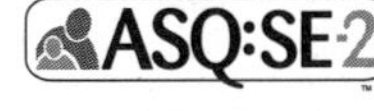

Figure 5.12. A sample Parent Feedback Letter: Monitoring for parents or guardians whose child's social-emotional development needs monitoring. Appendix D contains blank, photocopiable versions of this letter in English and Spanish.

Create a Community Referral Guide

A comprehensive community inventory that lists services available to parents of young children can be compiled during the planning phase or during the present phase to assist agencies when families request community resources and when a need for further assessment is indicated by ASQ:SE-2 results. In addition, agencies involved in screening need to keep an up-to-date list of local EI/ECSE agencies and mental health providers or agencies that provide social-emotional assessments and intervention services to infants and young children. The list should include the following information for each entry:

- Agency name and address
- Contact person
- Telephone number
- E-mail, web site
- Eligibility criteria for assessment and/or intervention the agency offers
- Services provided

Dear Dr. Yoshi:

Ages & Stages Questionnaires: Social-Emotional, Second Edition (ASQ:SE-2), is a series of nine parent-completed questionnaires developed for screening children from 1 month to 72 months (6 years). ASQ:SE-2 helps monitor children's social-emotional development and identify potential social-emotional/behavioral issues. ASQ:SE-2 is a companion tool to the Ages & Stages Questionnaires, Third Edition (ASQ-3), which is designed to screen children's developmental skills/milestones. More information on use of ASQ:SE-2 in a medical setting can be found at www.agesandstages.com.

An ASQ:SE-2 questionnaire was recently completed for your patient as follows:

Child's name: Luke Wallace

Child's date of birth: September 1, 2014

Date completed: September 8, 2015

Questionnaire completed by: Yvette Wallace

A copy of the ASQ:SE-2 Information Summary sheet is provided for your records.

The checked box below provides a brief summary of the results of that questionnaire:

☐ The child's ASQ:SE-2 score is **below the established cutoff,** indicating social-emotional development appears to be on schedule at this time.

☐ The child's ASQ:SE-2 score is **close to the established cutoff** (within the monitoring zone). We have provided information to the family and will monitor the child's development.

☒ The child's ASQ:SE-2 score is **above the established cutoff,** indicating a need for further social-emotional/behavioral evaluation. We have discussed referral options with the family.

The checked box below indicates the needed follow-up action:

☐ **No follow-up action needed.**

☒ **Follow-up action needed.** Attached is the completed ASQ:SE-2 with specific behavioral concerns highlighted. We hope you can discuss these concerns with the caregiver during the child's upcoming appointment to help the family determine the most effective next steps.

Please contact me if you have any questions.

Sincerely,

LaShanda Mason
Steps-Ahead

ASQ:SE-2

Figure 5.13. A sample Physician Results Letter for a child's heath care provider that indicates that the child's score is above the cutoff. Appendix D contains a blank, photocopiable version of this letter.

13. Articulate Screening Policies and Procedures

This step covers developing the necessary policies and procedures to ensure the effective and efficient operation of the screening/monitoring program. When planning the ASQ:SE-2 system, it is essential to create policies and procedures to ensure that the process of screening is reliable and valid, as well as culturally appropriate and respectful of families. It can be a useful exercise for an agency that is involved in screening children to create a system map that outlines and describes the steps involved in the screening program and who is responsible for which steps along the way (see Figure 5.14). Supervisors, mentors, and senior staff play important roles in any screening/monitoring program and may be involved at different steps in the process to ensure the integrity of the screening program. For example, although a staff member may have the skills necessary to support a family in completing ASQ:SE-2, he or she may need guidance from a more experienced staff person if ASQ:SE-2 indicates social-emotional concerns. In general, the necessary actions involved in questionnaire use include

1. *Introduce the screening program, obtain consent, and gather demographic information:* Provide a general introduction to the screening/monitoring program and its purpose either in writing or face to face. Although there are a variety of ways that consent may be obtained, identify who is responsible for this step in the process. Finally, specify how the demographic information will be collected and who is responsible for gathering this information.
2. *Distribute questionnaires in a timely manner:* Make clear who has responsibility for identifying which children need to be screened in any week, determining the appropriate age intervals, and preparing the questionnaires. Identify not only how this will occur but also who is responsible for reproducing and distributing questionnaires to parents. Depending on the type of setting/method, completing ASQ:SE-2 may be entirely the parents' responsibility or it may require a staff person to provide assistance during a home visit. Although it may be clear that a home visitor will assist parents in the home, it may be less clear who is responsible to support families in clinic settings. Stipulate which staff members within each agency or setting will provide support to families. At a minimum, program staff should have an understanding of the purpose of screening, ASQ:SE-2, and the necessary skills to support families as needed to complete ASQ:SE-2 (e.g., fluency in other languages).
3. *Score and interpret ASQ:SE-2 results:* ASQ:SE-2 is not a complicated tool. It is important, however, to know who is responsible for scoring. Identify who will score ASQ:SE-2, when scoring will occur, and who will interpret results. With supervision, paraprofessionals or clerical staff can reliably score questionnaires or input ASQ:SE-2 data for scoring in the ASQ Online management system. That said, a supervisor or other professionals, ideally a multidisciplinary team, needs to be available to interpret ASQ:SE-2 results that are in the monitoring zone or above the cutoff. Providing necessary support for less experienced staff during this step will ensure that referrals are appropriate and that consideration is given to other factors, such as a child's health, cultural context, and opportunity to practice skills that may influence screening results.
4. *Communicate screening results:* Decide whether results will be communicated through letters, e-mails, over the telephone, or in person. Any results that suggest a potential delay or any responses to a parent's concerns should be communicated in person by an experienced professional.
5. *Conduct screening follow-up:* Programs should have a policy that specifies what happens following screening. Decide how actions are recorded and who is responsible for the specified follow-up. For example, clearly specify who will identify appropriate activities and provide them to the family of children whose scores are within the monitoring zone. Specify who has responsibility for identifying appropriate community referrals and supporting families of children whose scores are above screening cutoff scores.

In planning these processes, it is useful to consider each step in relation to staff available for the screening/monitoring program. Table 5.2 contains a list of the procedures involved in the screening/monitoring process and the competencies and skills necessary for their successful completion.

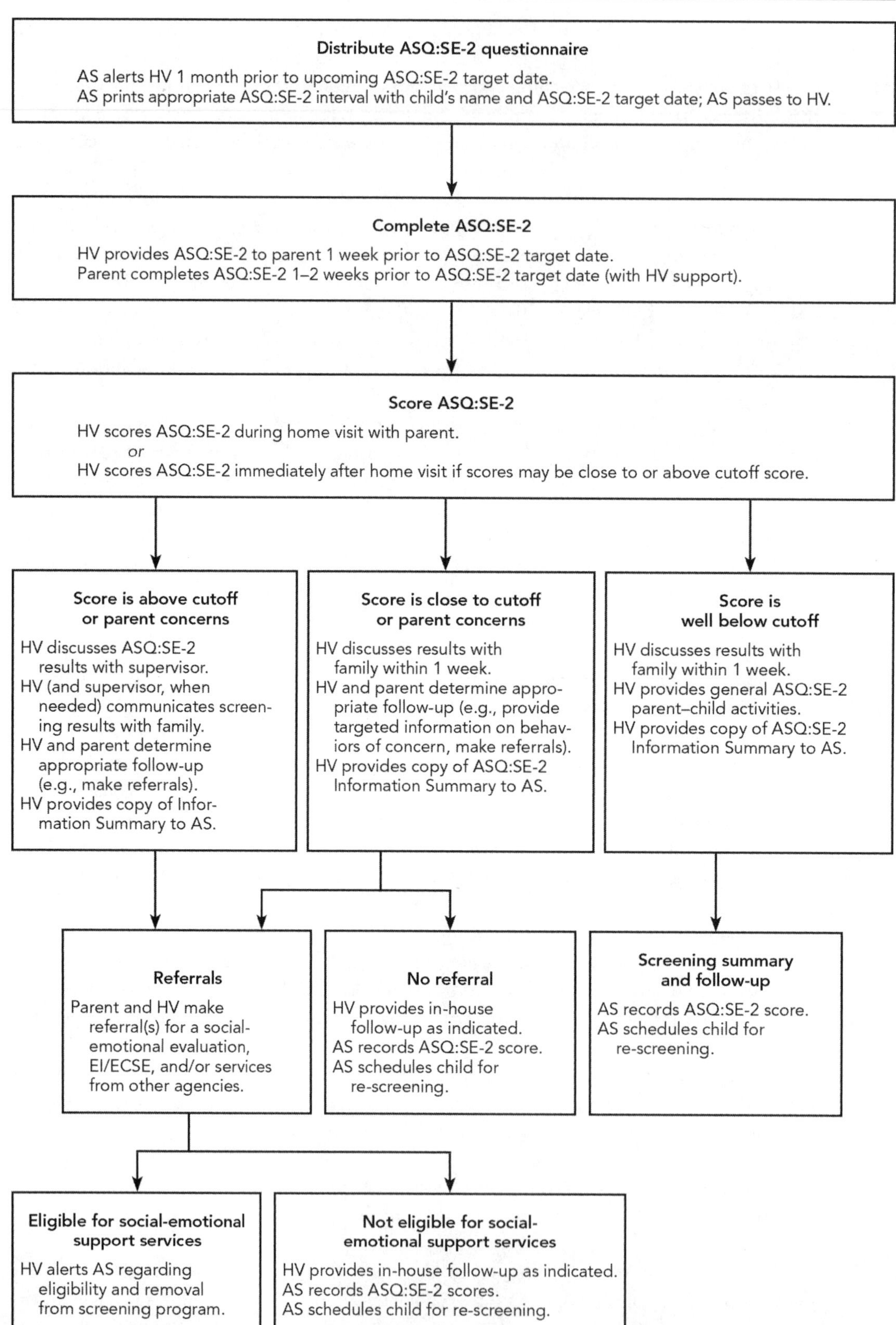

Figure 5.14. A sample ASQ:SE-2 system map. (*Key:* AS, administrative staff; EI/ECSE, early intervention/early childhood special education; HV, home visitor[s].)

Table 5.2. Procedures involved in the screening/monitoring process and the competencies and skills necessary for their successful completion

Procedure	Necessary competencies and skills
Introduce the screening program, obtain consent, and gather demographic information	Communicate purpose of screening to families. Understand how ASQ:SE-2 screening differs from other assessment processes. Describe features of ASQ:SE-2 to families. Obtain consent to screen. Provide support only as needed for families to complete ASQ:SE-2. Do not provide opinions on child's behaviors.
Distribute questionnaires in a timely manner	Calculate exact age of child, and choose appropriate ASQ:SE-2 interval to administer. Adjust for prematurity, if necessary. Use online, tickler, or informal management system.
Score ASQ:SE-2	Calculate results. Enter item-level responses in online management system.
Interpret ASQ:SE-2 results	Discuss factors with families that may affect a child's performance (e.g., time/settings, child's health, child's development, family/cultural values). Understand cutoff and interpret child's score. Understand gender differences in score distribution. Know how to expand on noted parent concerns through open-ended questions.
Communicate screening results	Sensitively discuss results that are in the monitoring zone or above cutoff.
Conduct screening follow-up	Be knowledgeable about local community resources and processes for referring children to primary health care providers, mental or behavioral health organizations, early childhood/early special education services, and/or parenting support or educational agencies. Be knowledgeable and have access to parenting resources for typical social-emotional development and behaviors of concern.

14. Provide Staff Training and Support

Screening and monitoring with ASQ:SE-2 (or any screening tool) is a potentially complicated process, requiring an understanding of the purposes and limitations of screening, effective communication skills (particularly when sharing sensitive and potentially difficult information with parents), the ability to consider what factors may be influencing a child's performance on ASQ:SE-2 (including cultural factors), and knowledge of community resources for appropriate referral. Users of ASQ:SE-2 should thoroughly read the User's Guide prior to initiating the screening/monitoring program. It is ideal to have at least one member of the program staff attend an ASQ training—the ASQ:SE-2 Introduction session, the ASQ Comprehensive session, and Train-the-Trainers session are available through Brookes On Location professional development seminars. Participants who attend Train-the-Trainers sessions will receive in-depth guidance as well as supporting materials that will assist in training others within their agency. Trainers can provide follow-up coaching and consultation with staff who are beginning to use ASQ:SE-2 as well as shadow newly trained staff during their first screening experiences with families. Users are encouraged to visit www.agesandstages.com for specific information about training materials and available training seminar options.

CONCLUSION

Phase III, administering and scoring ASQ:SE-2 and following up, is described in the following chapter. That phase addresses information that staff will need for scoring ASQ:SE-2, interpreting results, and sharing these results with families.

6

Phase III
Administering and Scoring ASQ:SE-2 and Following Up

ASQ:SE-2™

After the planning phase of the ASQ:SE-2 process is completed, program personnel can initiate Phase III of the ASQ:SE-2 system, which focuses on the actual screening of children, scoring the questionnaires, and determining follow-up activities.

STEPS IN THE ADMINISTRATION, SCORING, AND FOLLOW-UP PHASE

Phase III is composed of seven steps (see Figure 6.1):

15. Select the appropriate ASQ:SE-2 age interval
16. Support parent completion of ASQ:SE-2
17. Score ASQ:SE-2
18. Review written comments on scored and unscored sections of ASQ:SE-2
19. Interpret the ASQ:SE-2 score
20. Communicate results with families
21. Determine appropriate follow-up

15. Select the Appropriate ASQ:SE-2 Age Interval

Children must be screened using the correct questionnaire age intervals (e.g., a 12-month-old child should be screened using the 12 month ASQ:SE-2 questionnaire) to obtain accurate outcomes. To begin, it is essential to determine a child's exact age in years, months, and days. Calculating a child's exact age can be done by hand or using an age calculator. Figures 6.2 and 6.3 illustrate how to calculate a child's exact age by hand. Figure 6.2 shows how the child's

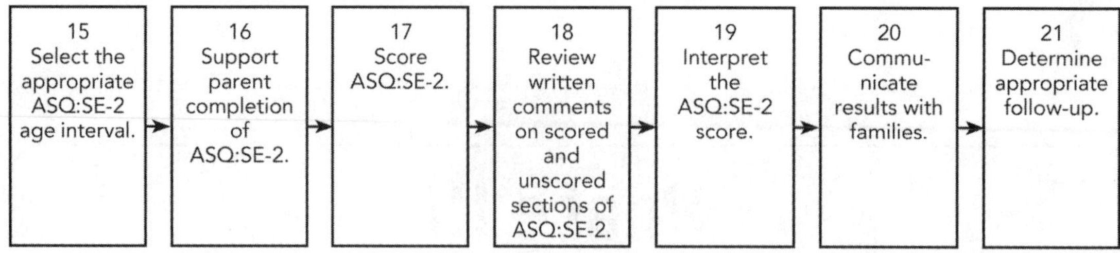

Figure 6.1. Phase III of ASQ:SE-2 implementation and associated steps.

exact age is calculated by subtracting the date of birth from the current date. Figure 6.3 shows how to calculate a child's exact age when it is necessary to borrow in subtraction. A number of age calculators are available for use, including one online at www.agesandstages.com and others available as apps for mobile devices and tablets through the App Store and Google Play (ASQ Calculator).

	Year	Month	Day
Administration date	2015	7	18
Date of birth	2012	4	9
Age of child	***3 years***	***3 months***	***9 days***

Figure 6.2. Calculating age. This example shows simple subtraction to calculate an exact age of 3 years, 3 months, and 9 days. The 36 month questionnaire will be used.

Adjusting for Prematurity

Programs administering ASQ:SE-2 should correct for prematurity for children younger than 24 months of age. This adjustment is important for three reasons:

1. The ASQ:SE-2 cutoffs were established using adjusted ages for premature children in the normative sample.
2. Not correcting for prematurity may overidentify children with regulatory issues that are a result of prematurity rather than social-emotional delays.
3. It is simpler to develop a comprehensive screening and monitoring schedule if processes for ASQ:SE-2 and ASQ-3 are on the same time frame. Most regulatory issues that result from prematurity have diminished by 24 months, and a child's social-emotional development is progressing at a typical pace. As with ASQ-3, a child's chronological age should be used at 24 months and older to determine the correct ASQ:SE-2 questionnaire to administer.

The following two methods can be used to correct for prematurity:

1. *Adjusted age:* The first method of accounting for prematurity is calculating adjusted age. The adjusted age is calculated by subtracting the number of weeks of prematurity from the child's chronological age. The resulting adjusted age is used to determine the appropriate ASQ:SE-2 questionnaire to administer on any given day.

	Year	Month	Day
Administration date	2014 201~~5~~	16 (4 + 12 months) ~~5~~	42 (12 + 30 days) ~~12~~
Date of birth	2013	10	30
Age of child	***1 year***	***6 months***	***12 days***

Figure 6.3. This example shows how to calculate exact age when it is necessary to borrow in subtraction—30 days can be borrowed from the month column, and 12 months can be borrowed from the year column. Starting in the right column and moving left, begin with the day. Because 30 days cannot be subtracted from 12, subtract 1 month from the month column and add 30 days to the day column, making 42 days in the day column and leaving 4 months in the month column. Subtract 30 days from 42 to get 12 days. Next, because 10 months cannot be subtracted from 4, subtract 1 year from the year column and add 12 months to the month column, making 16 months and leaving 2014 in the year column. Then, subtract 10 months from 16 to get 6 months. Finally, subtract 2013 from 2014 to get 1 year in the year column. This child is 1 year, 6 months, 12 days (or 18 months 12 days) old at the time of administration, so the 18 month questionnaire will be used.

2. *Corrected date of birth:* The second method of adjusting age for prematurity is corrected date of birth (CDOB) and is used to project an ongoing screening/monitoring schedule. CDOB is calculated by adding the number of weeks the infant was born premature to the child's date of birth—the CDOB is essentially the same date as the child's original due date. The target date (or dates) for administering ASQ:SE-2 is then determined by adding the desired number of months (e.g., 12 months for the 12 month ASQ:SE-2) to the child's CDOB.

After determining the child's exact age in months and days (or adjusted age if correcting for prematurity), check the age range listed at the top of the family information sheet and the first questionnaire page to be sure that the child's age is within this range. Table 6.1 can be used to determine which ASQ:SE-2 interval to select.

Table 6.1. ASQ:SE-2 age administration chart

Child's age	Use this ASQ:SE-2
1 month 0 days *through* 2 months 30 days	2 month
3 months 0 days *through* 8 months 30 days	6 month
9 months 0 days *through* 14 months 30 days	12 month
15 months 0 days *through* 20 months 30 days	18 month
21 months 0 days *through* 26 months 30 days	24 month
27 months 0 days *through* 32 months 30 days	30 month
33 months 0 days *through* 41 months 30 days	36 month
42 months 0 days *through* 53 months 30 days	48 month
54 months 0 days *through* 72 months 0 days	60 month

Note: A program may choose not to correct for prematurity for programmatic or other reasons. Program staff need to check in with families of premature infants early to ensure that they are getting adequate support and feel comfortable parenting their premature infants. If a program does not correct for prematurity, however, then scores in the monitoring zone or above the cutoff need to be interpreted with this consideration in mind.

16. Support Parent Completion of ASQ:SE-2

A program staff member ideally will do an initial introduction of ASQ:SE-2 to a family. It is important to explain the purpose of screening and describe ASQ:SE-2 to parents, regardless of the setting and administration methods chosen. Although some programs may not have the resources necessary to visit each family, staff should make every effort to ensure this process is as user friendly and personal as possible. If program staff cannot visit the home or meet with a parent in person, then they should schedule a telephone conversation. While introducing ASQ:SE-2, it is critical to set a positive tone and establish open communication with family members. The tone and sensitivity of this initial introduction may encourage or deter a parent's participation in the screening/monitoring program. The handout called What Is ASQ:SE-2? is useful in supporting this introduction.

A letter such as the one found in Figure 6.4 can be attached to the first ASQ:SE-2 questionnaire to remind parents about the purpose of the screening/monitoring program. The letter

Dear parent/caregiver:

Welcome to our social-emotional screening and monitoring program! The first 5 years of your child's life are very important. Social-emotional development within the first few years of life prepares your child to be confident, trusting, curious, and able to develop positive relationships with others. Your child's positive social-emotional development forms a foundation for learning throughout life.

As part of this service, we provide the Ages & Stages Questionnaires: Social-Emotional, Second Edition (ASQ:SE-2), to help you keep track of your child's social-emotional development. ASQ:SE-2 asks questions about your child's behaviors and social-emotional growth.

If the questionnaire shows that your child is developing without concerns, we will share some activities that you can do at home to encourage your child's social-emotional development. Then, we will give you a questionnaire every 6 months until your child is 3 years old, and then again at 4 and 5 years old.

If completing this questionnaire brings up any questions or concerns, we can talk about information and resources that can help. Information will be shared with other professionals or agencies only with your written consent.

We look forward to your participation in our program. Please call or e-mail me at any time if you have any questions or would like to discuss any concerns about your child's development.

Sincerely,

Carletta Duncan
Steps-Ahead

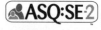

Figure 6.4. A sample Parent Welcome Letter for parents or guardians. Appendix D contains blank, photocopiable versions of this letter in English and Spanish.

contains a brief description of the importance of early social-emotional development, a description of the program, an explanation of the amount of parent participation expected, and a description of the program's activities.

Allay Fears About Screening

An important distinction between ASQ:SE-2 and some other social-emotional screening tools is that it can be used to identify a child's social-emotional strengths in addition to identifying problem behaviors that indicate the need for further evaluation or mental health or parenting support services. ASQ:SE-2 is an excellent universal resource for any parent, providing a springboard for discussion about what to expect at different stages of social-emotional development. This discussion can alleviate common concerns parents may have about children's typical behaviors and can extend to a conversation about what types of general parenting supports may be available in any given community to ease the parenting journey.

Be clear about the purpose of the screening program, about who will have access to screening information, and about how the screening results will be used. Some parents may have concerns about confidentiality issues or may worry that information will be used against them. For example, family members involved with child protective services may be concerned about how their answers will be interpreted. If parents admit that their child is out of control or has hurt other children, then they may be concerned about how this information will be used and who will have access to it. Establishing trust with parents is an important first step for program staff to gather reliable information. This may be a difficult path for program staff to walk, given mandatory reporting laws on child abuse and neglect, but any concerns about abuse and/or neglect need to be addressed and discussed with parents. Depending on the administering program, information gathered may be used to 1) make a referral for a social-emotional evaluation, 2) help monitor the child's social-emotional development, and 3) help determine information, resources, or support services the family may need. Consider the following language when discussing the purpose of screening with ASQ:SE-2:

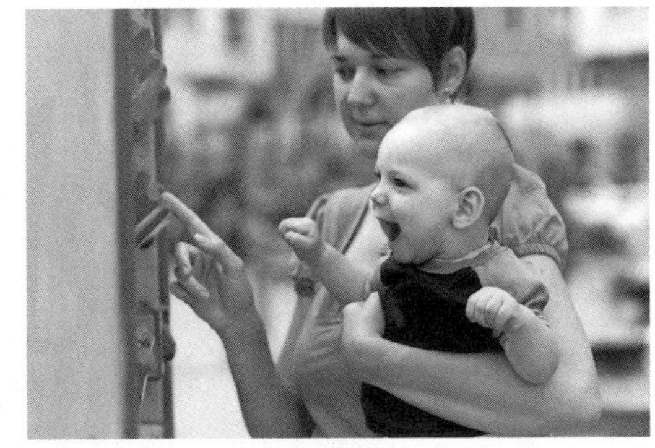

- "The ASQ:SE-2 questionnaire provides a quick check of your child's social-emotional development."
- "The information on this questionnaire will remain confidential. I will not share the information with anyone without your consent."
- "Your answers will show your child's strengths and if your child is showing behaviors you would like to talk about."
- "Your answers will help me know what type of information I may be able to gather for you."
- "Your answers will help me get to know your child better and how I can support him in the classroom."
- "If you have questions or concerns about any of your child's behaviors that are beyond my knowledge, then I will help you find other resources or agencies in our community that can help."

Review Important Points to Remember

It is important to give parents guidance and make them feel prepared to successfully complete a screening. Go over the instructions and items listed under "Important Points to Remember" at the top of the first page of the ASQ:SE-2 questionnaire.

- "Answer questions based on what you know about your baby's behavior."
- "Answer questions based on your baby's *usual* behavior, not behavior when your baby is sick, very tired, or hungry." The professional might explain further or offer some context: "For example, your child may become very clingy when ill but otherwise may be quite independent and outgoing."
- "Please return this questionnaire by [date]. If you have any questions or concerns about your child or about this questionnaire, contact [person]."

Tell Parents About the Possible Responses

With the exception of the open-ended questions at the end of the questionnaire, each question has three possible response options as well as a space for the parent to mark if the item is a concern. Staff should explain these choices and ask parents to check the most appropriate response.

- *Often or always* indicates the child does the behavior often or always does the behavior.
- *Sometimes* indicates the child does the behavior sometimes but not consistently.
- *Rarely or never* indicates the child rarely performs the behavior or has never performed the behavior.

Staff may show the parents how the questions and response options look on the questionnaire and should be sure to show parents the column where concerns can be indicated.

- *Item concerns:* Marking the circle in the far right column indicates that this behavior is a concern to the parent. Sometimes parents check only the Concern column but fail to check one of the response options. Encourage parents to check a response first and then indicate if the question reflects a concern about the child's behavior (see Figure 6.5).
- *Open-ended questions:* At the end of each questionnaire are three unscored, open-ended questions that ask about a parent's overall concerns—concerns related to the child's eating, sleeping, and with older children, toileting behaviors. The final question asks what parents enjoy most about their child. Parents should be encouraged to respond to these questions as appropriate.

Program staff should discuss response options before parents complete ASQ:SE-2, but staff should not provide their opinions about how to answer the questionnaire. If a parent asks for assistance to understand or interpret items, then staff should try to reflect the question back to the parent and encourage the parent to provide his or her best answer. Staff should provide as little interpretation about questions as possible, other than to help the parent understand what the question is asking.

	OFTEN OR ALWAYS	SOME-TIMES	RARELY OR NEVER	CHECK IF THIS IS A CONCERN
19. Does your child let you know how he is feeling with words or gestures? For example, does he let you know when he is hungry, hurt, or tired?	☐ z	☑ v	☐ x	✓ v

Figure 6.5. Marking behaviors of concern.

17. Score ASQ:SE-2

The questionnaires contain between 16 and 36 scored questions related to a child's behaviors and an additional set of open-ended (and unscored) questions about eating, sleeping, and toileting concerns; overall worries about the child; and what parents enjoy about their child. Simple step-by-step scoring instructions are outlined next. The sections following these basic instructions explain how to score questionnaires with missing items, how to calculate an adjusted score, and how to use the optional Item Response Sheet for recording and scoring questionnaires.

1. *Check for unanswered items.* Proceed to Step 2 if all items on the questionnaire are answered. If responses are missing, then first try to contact the parent to obtain answers. If it is not possible (e.g., the parent cannot be reached or does not wish to answer specific items), then proceed to Step 2. If one to three items remain missing, then review the options described in Scoring Questionnaires with Omitted Items, and Calculating an Adjusted Total Score. *Note:* If four or more scored items are unanswered or missing, the questionnaire is not valid.
2. *Review any parent comments.* Proceed to Step 3 if there are no parent comments. If the parent has written in a response, then see Section 18, Review Written Comments on Scored and Unscored Items, to determine if the response indicates a behavior that may be of concern.
3. *Score each item on the questionnaire.* Item points will range from 0 to 15 points and can be noted on the line to the right of each item (see Figure 6.6). Assign appropriate points for each item as follows:
   Z (for zero) next to the checked box = 0 points
   V (for Roman numeral V) next to the checked box = 5 points
   X (for Roman numeral X) next to the checked box = 10 points
   V (for Roman numeral V) next to checked concern circle = additional 5 points

	OFTEN OR ALWAYS	SOME-TIMES	RARELY OR NEVER	CHECK IF THIS IS A CONCERN	
18. Does your child follow simple directions? For example, does she sit down when asked?	☐ Z	☑ V	☐ X	✓ V	10

Figure 6.6. Recording item points. Sometimes (marked with a V) is given 5 points. A checked concern adds another 5 points. The total score for this item is 10 points.

4. *Add page totals and transfer to the Information Summary sheet* (see Figure 6.7).
5. *Record the child's total score on the Information Summary sheet.* The ASQ:SE-2 total score should be filled in on the scoring chart next to the cutoff score (see Figure 6.7). A total score may be above the cutoff, close to the cutoff (in the monitoring zone), or below the cutoff, which is illustrated on the scoring graphic on the Information Summary sheet. See Section 19, Interpret the ASQ:SE-2 Score, for more information about score interpretation. The following is a general guideline:
   - *Above the cutoff:* The dark shaded area is above the statistically derived cutoff score. A total score that is above the cutoff indicates a need for further evaluation and/or additional follow-up actions.
   - *Monitoring area:* The lightly shaded monitoring zone identifies children whose performance is close to the cutoff score. A total score that is in the lightly shaded area indicates a need for monitoring and may require follow-up actions.

TOTAL POINTS ON PAGE 1	15
TOTAL POINTS ON PAGE 2	20
TOTAL POINTS ON PAGE 3	10
TOTAL POINTS ON PAGE 4	5
Total score	50

Cutoff	**Total score**
65	50

Figure 6.7. Scoring chart section of the Information Summary sheet.

- *Well below the cutoff:* The white area indicates scores well below the cutoff. If there are no concerns about the child's behavior, then a total score in this area indicates that the child's social-emotional development appears to be on schedule at the time of administration.

Scoring Questionnaires with Omitted Items

Parents sometimes omit an item because they are unsure how to respond or have a concern about their child's behavior. Parents occasionally may not respond to an item because it is culturally inappropriate or inappropriate for their family's values. For example, some parents may feel uncomfortable answering questions related to a child's knowledge of "sexual language and activity," so the item about that topic may be left unanswered. It is important to attempt to reach parents as soon as possible to try to discern why items are unanswered. Responses should be obtained whenever possible, assuming that they do not compromise a family's culture or value system. If missing responses are provided, then the person scoring the questionnaire should follow the scoring steps outlined previously.

The following guidelines should be used to interpret ASQ:SE-2 scores when a parent cannot be contacted or a decision is made to omit the items. It is recommended that *no more than three items* are omitted on any questionnaire interval in order to accurately interpret ASQ:SE-2 results. Although it is possible to calculate an adjusted total score that provides credit for up to three missing items, this adjusted score will not influence the interpretation of the results in the majority of screenings (e.g., a child well below the cutoff will remain well below the cutoff). See the next section, however, if providers wish to create a precise adjusted total score so as not penalize a child for unanswered items.

It is recommended that providers follow these guidelines to interpret ASQ:SE-2 total scores with missing items.

- *One or two missing items:* If one or two items are missing, then proceed with the child's total score. Adjusting the total score will not change the interpretation of the child's score (i.e., the child's adjusted total will still be *above* the cutoff, *close to* the cutoff in the monitoring zone, or *below* the cutoff). No additional calculations are needed.
- *Three missing items:* If three items are missing *and* the total score of completed items is within 5 points of a cutoff, then adjusting the total score *will* change the child's results (i.e., results will move from below the cutoff to the monitoring zone, or from the monitoring zone to above the cutoff). For example, if three items are missing, and the unadjusted score is 45 and the monitoring zone starts at 50, then adjusting the child's total score would move the results from below the cutoff into the monitoring zone.

Calculating an Adjusted Total Score

An average item score is computed by dividing the questionnaire's total points (child's total score for answered items) *by* the number of items answered. This formula yields an average item score between 0 and 15. The average item score is then multiplied by the number of unanswered questions and added to the child's total score, giving an adjusted total score to compare with the cutoff on the ASQ:SE-2 Information Summary sheet. Figure 6.8 shows an example of calculating an adjusted total score.

Recording Individual Item Responses (Optional)

If program staff wish to return completed questionnaires to parents but still want to keep a summary of responses, then staff can use the optional ASQ:SE-2 Item Response Sheet to record questionnaire information, including individual item responses, parent concerns, and parent comments. This form, as well as the ASQ:SE-2 Information Summary sheet, may be useful for sharing results with health care providers or developmental specialists. The Item Response Sheet also may be used by the professional to score the parent responses. See Figure 6.9 for an example of an Item Response Sheet.

18. Review Written Comments on Scored and Unscored Sections of ASQ:SE-2

A few ASQ:SE-2 scored questions include space for additional comments. These questions are discussed next, along with some guidelines for interpreting parent answers.

1. Calculate average score:

$$\frac{\text{Total points of questionnaire (child's total score for items answered)}}{\text{Total number of items answered}} = \text{average score}$$

2. Calculate final total score:

$$\text{Total points of questionnaire} + (\text{average score} \times \text{number of items unanswered}) = \text{final total score}$$

Example: There are 35 scored items on the 36 month ASQ:SE-2. A parent answered 32 of 35 questions. The parent checked 24 items with 0 points; 2 items with 10 points; 6 items with 5 points; identified 1 concern (5 points); and left 3 items blank. The child's total score (for answered items) for the questionnaire is 55 points (20 + 30 + 5). The average score (55 points ÷ 32 items) equals 1.72. This number is the "best-guess point value" for each of the missing items. Because there are three missing items, 1.72 is multiplied by 3 and then added to the child's total score. The final total score (55 + [1.72 × 3]) is 60.16 points.

Average score:

$$\frac{\text{55 (child's total score for items answered)}}{\text{32 (number of items answered)}} = \text{1.72 points}$$

Final total score:

$$\text{55 (total score)} + [\text{1.72 (average score)} \times \text{3 (number of items unanswered)}] = \text{60.16 points}$$

The cutoff for the 36 month ASQ:SE-2 questionnaire is 105; therefore, this score is below the cutoff point. This child's social-emotional development appears to be on schedule at the time of administration. The monitoring program will ask the parent to complete the 48 month ASQ:SE-2 in 6–12 months to continue monitoring the child's social-emotional status. Rather than use the average score, however, it is preferable to contact the parent to obtain the answers to unmarked questions or find out why the parent did not complete specific items.

Figure 6.8. Formulas to calculate an adjusted total score from an average score on ASQ:SE-2.

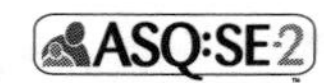

6 Month Item Response Sheet *3 months 0 days through 8 months 30 days*

ASQ:SE-2

Baby's name: Dejohn Carson — Date ASQ:SE-2 completed: 7/7/15

Baby's ID #: 03352 — Baby's date of birth: 1/3/15

Person who completed ASQ:SE-2: Marcus Carson — Baby's age/adjusted age in months and days: 6 months 14 days

Administering program/provider: Steps-Ahead — Baby's gender: ● Male ○ Female

This optional sheet is intended for **program use only** and should not be used for questionnaire completion.

To record item responses:
1. Transfer item response points to the Item score column.
2. Enter 5 points in the Concern score column for each item checked as a Concern.
3. Circle YES or no for Overall items.
4. Record any item comments or notes.

Item score key:
Z = 0
V = 5
X = 10

Concern score key:
No Concern marked = 0
Concern marked = 5

Item no.	Item description	Item score	Concern score	Comments/notes
1.	Calms within half hour when upset?	5	0	
2.	Smiles at you and family members?	0	0	
3.	Likes to be picked up and held?	0	0	
4.	Stiffens and arches back when picked up?	0	0	
5.	Looks at you and seems to listen when you talk?	0	0	
6.	Lets you know when hungry or sick?	0	0	
7.	Seems to enjoy watching or listening to people?	0	0	
8.	Can calm self?	5	0	
9.	Cries for long periods of time?	5	0	
10.	Body relaxed?	0	0	
11.	Trouble sucking from breast or bottle?	0	0	
12.	Feeding takes longer than 30 minutes?	0	0	
13.	Enjoy feeding times together?	0	0	
14.	Eating problems?	0	0	
15.	Stays awake for hour or more at one time during the day?	0	0	
16.	Trouble falling asleep at naptime or night?	5	0	
17.	Sleeps at least 10 hours in a 24-hour period?	5	0	
18.	Gets constipated or has diarrhea?	0	0	

(continued)

6 Month Item Response Sheet *(continued)*

ASQ:SE-2

Item no.	Item description	Item score	Concern score	Comments/notes
19.	Makes sounds and looks at you while playing with you?	0	0	
20.	Makes sounds or gestures to get attention?	0	0	
21.	Smiles back at you?	0	0	
22.	Makes sounds back when you talk?	0	0	
23.	Anyone shared concerns about behaviors?	0	0	
24.	Parent concerns about eating or sleeping behaviors?	YES (no)		
25.	Parent worries about baby?	YES (no)		
26.	What parent enjoys about baby?			He smiles and laughs a lot.

Item score subtotal		Concern score subtotal		Total score	Cutoff
25	+	0	=	25	45

Figure 6.9. A sample Item Response Sheet.

- *Eating problems (all intervals):* On the 2 month and 6 month questionnaires, the question "Does your baby have any eating problems such as gagging, vomiting, or ___?" provides a space for parents to write in another problem their child may be experiencing (e.g., refuses solid foods). This question is modified in the older age intervals as "Does your child have eating problems? For example, does she stuff food, vomit, eat things that are not food, or ___?" This question is targeting severe eating difficulties, such as eating only one food item or food texture. If the parent writes comments that seem within developmental norms (e.g., child is a picky eater) and has no concerns about the child's behavior, then program staff can inform the parent that the child's eating habits are typical of children that age and provide information or resources on this subject. If the parent writes comments that seem atypical for a child that age, then program staff may want to refer the parents to the pediatrician or seek advice from a feeding or nutritional expert.
- *Perseverative behaviors (18 months and older):* The question "Does your child do things over and over and get upset when you try to stop him? For example, does he rock, flap his hands, spin, or ___?" is designed to identify stereotypic or perseverative behaviors. A parent may write in a behavior that is a favored activity of the child (e.g., reading books, singing songs, playing tea party), and that behavior may not be of concern to the parent. When interpreting responses to this item, staff may use professional judgment to determine whether the behavior is atypical or can ask the parent for more information. Questions that may help distinguish a true perseverative behavior include "How difficult is it for your child to stop the behavior?" or "What happens when you try to stop your child from doing this behavior?"
- *Others' concerns (all intervals):* "Has anyone shared concerns about your baby's/child's behavior?" appears as the last scored item on all questionnaires. This question provides a glimpse into others' perceptions of the child's behavior. In many cases, a child care provider or a relative may have commented on a child's behavior, even though a parent may not have any concerns. This item provides an opportunity for parents to describe the comments of friends and relatives about their child's behavior.

Overall Questions Every questionnaire includes an unscored, open-ended section of Overall items with questions about general concerns related to eating and sleeping behaviors, and a question about concerns related to toilet training or toileting behaviors is included on the 30, 36, 48, and 60 month questionnaires. "Is there anything that worries you about your baby/child?" also is included on each questionnaire. These Overall questions are not scored but should serve as general indicators of parental concerns. Program staff should respond to any concerns noted in this section. A referral may be made based solely on a parent's response to an open-ended question, even if a child's ASQ:SE-2 score is below the cutoff. For instance, a child had a score of 65 on the 36 month ASQ:SE-2, 40 points below the cutoff score, indicating typical social-emotional development. However, on the open-ended questions, the parents indicated a concern about the child's regression in her toileting skills. Based on this parent concern, the child and parents were referred to the child's primary health care provider as a first step to gathering more information about this regression. Finally, each ASQ:SE-2 questionnaire asks what the parent enjoys about the child. This final question lets the parent finish the questionnaire on a positive note and gives the professional a positive place to begin a conversation about results.

19. Interpret the ASQ:SE-2 Score

After totaling the items and considering parent comments and concerns, program staff need to understand how to interpret a score and what additional information they need to gather to determine, together with the child's family, appropriate follow-up steps. This section describes the Information Summary sheet and also provides information on ASQ:SE-2 cutoffs, referral criteria, and additional factors that need to be considered prior to making a referral.

Using the ASQ:SE-2 Information Summary Sheet

The final page of each questionnaire is the ASQ:SE-2 Information Summary sheet (see Figure 6.10). The Information Summary sheet includes a top area to record identifying information about the child and family as well as five sections:

1. *Scoring Chart:* This section provides a place to document the child's total ASQ:SE-2 score and compare it with the established cutoff for that ASQ:SE-2 interval (see Figure 6.7).

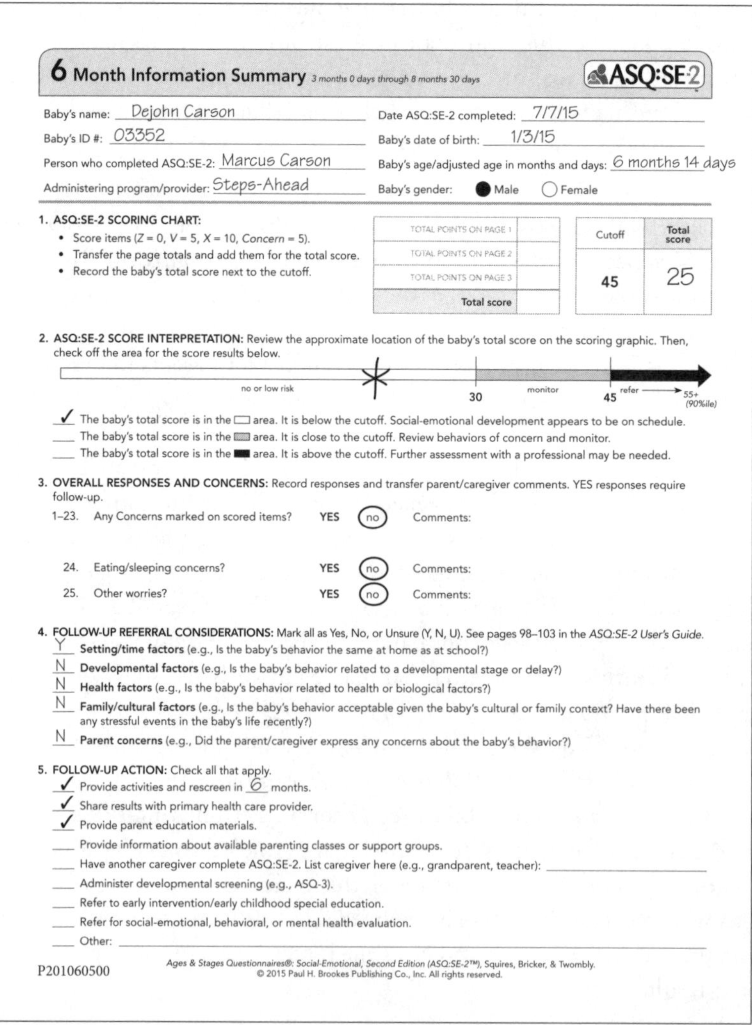

6 Month Information Summary *3 months 0 days through 8 months 30 days* ASQ:SE-2

Baby's name: Dejohn Carson
Date ASQ:SE-2 completed: 7/7/15
Baby's ID #: 03352
Baby's date of birth: 1/3/15
Person who completed ASQ:SE-2: Marcus Carson
Baby's age/adjusted age in months and days: 6 months 14 days
Administering program/provider: Steps-Ahead
Baby's gender: ● Male ○ Female

1. ASQ:SE-2 SCORING CHART:
- Score items (*Z* = 0, *V* = 5, *X* = 10, *Concern* = 5).
- Transfer the page totals and add them for the total score.
- Record the baby's total score next to the cutoff.

TOTAL POINTS ON PAGE 1	
TOTAL POINTS ON PAGE 2	
TOTAL POINTS ON PAGE 3	
Total score	

Cutoff	Total score
45	25

2. ASQ:SE-2 SCORE INTERPRETATION: Review the approximate location of the baby's total score on the scoring graphic. Then, check off the area for the score results below.

✓ The baby's total score is in the □ area. It is below the cutoff. Social-emotional development appears to be on schedule.
___ The baby's total score is in the ▒ area. It is close to the cutoff. Review behaviors of concern and monitor.
___ The baby's total score is in the ■ area. It is above the cutoff. Further assessment with a professional may be needed.

3. OVERALL RESPONSES AND CONCERNS: Record responses and transfer parent/caregiver comments. YES responses require follow-up.

1–23. Any Concerns marked on scored items? YES (no) Comments:

24. Eating/sleeping concerns? YES (no) Comments:

25. Other worries? YES (no) Comments:

4. FOLLOW-UP REFERRAL CONSIDERATIONS: Mark all as Yes, No, or Unsure (Y, N, U). See pages 98–103 in the *ASQ:SE-2 User's Guide.*

Y **Setting/time factors** (e.g., Is the baby's behavior the same at home as at school?)
N **Developmental factors** (e.g., Is the baby's behavior related to a developmental stage or delay?)
N **Health factors** (e.g., Is the baby's behavior related to health or biological factors?)
N **Family/cultural factors** (e.g., Is the baby's behavior acceptable given the baby's cultural or family context? Have there been any stressful events in the baby's life recently?)
N **Parent concerns** (e.g., Did the parent/caregiver express any concerns about the baby's behavior?)

5. FOLLOW-UP ACTION: Check all that apply.

✓ Provide activities and rescreen in 6 months.
✓ Share results with primary health care provider.
✓ Provide parent education materials.
___ Provide information about available parenting classes or support groups.
___ Have another caregiver complete ASQ:SE-2. List caregiver here (e.g., grandparent, teacher): ______
___ Administer developmental screening (e.g., ASQ-3).
___ Refer to early intervention/early childhood special education.
___ Refer for social-emotional, behavioral, or mental health evaluation.
___ Other: ______

P201060500

Ages & Stages Questionnaires®: Social-Emotional, Second Edition (ASQ:SE-2™), Squires, Bricker, & Twombly.

Figure 6.10. Dejohn's score on his 6 month ASQ:SE-2 indicates that his social-emotional development appears to be on schedule, and his father did not list any concerns in the Overall section. Steps-Ahead will continue to monitor Dejohn's progress.

Information about item point values and a table to tally page totals are included here in addition to the scoring chart with cutoff.

2. *Score Interpretation:* This section includes a scoring graphic with a place to visually review the general placement of a child's total score (see Figure 6.11). *Note:* The scoring graphic displays only up to the 90th percentile of ASQ:SE-2 scores gathered in the normative sample (i.e., not all of the scores are indicated, due to limited space.) After looking to see whether the child's total score is in the dark shaded, lightly shaded, or unshaded area, the professional should mark the appropriate line next to the scoring interpretation that reflects the child's numerical score.
3. *Overall Responses and Concerns:* Section 3 provides a space for noting parent concerns and comments, including which scored items were marked as concerns as well as responses to Overall items. These concerns should be discussed with the family, regardless of child's total score, and follow-up should be provided as indicated.
4. *Follow-Up/Referral Considerations:* Section 4 outlines factors that influence a child's behavior (e.g., health). Providers should review and discuss these with parents prior to determining appropriate follow-up, marking each factor as *Yes, No,* or *Unsure.*
5. *Follow-Up Action:* Section 5 provides a place to document follow-up actions.

Program staff will use the ASQ:SE-2 Information Summary sheet to summarize assessment information and help with the decision-making process. If parent consent has been provided, then this form can be shared with a child's health care provider (or other professional, as appropriate). If the Information Summary sheet is shared, then it is important that the professional who receives it is familiar with ASQ:SE-2 or has been given information about the purpose, scoring, and interpretation of ASQ:SE-2. Resources such as the ASQ:SE-2 Information for Health Care Providers (see Appendix D) can be shared with the ASQ:SE-2 Information Summary sheet.

The Information Summary sheet is for professional use and not for parent completion. Parents should not complete this form themselves. Programs using a mail-out method to administer ASQ:SE-2 should be sure to remove the Information Summary sheet from the materials sent to the family. It is recommended that program staff use the sheet to score questionnaires and review cutoffs. Professionals can use the Information Summary sheet to share results with families through a guided interview format, gather information related to referrals as needed, and work together with parents to determine appropriate follow-up actions.

ASQ:SE-2 Cutoff Points, Monitoring Area, and Referral Criteria

ASQ:SE-2 questionnaires are useful only if they identify children who may require further evaluation (i.e., children who score above the cutoff) and accurately exclude children who do not (i.e., children who score below the cutoff). Questionnaire cutoff points provide an index to do this. A standard cutoff point, or referral criterion, for each age interval was determined statistically using a variety of best-fit measures to obtain the ideal balance between overreferral and underreferral and maximize sensitivity and specificity (see Appendix C for the full ASQ:SE-2 technical report). Other analyses looked at general scoring trends in the normative

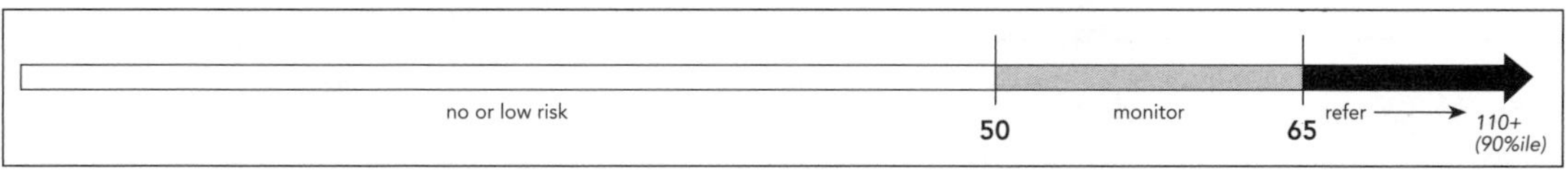

Figure 6.11. Score interpretation section of the Information Summary sheet.

sample. Monitoring zones were developed based on these data, with the monitoring area beginning at the 65th percentile point up to the standard cutoff, which tends to be closer to the 80th percentile point. See Table 6.2 for ASQ:SE-2 monitoring zone ranges, standard cutoff points, 90th percentile points by age interval, and percent of children identified with scores above the cutoff, indicating the need for referral.

It is often difficult to look at assessment results as "black and white" when assessing social-emotional concerns. Although the cutoff score and monitoring zone provide guidelines for how to interpret the ASQ:SE-2 score, program staff must look at the larger picture prior to making decisions about referrals and follow-up. For example, staff should consider the setting/time, the child's health and development in other areas, and the child's family/cultural factors that may have influenced a score. Staff may also consider a referral for further evaluation for a child's score in the monitoring zone. These factors are discussed in more depth in the next section. In addition, the referral resources that are available to a program may require the program to modify its referral criteria. Many programs and locales may find it challenging to find services for young children with social-emotional delays. A program's access to resources may influence its referral criteria and process.

ASQ:SE-2 scores provide staff with direction but do not provide all the information needed to make informed decisions about next steps. Additional factors that need to be considered and common follow-up activities when using ASQ:SE-2 are presented in Table 6.3. In general terms, the ASQ:SE-2 recommended referral criteria are as follows:

- *Score is **above the cutoff**, indicating the child needs a referral.* The dark shading on the scoring graphic indicates the area above the statistically derived cutoff score. Total scores that are above the cutoff indicate a need for further evaluation and/or additional follow-up actions.
- *Score is in the **monitoring zone**, indicating the child may have a problem.* The lightly shaded monitoring zone was developed to identify children whose performance is close to the cutoff score. Scores in the lightly shaded area indicate a need for monitoring and may require follow-up actions for items of concern. If the child being screened is a girl, then consider a

Table 6.2. ASQ:SE-2 intervals, monitor areas, standard cutoff scores, 90th percentile points, and percentages of children identified by referral cutoff

ASQ:SE-2 interval	Monitoring zone[a, b]	Referral above cutoff[c]	90th percentile[d]	Percent of children identified
2	25–35	35	55	18.4
6	30–45	45	55	14.7
12	40–50	50	75	24.0
18	50–65	65	105	23.3
24	50–65	65	110	22.8
30	65–85	85	135	23.7
36	75–105	105	155	22.0
48	70–85	85	150	26.0
60	70–95	95	155	22.6

[a]Scores lower than monitoring zone indicate typical development.

[b]Scores in monitoring zone may need further investigation.

[c]Scores above referral cutoff indicate a possible delay in social-emotional development (further evaluation with a professional is recommended).

[d]At this point, a child's score is higher than 90% of scores gathered in the normative sample.

referral for further evaluation. Data collected in the renorming of ASQ:SE-2 indicated that girls' total scores overall were significantly lower than boys' scores. See the technical report in Appendix C for further discussion on the differences between boys' and girls' performance on ASQ:SE-2. *Note:* The monitoring zone begins at the 65th percentile of ASQ:SE-2 scores gathered in the normative sample and ends at the established cutoff score.

- *Score is **well below the cutoff**, indicating the child's social-emotional development appears to be on schedule.* The white area on the scoring graphic indicates scores well below the cutoff score. If there are no concerns about the child's behavior, then total scores in this area indicate that the child's social-emotional development appears to be on schedule at the time of administration.

Table 6.3. Factors to consider before referral, sample questions, and examples of follow-up action options

Factors to consider before referral	Sample questions	Examples of follow-up action options
Setting/time	Does the child act the same way at home and in child care or preschool? (i.e., Is the behavior consistent across settings?) How long has the problem behavior been occurring? Is the setting new or unfamiliar to the child or family? Is the setting a good match for the child's temperament (e.g., large versus small child care settings)? Where, when, and under what environmental conditions does the behavior occur? Is the child being reinforced for this behavior or gaining access to reinforcers, such as preferred foods or activities, special time with a parent or teacher, or time alone?	Have another caregiver complete ASQ:SE-2 to determine the consistency of behavior across settings. If the child's behavior is not consistent, consider developing a behavior support plan in the setting where the behavior is problematic. Analyze caregiving environments to determine in what ways the environment is supporting or compromising the child's positive behaviors. (See Appendix F for examples of environmental assessments.) Provide parenting support and education to the parent in the home environment. Conduct a functional behavioral analysis (Dunlap et al., 2014) to determine the function of the behavior for the child. Use the results to create a positive behavior support plan for the child. (See Appendix F for examples.) Refer the child for an early childhood behavioral or mental health evaluation if concerns persist.
Development	Is the behavior related to a developmental stage? Are individual factors (e.g., temperament) related to the child's behavior? Can the behavior be attributed to a developmental delay or a sensory processing disorder? Are the child's skills at age level in the following domains? • Fine and gross motor • Cognitive/problem solving • Personal-social • Expressive and receptive communication	Provide developmental information (e.g., ASQ:SE-2 Social-Emotional Development Guides and Activities in Appendix E), positive behavior management suggestions, and so forth. Screen the child using a developmental screening tool such as ASQ-3. Refer the child to local Part C (early intervention) or Part B (early childhood special education) agency if concerned and/or if developmental screening tool indicates a need for further evaluation. Refer the child for an early childhood behavioral or mental health evaluation if concerns persist.
Health	Is the child's behavior related to health or biological factors? Has the child had a recent medical checkup? Have the following been considered as behavioral influences? • Lack of sleep or hunger • Medications or allergies • Exposure to drugs in utero	Refer the child to his or her primary health care provider. Address behavior of concern to determine if there is a biological/medical cause, and make referrals or provide follow-up as indicated within the health system. Keep in close contact with the family regarding all aspects of the child's health. Refer the child for an early childhood behavioral or mental health evaluation if concerns persist.

(continued)

Table 6.3. *(continued)*

Factors to consider before referral	Sample questions	Examples of follow-up action options
Family/cultural	What is the child's home (native) language? Is the "problem" behavior within the cultural norm for this child's family? Is the parent–child relationship influencing the child's ASQ:SE-2 results? Has the child been affected by stressful or traumatic events (ongoing, past, or present)? • Has the child witnessed violence in the home or in the community? • Has the child been involved in abusive or neglectful situations? • Has the child recently been moved from his or her home? • Are there family issues that are stressful (e.g., parent mental health issues, drug and alcohol issues)?	Determine if language or translation issues may be influencing parent responses to items (e.g., misunderstanding the intent of items). Talk to family members about the behavior and whether they consider it to be problematic. Work with the family to determine appropriate follow-up action. Seek advice from community health workers or "cultural brokers" (i.e., professionals who are familiar with or a member of the culture of the family) to determine if the behavior is within the cultural "norm." Use a professionally administered parent–child interaction measure (see Appendix F). Support the parent's understanding of responses to the social-emotional needs of the young child. If necessary, refer the child to early childhood mental health specialists to assess needs and provide therapeutic services to the parent–child dyad. If the child recently has moved to a new caregiving environment that is safe and nurturing, it may be appropriate to wait a short time before referring. If the child is in an unsafe or neglectful environment, refer to child protective or other services. Refer the child for an early childhood behavioral or mental health evaluation if concerns persist.
Parent concerns	Did the parent or caregiver express any concerns about the child's behavior? What is the *intensity* and *frequency* of the behavior of concern? Is the behavior of concern typical or atypical given the child's developmental stage? Are individual factors of parent or child (e.g., temperament) related to the parent's concern about the child's behavior?	Obtain more information from the parent or caregiver about any concerns noted on ASQ:SE-2; ask, "Can you tell me more about . . . ?" Provide developmental information (e.g., ASQ:SE-2 Social-Emotional Development Guides and Activities in Appendix E, *ASQ:SE-2™ Learning Activities*), parenting education or support, and so forth. Listen carefully to all parent concerns. Support the parent in identifying and accessing resources and supports within the community to address any priority concerns (e.g., support agencies to access basic needs such as housing/food, quality child care, respite care, drug/alcohol counseling, adult mental health counseling). Refer the child for an early childhood behavioral or mental health evaluation if concerns persist and are atypical for the child's age.

- *Parent concerns, indicating the need for follow-up.* Follow up on *any* concern parents indicate on questionnaires. Provide information or referrals to appropriate agencies for areas of concern. For example, staff can refer the parent who is struggling with toilet training or age-appropriate discipline to a parenting group. Although a child's score may not be above or near the ASQ:SE-2 cutoff, a decision to refer a child may be made based solely on parent concerns or the presence of a single behavior that is particularly problematic (e.g., a behavior that affects the safety of the child or others) or the parent's level of frustration with the behavior.

Professional Judgment Given the lack of professional and financial resources currently available in the field of infant and early childhood mental health, early childhood professionals may often feel alone and burdened with the enormous responsibility of determining the state of a young child's mental health. ASQ:SE-2 can assist practitioners in their decision-making process and can provide validity to referrals made to mental health professionals. If ASQ:SE-2 results do not validate concerns about a young child's behavior—either because the parent was unable to provide an accurate report or because the tool was not sensitive in a specific circumstance (e.g., picking up a child who seems unusually withdrawn or depressed)—then practitioners should seek alternative ways to identify children with potential problems and provide them with services.

Professionals should consider optional strategies to get information that can validate the need for referrals, such as having an alternative caregiver complete ASQ:SE-2, using a professionally administered screening tool, or administering a parent–child interaction measure. (Examples of parent–child interaction measures are included in Appendix F.) On the flip side, professionals also should look carefully at ASQ:SE-2 scores and consider the possibility of an inflated score, such as when parents frequently mark the *sometimes* option. If your professional judgment tells you that the score may be inflated, then consider the following section, Looking at Assessment Information in Context, which describes variables that might influence a parent's interpretation of a child's behavior. It is important to determine why an inflated score is occurring.

If a referral is made and a child is determined not to have a social-emotional delay (at least not to the extent that makes the child eligible for services), then it is still critically important to listen to parent concerns and provide information and support related to behaviors of concern. Discuss assessment results and gather information and resources from colleagues and specialists in early childhood, family service, health, and mental health fields. Infant/early childhood mental health is a new and developing field, and practitioners should not feel that they must have all of the answers to the complex questions and situations that arise.

Orletta's teacher and adoptive parents were concerned about her behavior at the Kool Kids Preschool. Although she sought out other children as playmates, Orletta often hit or made hurtful statements to playmates. The preschool director asked both Clay, Orletta's teacher, and her adoptive parents, Juan and Patrice, to complete a 48 month ASQ:SE-2 when Orletta was 43 months old. The score on the questionnaire completed by Clay was 148 points, compared with a score of 85 on the questionnaire completed jointly by Orletta's parents. Although the parents did not see as many aggressive behaviors at home, they were concerned about her tantrums and poor sleep habits. Because both ASQ:SE-2 scores were above the cutoff point, Orletta's parents decided to take her to a county mental health specialist who could conduct an in-depth social-emotional assessment and make recommendations for further intervention.

Looking at Assessment Information in Context It is always important to look at assessment information in the context of other factors influencing a child's life. ASQ:SE-2 is designed to gather information about a child's social-emotional development and help guide referral decisions, but it is not the only information that should be considered prior to making

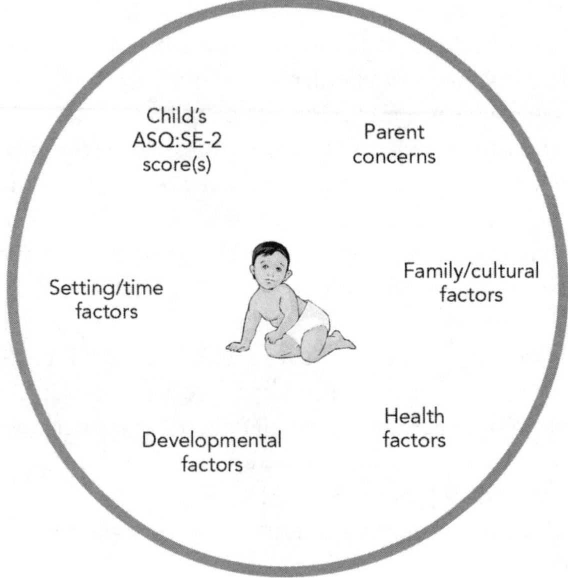

Figure 6.12. Factors to consider prior to referral.

decisions. When analyzing a young child's behavior, there are three reasons why it is critical to gather additional information other than assessment scores before making a referral decision.

1. A young child's behavior may depend on a variety of setting/time, developmental, health, and family/cultural factors. For example, a child with a speech delay may feel frustrated when unable to communicate his or her needs and react negatively (e.g., by hitting other children). Rather than immediately referring the child to a mental health professional, a more appropriate first step may be a referral to a speech-language pathologist (SLP).
2. Using diagnostic assessments is an expensive and time-consuming process. As previously mentioned, the field of early childhood mental health is new and growing, but resources are lacking. Program staff should make referrals only when necessary and for services that are the most appropriate and accessible.
3. The referral process can be stressful for the child and family. It may be more appropriate for staff to use preventive measures and closely monitor the child's behavior while attempting minimal interventions or providing family support.

Figure 6.12 provides an illustration of the factors that should be explored prior to making follow-up decisions.

A foster parent completed an ASQ:SE-2 for 4-year-old Aisha soon after Aisha entered her care. Aisha's total score was close to the cutoff, with the foster parent noting that Aisha was wetting her pants during the day, did not seem to be happy, was not using words to get her needs met, and was not playing with other children. After the caseworker reviewed the ASQ:SE-2 results, she met and talked with the foster parent about Aisha's behavior. The caseworker noted that Aisha had only been in foster care for 3 weeks when the questionnaire was completed and felt that Aisha was still adjusting to a new home. At a follow-up meeting, the foster parent indicated that Aisha seemed to be more relaxed in the 2 weeks since she had completed the questionnaire. The caseworker and the foster parent decided together to wait a month before administering the questionnaire again in order to allow Aisha to settle in at her new home. During that time the caseworker would enroll Aisha in a therapeutic playgroup for young children in foster care. The caseworker advised Aisha's foster parent to continue being warm and supportive and to encourage Aisha to talk about her feelings.

The ASQ:SE-2 Information Summary sheet has a section to indicate that these factors have been considered, which includes example questions that parents and providers can use as prompts. Table 6.3 shows a list of these factors, with examples of questions that could be explored if a child's score is in the monitoring zone or above the cutoff, and potential follow-up suggestions for referrals or preventive interventions. The table outlines follow-up options that program staff should consider while making decisions about referrals for young children. *These considerations are not intended to discourage professionals from making referrals for mental health evaluations or services. Rather, these considerations may help guide appropriate referrals or, when appropriate, guide preventive interventions.*

20. Communicate Results with Families

When an ASQ:SE-2 score is above the cutoff or in the monitoring zone, or when a parent has expressed concerns about behaviors the child is exhibiting, it is important to have a conversation in person to discuss results. It is important to have this conversation for two reasons: 1) parents will need to inform and direct any referral process, and 2) parents are a critical source of information about factors discussed in the previous section that may affect a child's ASQ:SE-2 results. Gathering information on these factors will help staff make informed decisions about what follow-up steps need to be taken. The Parent Conference Sheet can be a useful tool for organizing conversations with parents about results and next steps. (A blank, photocopiable version of this sheet appears in Appendix D and in PDF format on the CD-ROM included with the ASQ:SE-2 questionnaires box.)

Suggestions for Talking to Parents When Results Indicate the Need for Further Investigation

Sharing ASQ:SE-2 results requires sensitivity and attention to a family's needs or situation when scores are above the cutoff, in the monitoring zone, when parents have indicated behavioral concerns, or when providers may have concerns about a child's behavior. Program personnel need to carefully prepare for these discussions and should conduct them with compassion and empathy. Parents may react defensively or become angry at the person who is delivering the information. It may be helpful to role-play with a trusted peer or supervisor before communicating screening results with parents. The setting for the conversation should be private, and the meeting should take place at a time that is convenient for the family. Consider cultural practices (e.g., whether other family members should be invited to the meeting) and language issues (e.g., whether an interpreter is needed). Delivering ASQ:SE-2 results for a child whose score is above the cutoff should always be done in person or, alternatively, over the telephone; parents should never receive results of this type by mail or e-mail. Keep in mind the following points when sharing results with parents:

- Share screening results as quickly as possible.
- Make sure the meeting occurs in a private place and assure parents that the conversation is confidential.
- Remind parents about the purpose of screening. Make sure they understand that screening only indicates the need for further assessment and does not diagnose a child.
- Emphasize the child's social-emotional strengths while reviewing ASQ:SE-2 results. (Hint: All items with a score of 0 points are strengths for that child.) Regardless of a child's total score, it is important to begin by highlighting some of these positive items when communicating results with families.
- Discuss parent concerns and provide specific, nonjudgmental, objective examples of your concerns.
- Listen to parents' perceptions of their child, and be open to new ideas and viewpoints.
- Emphasize parents' current skills and resources. For example, if the family includes a grandparent who is willing to help, this resource can be mentioned as part of future steps to address the child's tantrums and self-regulation difficulties.
- Use phrases such as *well above the cutoff, close to the cutoff,* and *below the cutoff* when explaining cutoffs and a child's score. Avoid terms such as *test, fail, normal,* or *abnormal.*
- Discuss the fourth section of the Information Summary sheet, which includes important factors that may have affected scores (e.g., time/setting, developmental, health, family/cultural factors). Read the next sections for more information on follow-up and referral.
- If parents are interested, provide information about community resources and referral options. See the next section for more information.
- Remember that you are there to help parents take the next steps and facilitate the process.

Community Referral Information

To assist in making appropriate, timely referrals, it is helpful to keep updated lists of community agencies that provide developmental assessments and programs that provide intervention services to infants and young children. The list should include the following information for each entry:

- Agency name and address
- Contact person
- E-mail, web site
- Telephone number
- Eligibility criteria for assessment and/or intervention
- Services provided and cost of services

21. Determine Appropriate Follow-Up

Parents should inform and direct the referral process and decide the specific next steps and a time line for taking these actions. Several follow-up options should be considered based on the child's screening results and subsequent conversations with parents about factors that may influence a child's behavior.

Common Follow-Up Activities When Using ASQ:SE-2

The fifth section of the ASQ:SE-2 Information Summary sheet provides a list of potential actions that may follow the administration of ASQ:SE-2, based on the child's score and/or the parent's concerns (see Figure 6.13).

5. FOLLOW-UP ACTION: Check all that apply.

✓ Provide activities and rescreen in _6_ months.

✓ Share results with primary health care provider.

____ Provide parent education materials.

____ Provide information about available parenting classes or support groups.

____ Have another caregiver complete ASQ:SE-2. List caregiver here (e.g., grandparent, teacher): ____

____ Administer developmental screening (e.g., ASQ-3).

____ Refer to early intervention/early childhood special education.

____ Refer for social-emotional, behavioral, or mental health evaluation.

____ Other: ____________________

Figure 6.13. Follow-up action section of the Information Summary sheet.

- *Provide activities and monitor (rescreen) child.* Appendix E provides a set of social-emotional development guides that describe behaviors that are typical at different ages and correspond with ASQ:SE-2 screening intervals. In addition, parent–child activity sheets, which provide examples of age-appropriate activities that parents can do together with their children, can be shared with parents after screening. It also is recommended to monitor (rescreen) a child every 6–12 months, using available ASQ:SE-2 age intervals (e.g., 2, 6, 12, 18, 24, 30, 36, 48, 60 months), because of rapid changes in a child's social-emotional development over the first 5 years of life. Providing activities and monitoring a child's social-emotional development are recommended follow-up for all children who have been screened using ASQ:SE-2.
- *Share results with the primary health care provider.* Sharing results of the child's ASQ:SE-2 screening is considered best practice, and health care providers will appreciate having this information available during well-child checkups. When sharing results, providers should include information about ASQ:SE-2 and how to interpret scores (see ASQ:SE-2 Information for Health Care Providers and other letters in Appendix D) in addition to a copy of the child's ASQ:SE-2 Information Summary sheet and Item Response Sheet. If the ASQ:SE-2 score indicates a potential behavior problem, then sharing results of ASQ:SE-2 provides an opportunity for health care providers to talk to parents and determine if any problem behaviors may have a medical or health root.
- *Provide parent education materials.* The *ASQ:SE-2 Learning Activities* includes age-by-age handouts and activities to support parents. In addition, there are numerous parent education materials available, many on the Internet, that cover topics that may come up during the process of screening with ASQ:SE-2 (e.g., toileting, sleeping). ZERO TO THREE is one example of a national organization that provides excellent resources on parenting young children. See Appendix F for other helpful resources for parents about children's social-emotional development.
- *Provide information about available parenting classes or support groups.* Parents or caregivers may ask for community resources such as classes about behavioral management or guidance about supporting foster children who have experienced trauma. Keeping an up-to-date list of these resources will help providers make appropriate referrals when caregivers need additional supports.
- *Have another caregiver complete ASQ:SE-2.* Children's behavior varies across environments and with different caregivers (e.g., mother, father, grandparent, teacher). A child with a

serious mental health/social-emotional delay will generally exhibit similar behaviors across environments and caregivers. Follow-up steps for a child who exhibits problematic behaviors with only one caregiver or in only one setting, however, may be more specific (e.g., geared toward the caregiver or setting). In addition, providers may want to gather another perspective when working with parents with mental illness or those who may not trust why information is being gathered or how information will be used (e.g., parents involved with child protective services). Multiple perspectives, especially when caregivers or providers have concerns about a child's behavior, will provide more information to help determine appropriate follow-up.

- *Administer developmental screening.* It is imperative to conduct a screening for the child's overall development at the same time as the child's social-emotional development. Children with developmental delays are at increased risk for social-emotional delays, with approximately 40% of children with developmental delays identified as having a social-emotional delay compared with approximately 20% in the general population (AAP, 2014; Freeman, 2014; Merrell & Holland, 1997; Sameroff, Seifer, & McDonough, 2004). These children need services to address their developmental needs in conjunction with any behavioral-focused services. In addition, a child may have a developmental delay that is the root cause of the child's social-emotional delay; addressing overall development may remediate behavioral issues. For example, a child with a motor delay may react emotionally when unable to join in a game of kickball (e.g., by hitting other children). It is important to rule out a potential developmental delay as a cause of a high ASQ:SE-2 score. The appropriate intervention for a child with a motor delay is physical therapy, not mental health services.
- *Refer to EI/ECSE.* Under the IDEA Part C early intervention program (for infants and toddlers), all areas of development, including social-emotional/behavioral areas, must be assessed to determine delays and disabilities. Under IDEA Part B, Section 619 (early childhood special education), social and social-emotional development must be assessed if there is an area of concern or suspected delay. Eligibility criteria for these programs is so stringent in many states, however, that it can be very difficult to ensure a child's eligibility for services based on the child's social-emotional development alone if a child is developmentally on track in areas such as communication and cognitive development. IDEA clearly points to the importance of evaluating and serving a child based on this area of development, however, and Part C early intervention includes attachment disorders among a list of established conditions that automatically make an infant or toddler eligible for Part C services. Referral to the local EI/ECSE provider is always a good idea when ASQ:SE-2 scores are above cutoffs because social-emotional delays and behavior problems will ultimately interfere with a child's ability to learn and readiness for school (Jones & Bouffard, 2012). If the child is not eligible for EI/ECSE services, then staff can also point caregivers to other community services.
- *Refer for social-emotional, behavioral health, or mental health evaluation.* Mental health agency staff and providers in many communities are becoming more knowledgeable and have more tools to evaluate very young children's social-emotional development. Talk to local mental health providers to determine where referrals can be made for social-emotional evaluations.
- *Follow up about items of concern.* Any concern that a parent indicates or expresses during the process of screening with ASQ:SE-2 should be addressed by program staff administering ASQ:SE-2 (see Section 3 on the Information Summary sheet). Many concerns can be addressed easily through a conversation with parents about common behaviors seen

at different ages (e.g., fear of loud noises is common among toddlers). Other behaviors of concern may require more follow-up from program staff in upcoming weeks to support the parents' understanding of the behavior and strategize ways to decrease or minimize challenging behaviors. For example, parents who are struggling with their 3-year-old's trouble with falling asleep may need to learn about the importance of bedtime routines and may need to try out a new routine over the next few weeks.

- *Other.* Program staff and parents may have to be creative when determining possible follow-up to screening with ASQ:SE-2. Referrals may include community agencies that provide concrete support services to families and help ease a parent's stress or community agencies that provide parenting support or early childhood services, such as Early Head Start or Head Start.

CONCLUSION

Phase III describes the steps necessary for using the questionnaires. This User's Guide is intended to be a reference; there are many sections in this chapter that will need to be reviewed as screening/monitoring program operations begin. For example, although the scoring instructions may seem complicated during the first reading, a short practice session with two or three questionnaires should clarify the process. In addition, staff may need to exercise best judgment in certain circumstances, such as when first using questionnaires and ways to give parents feedback, until a system is established that fits individual program needs and outlines specific program guidelines. Chapter 7 describes the final phase of the ASQ:SE-2 system—evaluating the screening/monitoring program.

7

Phase IV
Evaluating the ASQ:SE-2 Screening/ Monitoring Program

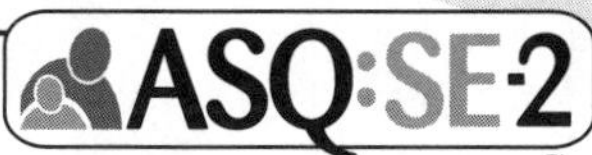

Phase IV of implementing an ASQ:SE-2 screening/monitoring program focuses on evaluating the program in terms of its implementation progress as well as the effectiveness of the screening tool. This phase has two steps, shown in the shaded portion of Figure 7.1. As with any screening/monitoring program, each step in implementing an ASQ:SE-2 program should lead to the next one.

The evaluation stage involves systematically collecting data on screening activities to measure the accuracy and overall success of the program. Evaluation data will assist in decision making about program operations as well as measure the program's effectiveness in identifying children who need intervention services. Funding sources, parents, boards of directors, lawmakers, community members, and the medical community are examples of potential audiences for evaluation reports.

STEPS IN THE EVALUATION PHASE

As indicated in Figure 7.1, the evaluation of the ASQ:SE-2 screening/monitoring program provides information about the attainment of program goals and also may suggest new goals. Ongoing evaluation may result in the modification of procedures and steps in all four phases of the program.

22. Assess Progress in Establishing and Maintaining the Screening/Monitoring Program

Contemplating the evaluation of the screening process should not begin at the end of Phase II. Rather, knowing the goals of the evaluation process facilitates the collection of necessary

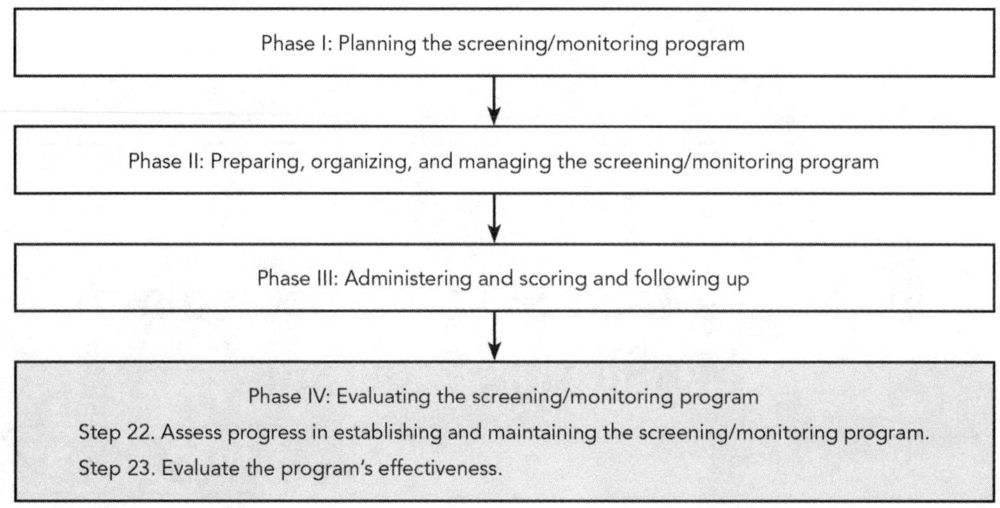

Figure 7.1. The four phases of ASQ:SE-2 implementation, including the two steps of Phase IV. (Phases I–III are discussed in Chapters 4–6.)

information as the program progresses. Setting up and maintaining a screening/monitoring program for a large number of children requires a range of activities. The Implementation Progress Worksheet (see Figure 7.2; a full-size, photocopiable version of this worksheet appears in Appendix D) was developed to assist program personnel in efficiently monitoring the required phases and steps for program initiation and maintenance. The items on this worksheet mirror the four phases and 23 steps that are necessary for implementing an ASQ:SE-2 screening/monitoring program. The worksheet is intended to be of assistance during the initiation and early stages of developing the program; however, staff may find it useful to refer back to the worksheet at designated intervals (e.g., quarterly) even after the program has been institutionalized.

Tasks

The left column of the Implementation Progress Worksheet lists each of the steps necessary to establish the ASQ:SE-2 system (e.g., finalize goals and objectives, determine program resources) in the order in which they are described in this User's Guide.

Actions

To the right of the Tasks column are five "action" columns: personnel needs, information needs, supplies and equipment needs, person/agency responsible, and projected completion date. Personnel can enter information for the individual steps in each column. For the "include parent perspectives" step, personnel from a program might enter the following information:

- *Personnel needs:* Social workers to make individual contacts with parents of infants identified from birth certificates; clerical staff to prepare letters to parents and take telephone messages
- *Information needs:* Current names, addresses, e-mail, and telephone numbers (if available) of families
- *Supplies and equipment needs:* Office supplies, including stamps, a computer and software for word processing, letterhead, and a telephone with two lines

ASQ:SE-2 Implementation Progress Worksheet

Program name/site: ______

Use the following scale for progress rating(s): 0 = not applicable; 1 = not begun; 2 = partially begun or implemented; 3 = fully completed or implemented.

Tasks	Actions					Progress rating			
	Personnel needs	Information needs	Supplies and equipment needs	Person/agency responsible	Projected completion date				
Phase I: Planning the screening/monitoring program						10/1	3/1	6/1	9/1
1. Communicate with community partners.		Contacts	Database	DL	1/15	2	3		
2. Include parent perspectives.	Parents	Contacts		MR/DL	Ongoing	2	2		
3. Involve health and mental health providers.	Providers	Contacts		KF	Ongoing	1	2		
4. Determine target population.				Board		3	3		
5. Finalize goals and objectives.				Board	2/1	2	3		
6. Determine program resources.	Accounting	Fiscal reports		Fiscal	11/30	3	3		
7. Determine administration methods and settings.				Board	11/30	3	3		
8. Determine depth and breadth of program.				Board	2/1	2	3		
9. Select referral criteria.				Board	11/30	3	3		

(continued)

ASQ:SE-2 Implementation Progress Worksheet *(continued)*

Tasks	Actions					Progress rating			
	Personnel needs	Information needs	Supplies and equipment needs	Person/agency responsible	Projected completion date				
Phase II: Preparing, organizing, and managing the screening/monitoring program						10/1	3/1	6/1	9/1
10. Create a management system.	0.02 FTE		Database	ST	1/15	1	3		
11. Prepare questionnaires.			ASQ:SE-2	BC	2/15	1	3		
12. Develop forms, letters, and a referral guide.			ASQ:SE-2	DL	12/15	1	2		
13. Articulate screening policies and procedures.	Board			MR/DL	3/1	1	3		
14. Provide staff training and support.	DL	Dates	Training materials	DL/LO	Ongoing	1	2		
Phase III: Administering and scoring ASQ:SE-2 and following up						10/1	3/1	6/1	9/1
15. Select the appropriate ASQ:SE-2 age interval.	Clerical		ASQ:SE-2	LO	Ongoing	1	3		
16. Support parent completion of ASQ:SE-2.	Home visitor			MR/home visitor	Ongoing	1	3		
17. Score ASQ:SE-2.	Home visitor			Home visitor	Ongoing	1	2		
18. Review written comments on scored and unscored sections of ASQ:SE-2.				Home visitor	Ongoing	2	2		
19. Interpret ASQ:SE-2 score.	Home visitor			Home visitor	Ongoing	1	2		
20. Communicate results with families.	Home visitor	Community resources	Resource guide	Home visitor	Ongoing	1	2		
21. Determine appropriate follow-up.	Home visitor	Community resources	Resource guide	Home visitor	Ongoing	1	2		
Phase IV: Evaluating the screening/monitoring program						10/1	3/1	6/1	9/1
22. Assess progress in establishing and maintaining the screening/monitoring program.	Board	Board		DL/Board	Quarterly	2	2		
23. Evaluate the program's effectiveness.	Evaluator	Reports		DL/Board	Quarterly	1	2		

page 2 of 2

ASQ:SE-2

Figure 7.2. A sample Implementation Progress Worksheet. The items on this worksheet mirror the steps in the four phases of the ASQ:SE-2 system. Appendix D contains a blank, photocopiable version of this worksheet.

- *Person/agency responsible:* Social workers to be responsible for obtaining consent to participate from parents; thereafter, social workers to be responsible for ongoing contact with participating parents for feedback and for altering the ASQ:SE-2 method of completion when requested
- *Projected completion date:* Parents to be contacted for consent within 1 month after birth of child or within 1 month after child returns home from the hospital

Progress Rating

The final column provides four spaces to indicate the quantitative level of progress attained toward completing the specific step. The rating scale includes the following numeric values:

0 = Not applicable
1 = Not begun
2 = Partially begun or implemented
3 = Fully completed or implemented

During initial start-up, program staff may want to evaluate progress weekly using the Implementation Progress Worksheet. Later, monthly or quarterly evaluations of progress may be sufficient. Tasks to evaluate will change as a program matures and as more children are monitored. As program objectives are modified, it may be necessary to begin a new worksheet reflecting these new objectives.

For example, for Step 2, "include parent perspectives," the goal of garnering parents' support of the monitoring program 1 month after the birth of their child may not allow sufficient time. This task may need to be changed to contacting and mailing information to parents at 1 month and waiting until the infant is 2 months or older to make a home visit and explain the ASQ:SE-2 system.

Although most programs will strive for ratings of 3 on targeted steps, there may be instances in which a rating of 2 is sufficient. Limited resources, differing priorities, or modification of steps may be reasons for these lower ratings. If a modification occurs, then steps should be rewritten and reevaluated.

23. Evaluate the Program's Effectiveness

Evaluating the program's effectiveness is the final step shown in Figure 7.1. Every monitoring program, even those with limited resources, should conduct some form of evaluation to determine the effectiveness of the program and the procedures used. Recommended areas of evaluation are as follows:

- Parent feedback
- Effectiveness of questionnaires in accurately identifying children who need further assessment
- Effectiveness of questionnaires in facilitating the referral (and receipt) of support services to children and families
- Feedback from personnel using the questionnaires

How extensively each of these areas can be evaluated will depend on the program's resources and staff expertise. The evaluation procedures described next are simple and straightforward; they represent the basic, minimal amount of evaluation data that program personnel should collect.

Parent Feedback

The program should seek parent feedback *at least* yearly. A simple, short survey can be included with a questionnaire once a year (e.g., at 12, 24, 36, 48, 60 months). Figure 7.3 shows a sample Parent Feedback Survey. (Appendix D contains blank, photocopiable versions of this survey in English and Spanish.) This type of feedback will assist program personnel in making appropriate adjustments to procedures to help ensure parent participation and satisfaction.

Questionnaire Effectiveness

It is imperative to keep records of the number of children identified as needing further evaluation and the outcomes of their subsequent social-emotional evaluations in order to examine the effectiveness of the questionnaires. By recording this information, it is possible to determine

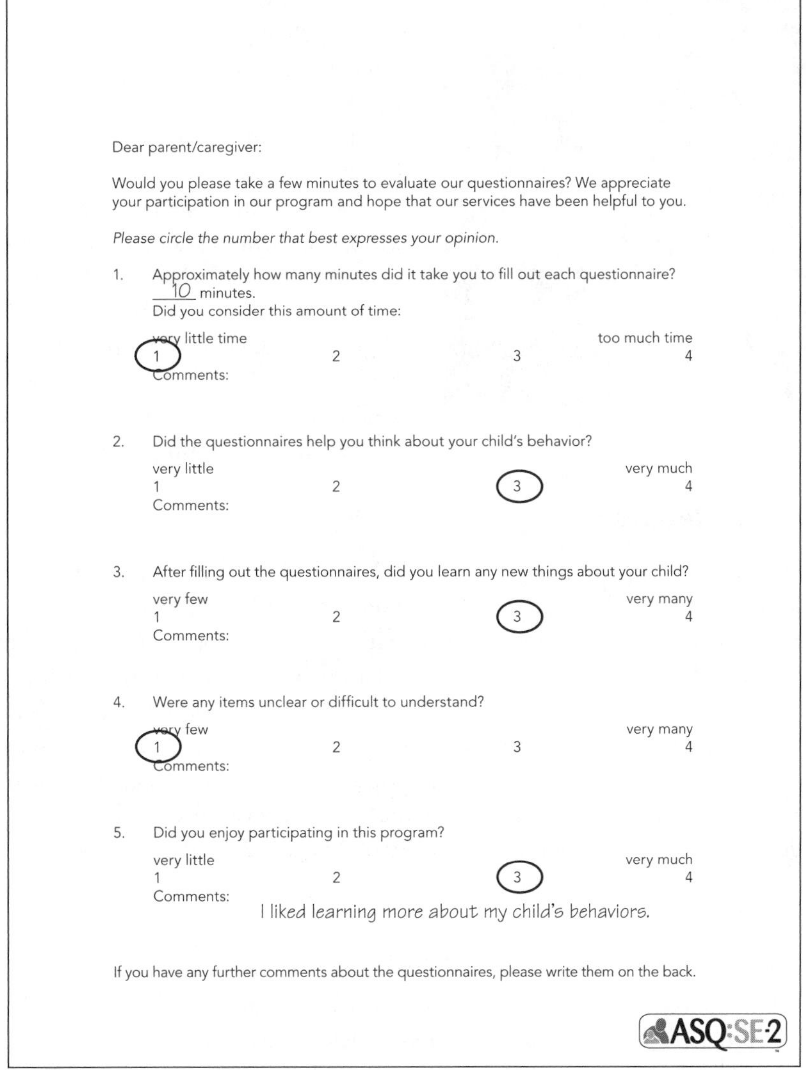

Dear parent/caregiver:

Would you please take a few minutes to evaluate our questionnaires? We appreciate your participation in our program and hope that our services have been helpful to you.

Please circle the number that best expresses your opinion.

1. Approximately how many minutes did it take you to fill out each questionnaire? 10 minutes.
   Did you consider this amount of time:
   very little time — too much time
   (1) 2 3 4
   Comments:

2. Did the questionnaires help you think about your child's behavior?
   very little — very much
   1 2 (3) 4
   Comments:

3. After filling out the questionnaires, did you learn any new things about your child?
   very few — very many
   1 2 (3) 4
   Comments:

4. Were any items unclear or difficult to understand?
   very few — very many
   (1) 2 3 4
   Comments:

5. Did you enjoy participating in this program?
   very little — very much
   1 2 (3) 4
   Comments: I liked learning more about my child's behaviors.

If you have any further comments about the questionnaires, please write them on the back.

ASQ:SE-2

Figure 7.3. A sample Parent Feedback Survey. Feedback from parents should be sought at least yearly. Appendix D contains blank, photocopiable versions of this survey in English and Spanish.

the percentages of children accurately identified by the questionnaires as having delays and those who were incorrectly recommended for further evaluation. These calculations provide information on the sensitivity and overidentification rates for the group of children being monitored. Providing information on the effectiveness of a screening program may help the program in a variety of ways. First, data on the effectiveness of the screening/monitoring program may be needed to maintain or extend funding; funding sources may request data and will appreciate reports of program outcomes and effectiveness. Second, these data may yield information useful for monitoring and adjusting implementation goals. For example, a program may project a screening rate of 10%. If the program's goal of 10% is not realized (i.e., percent screened is significantly higher or lower), then the criteria used to include children in the program may need to be modified.

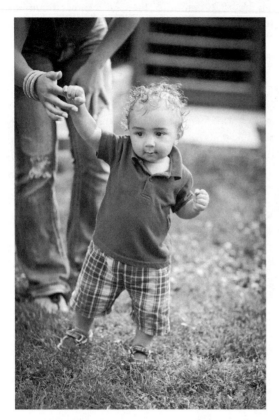

Figure 7.4 provides formulas for calculating the percentage of children appropriately identified as needing further assessment and sensitivity, specificity, overidentification, underidentification, and positive predictive value rates. Specificity and underidentification rates cannot be calculated unless a program conducts follow-up evaluations both with children who are *not* identified by ASQ:SE-2 as needing further evaluation and with children who *are* identified as needing further evaluation.

Support Services Received

Although the primary purpose of ASQ:SE-2 is to identify children needing further social-emotional evaluation, the use of these questionnaires with families often identifies other community services parents may find supportive in their parenting journey. For example, a child's score on ASQ:SE-2 may not indicate the need for further evaluation. During the process of discussing the ASQ:SE-2 results, however, the parent may have voiced concerns about the child's specific behaviors or expressed an interest in attending a parenting support group to learn more strategies to support the child's social-emotional development. Documenting these "other" community referrals and tracking the actual services received by families and children provide additional information on the utility of ASQ:SE-2 questionnaires.

Personnel Feedback

It is important to seek formal or informal feedback from personnel using the questionnaires to learn which procedural steps work well and which ones do not. The ASQ:SE-2 system is flexible, and program personnel can and should make adjustments in its use to ensure efficient, effective application.

		Follow-up assessment	
		Intervention needs	No intervention needs
ASQ:SE-2	Identified by questionnaires as needing further assessment	True positives A	False positives (overidentification) B
	Not identified by questionnaires; developing typically	False negatives (underidentification) C	True negatives D

Percentage of children identified as needing further assessment:

$$\frac{A + B}{A + B + C + D}$$

Sensitivity The proportion of children correctly identified by the questionnaires as needing further assessment:

$$\frac{A}{A + C}$$

Specificity The proportion of children correctly identified by the questionnaires as developing typically:

$$\frac{D}{B + D}$$

Overidentification The proportion of children (of the total number of children for whom a questionnaire was completed) incorrectly identified by the questionnaires as needing further assessment:

$$\frac{B}{A + B + C + D}$$

Underidentification The proportion of children (of the total number of children for whom a questionnaire was completed) incorrectly excluded by the questionnaires:

$$\frac{C}{A + B + C + D}$$

Positive predictive value The proportion of children identified by the questionnaires as needing further assessment who will, in fact, have intervention needs:

$$\frac{A}{A + B}$$

Figure 7.4. Formulas for calculating the percentage of children appropriately identified as needing further assessment and the sensitivity, specificity, over- and underidentified rates, and positive predictive value.

Determining Next Steps

Once the evaluation of the screening/monitoring program has been completed, program staff should review and discuss results and then take appropriate action. For example, an action based on evaluation results might include having staff review questionnaires to check that 1) parent concerns are reviewed and discussed with families and 2) questionnaires are accurately scored. Another action might be to modify referral criteria so that more (or fewer) children are referred for further assessment. Staff should meet at least once a year to examine ways to improve the activities associated with the screening/monitoring program. Parents and other stakeholders also should be invited to review program evaluation results and suggest improvements and modifications to the system.

Foundations for Success was a 5-year initiative designed to develop and implement a countywide system for early childhood mental health services in Ramsey County, Minnesota. Funded by the John S. and James L. Knight Foundation and coordinated by the Community Action Partnership of Ramsey and Washington Counties, the initiative promoted culturally competent and family-friendly services. Services were developed and implemented by a collaborative of more than 100 community agencies, representing local foundations, government, parents, school districts, health, mental health, early childhood professionals, and staff from the University of Minnesota. The initiative was evaluated by Wilder Research, and one component of the research included an analysis of the results of ASQ:SE.

Analysis of ASQ:SE included the following:

- Percentage of screenings completed at different age intervals (e.g., 36 month, 48 month)
- Percentage of screenings completed by language (e.g., English, Spanish, Hmong, Somali)
- Percentage of screenings with scores above the cutoff (by program, child age, race/ethnicity, language, mother's education, family income, disability, and receipt of specialized services)

ASQ:SE administration/completion data:

- Percentage of children receiving the correct age ASQ:SE interval
- Percentage of ASQ:SE questionnaires scored correctly

In addition, Wilder Research randomly selected a group of parents who had a child with a screening score at or above the clinical cutoff for ASQ:SE. These parents were interviewed and information was gathered to determine the parents' perception of the screening process and subsequent receipt of appropriate services. *For more information about Foundations for Success, visit www.wilder.org. For information about Minnesota's early childhood screening efforts, visit www.dhs.state.mn.us/main/idcplg?IdcService=GET_DYNAMIC_CONVERSION&RevisionSelectionMethod=LatestReleased&dDocName=dhs16_149102.*

SCREENING TESTS AND EVALUATION

Screening tests, as defined in Chapter 1, provide a brief snapshot of a child's current developmental skills and are designed for use with large groups of children at relatively low cost. These brief tests contain few items and thus do not offer comprehensive assessments of children's development. These features, although appropriate for screening, make such brief tests inappropriate for most other assessment purposes. Results of a screening test such as ASQ:SE-2 are not designed to diagnose a child or measure a child's progress over time, just as diagnostic social-emotional assessments are not designed for screening purposes.

Conducting an appropriate assessment requires using measures and/or procedures designed to fit or meet the purposes of the assessment. The types of assessment purposes and their associated assessments are shown in Table 7.1. Screening requires the use of a screening measure; determining eligibility for services usually requires a measure that provides an in-depth, diagnostic social-emotional assessment that compares children against established norms. Curriculum-based assessment, such as the Social-Emotional Assessment/Evaluation Measure

Table 7.1. Purposes and types of assessment

Type	Purpose	Examples
Screening test	Is the child in need of further testing?	ASQ:SE-2; Survey of Wellbeing of Young Children (Sheldrick & Perrin, 2013)
Eligibility test/diagnostic assessment	Is the child eligible for special services?	Child Behavior Checklist (Achenbach & Rescorla, 2001)
Programmatic/curriculum-based assessment	Is the child making progress?	Social-Emotional Assessment/Evaluation Measure (Squires, Bricker, Waddell, Funk, Clifford, & Hoselton, 2014).

(SEAM; Squires & Bricker 2014), should be used to evaluate child progress. Curriculum-based measures such as the SEAM are ideal for delineating step-by-step objectives that can be used for measuring child progress toward long-range goals, especially for children with delays in social-emotional development. *Screening tests are not sensitive enough to show progress toward outcomes; these tests are designed only to identify those children who need further assessment.*

Although not an evaluative tool, some child care and early childhood programs may use ASQ:SE-2 to reflect a general status of a population and to look at trends over time. For example, programs have reported percentages of children in a given population scoring above designated cutoff scores, in the monitoring zone, or below cutoff scores. Other programs may choose to monitor a child's development using the three general outcomes of ASQ:SE-2 (e.g., above cutoff, monitoring zone, below cutoff), tracking a child's progress from one ASQ:SE-2 administration to the next. See Figure 7.5 for an example of the ASQ:SE-2 Child Monitoring Sheet. (A blank, photocopiable version of this sheet appears in Appendix D, and in paper as well as in PDF format on CD-ROM with the ASQ:SE-2 questionnaires box.) Intervention programs have reported tracking children's total scores on ASQ:SE intervals over time, reporting that a decline of 25 points in a child's total score appears to be clinically significant. Results from ASQ:SE-2 questionnaires also may show improvement in a child's behavior. Finally, some programs may use an "average item score" to look at trends in scores over time. An average item score is required (rather than a total score) because the number of scored items on ASQ:SE-2 is different with each interval. To calculate average item scores, the ASQ:SE-2 total score is divided by the number of scored items on the ASQ:SE-2 interval.

$$\text{Average Item Score} = \frac{\text{Total ASQ:SE-2 Score}}{\text{\# of Scored Items}}$$

The average item scores are then compared from the first administration to the second administration (e.g., average item score = 5.8 points on the 24 month ASQ:SE-2 compared with average item score = 2.6 points on the 36 month ASQ:SE-2). An improvement in a child's social-emotional behavior would be reflected in a lower average item score at the second administration because ASQ:SE-2 tracks the number of problem behaviors.

As a social-emotional screening tool, the results of ASQ:SE-2 are designed to identify children who need further social-emotional evaluation. General information may be gained, however, if there are no other means of evaluation available to programs (Squires, Bricker, & Clifford, 2010). Normative and curriculum-based assessments will assist in measuring reliable improvements in behavior and help caregivers draw conclusions about individual child progress.

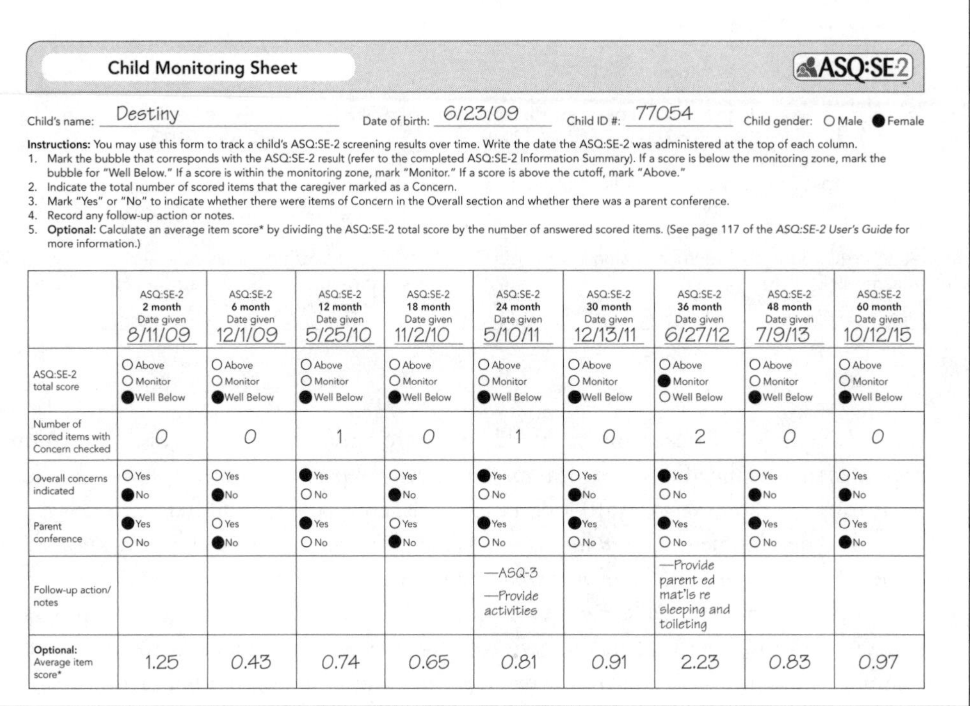

Child Monitoring Sheet ASQ:SE-2

Child's name: Destiny Date of birth: 6/23/09 Child ID #: 77054 Child gender: ○ Male ● Female

Instructions: You may use this form to track a child's ASQ:SE-2 screening results over time. Write the date the ASQ:SE-2 was administered at the top of each column.

1. Mark the bubble that corresponds with the ASQ:SE-2 result (refer to the completed ASQ:SE-2 Information Summary). If a score is below the monitoring zone, mark the bubble for "Well Below." If a score is within the monitoring zone, mark "Monitor." If a score is above the cutoff, mark "Above."
2. Indicate the total number of scored items that the caregiver marked as a Concern.
3. Mark "Yes" or "No" to indicate whether there were items of Concern in the Overall section and whether there was a parent conference.
4. Record any follow-up action or notes.
5. **Optional:** Calculate an average item score* by dividing the ASQ:SE-2 total score by the number of answered scored items. (See page 117 of the *ASQ:SE-2 User's Guide* for more information.)

	ASQ:SE-2 **2 month** Date given 8/11/09	ASQ:SE-2 **6 month** Date given 12/1/09	ASQ:SE-2 **12 month** Date given 5/25/10	ASQ:SE-2 **18 month** Date given 11/2/10	ASQ:SE-2 **24 month** Date given 5/10/11	ASQ:SE-2 **30 month** Date given 12/13/11	ASQ:SE-2 **36 month** Date given 6/27/12	ASQ:SE-2 **48 month** Date given 7/9/13	ASQ:SE-2 **60 month** Date given 10/12/15
ASQ:SE-2 total score	○ Above ○ Monitor ● Well Below	○ Above ○ Monitor ● Well Below	○ Above ○ Monitor ● Well Below	○ Above ○ Monitor ● Well Below	○ Above ○ Monitor ● Well Below	○ Above ○ Monitor ● Well Below	○ Above ● Monitor ○ Well Below	○ Above ○ Monitor ● Well Below	○ Above ○ Monitor ● Well Below
Number of scored items with Concern checked	0	0	1	0	1	0	2	0	0
Overall concerns indicated	○ Yes ● No	○ Yes ● No	● Yes ○ No	○ Yes ● No	● Yes ○ No	○ Yes ● No	● Yes ○ No	○ Yes ● No	○ Yes ● No
Parent conference	● Yes ○ No	○ Yes ● No	● Yes ○ No	○ Yes ● No	● Yes ○ No	● Yes ○ No	● Yes ○ No	● Yes ○ No	○ Yes ● No
Follow-up action/ notes					—ASQ-3 —Provide activities		—Provide parent ed mat'ls re sleeping and toileting		
Optional: Average item score*	1.25	0.43	0.74	0.65	0.81	0.91	2.23	0.83	0.97

Figure 7.5. A sample Child Monitoring Sheet. Blank, photocopiable versions of this sheet in English and Spanish appear in Appendix D. The sheet is also included with the ASQ:SE-2 questionnaires box.

The Kids First staff developed a plan to assess their progress in implementing their screening program every 3 months. The following scale was used to track the progress of each step of the screening system (*0* = not applicable, *1* = not begun, *2* = partially begun or implemented, *3* = fully completed or implemented; see Figure 7.2). A number of steps in the planning phase (Phase I) were complete at 6 months, although more work was needed to create a system for sharing screening results with primary health care providers. Advisory board staff and social workers were designated to continue to work with private pediatric groups and health care organizations to develop a system for information sharing. In addition, a decision was made to appoint parents and representatives from the health and behavioral community to the advisory board so that their input would be ongoing.

In terms of Phase II activities, a system to set up and maintain child files had been completed. Procedures for the tickler system and the recording of questionnaire results appeared to be working well. The development of forms and procedures for sharing results with health and behavioral health providers were still in progress. Although training had been provided for staff who would administer ASQ:SE-2, a system was set up to provide ongoing coaching and support for communicating results and determining appropriate follow-up—particularly for communicating results that indicated some potential behavioral concerns.

A number of Phase III steps were ongoing and would require more attention. One hundred randomly selected ASQ:SE-2 questionnaires were reviewed, and it was determined that 23% of these were incorrectly scored. In addition, 20% of questionnaires indicating a need for referral had no documented follow-up. Supervising staff were asked to review scoring and referral procedures with staff and develop a system of cross-checking to minimize errors and lack of follow-up. Progress toward fully implementing these steps was to be evaluated during monthly staff meetings. The next program evaluation meeting was scheduled for 3 months later.

Phase IV was just beginning. For the task of determining follow-up for children identified as needing further evaluation, staff believed that there were insufficient numbers to date to rate progress. They had screened 113 children, and 28 children had received elevated scores. Parents of 10 of the children had requested further monitoring with the questionnaires before referral. The additional 18 children had been referred for further evaluation based on their ASQ:SE-2 results. A decision was made to refer infants and toddlers to the local Part C early intervention provider and 3- to 5-year-olds to the Part B early childhood special education provider. Seven children had been referred to early intervention, and four of these children had been determined eligible for services based on a general developmental delay. Two were not eligible, and one family could not be contacted to schedule a further evaluation. Eleven children were referred to early childhood special education services, three were determined to be eligible for services, and two children did not qualify. Another four were in the process of being evaluated, and two were unable to be contacted to schedule an evaluation.

Kids First started a system for gathering parent feedback by adding a simple satisfaction survey to the screening process. In addition, the project evaluator had set a time to attend staff meetings and interview staff to gather feedback on the ease and utility of ASQ:SE-2. A plan was in place to conduct a follow-up phone interview with families who had been referred to services based on ASQ:SE-2 results. These follow-up phone calls would begin in 3 months.

CONCLUSION

Phase IV, evaluating the screening and monitoring program, involves two goals—assessing progress in establishing and maintaining the screening and monitoring program and determining the screening and monitoring program's effectiveness. Progress can be assessed by monitoring staff accomplishments during monthly or quarterly staff meetings and should not require extensive information or data that go beyond day-to-day operations of the program.

The second step, determining the system's effectiveness, is also of prime importance. Information may be needed from outside referral agencies to determine child evaluation outcomes. These data are necessary in order to determine whether the program is effective: Are the right children being identified for further evaluation? Are these children then referred for appropriate services? Evaluation of the monitoring program should be ongoing, and revision of steps and activities will be necessary as the program grows and changes.

III

ASQ:SE-2 in Practice

8

ASQ:SE-2 Completion Methods

ASQ:SE-2™

This chapter expands on the question of who should complete ASQ:SE-2 as well as the methods for obtaining completed ASQ:SE-2 questionnaires that are introduced in Chapter 4. Mail-out, online, interview, home visit, and on-site completion options are discussed. The material in this chapter underlines the questionnaires' flexibility and adaptability—an important advantage of using ASQ:SE-2 to monitor children's development. Accompanying the descriptions are examples of how different agencies and programs are using ASQ:SE-2.

There are also two appendixes that follow this chapter. Appendix 8A contains procedures for using a card file tickler system. Appendix 8B details the steps and decisions involved in implementing ASQ:SE-2 while on a home visit.

WHO SHOULD COMPLETE ASQ:SE-2?

Parents, extended family, caregivers, child care providers, preschool teachers, and others can complete an ASQ:SE-2 questionnaire for a child. One important guideline is that the person completing it should have a sustained, significant relationship with the child, including a minimum of 15–20 hours per week with the child. In addition, the person should have spent enough time with the child over a period of weeks to know the child's typical behavior in order to respond to the questions—that is, a child care provider or Head Start teacher may not be able to accurately respond within the first weeks of meeting a child but should have enough knowledge after a month or so. And even with this level of contact, there may be items that will need to be omitted. For example, a preschool teacher may be with a child for 30 hours a week but may have no opportunity to observe sleeping behaviors. These items should be omitted and the score adjusted. See Chapter 6 for more information on adjusting scores on ASQ:SE-2 with missing items.

Andrew is a 4-year-old child who was removed from his mother's home due to suspected neglect. He has been in foster care for 6 months and was recently screened using ASQ-3 and ASQ:SE-2. Andrew's foster mother was asked to complete the ASQ:SE-2 questionnaire because Andrew's mother currently has visitation rights with him for only 1 hour once a week. The caseworker chose to share results from the screening with Andrew's mother so that she could be kept informed of Andrew's development and behavior from the foster mother's perspective.

ASQ:SE-2 can be completed by parents independently or with assistance as needed. Interviewers or translators who help administer ASQ:SE-2 should be careful to clarify their role, which is to read and support parent understanding of items and gather information from the parent. ASQ:SE-2 has some items that some parents may consider subjective. For example, the question "Does your child scream, cry, or have tantrums for long periods of time?" may cause a parent to inquire about what might be considered a "long period." To the extent possible, interviewers should not advise or lead parents but should encourage parents to use their own judgment in answering questionnaire items.

Parents

ASQ:SE-2 was developed as a parent-completed screening tool, and, in general, having parents complete the tool is the preferred method of use. ASQ:SE-2 can be independently completed by most parents, which accounts for its low cost per child, or staff can provide support as necessary to complete screening information. There are many compelling reasons to include parents in the screening process, including the knowledge parents have about their children, the importance of understanding parents' perspectives, and the ability to respond to parents' behavioral concerns. A significant need exists for program staff to identify parent concerns and respond to these concerns in a timely and supportive manner. It may also be helpful to gather perspectives from both of the child's parents, especially while assessing social-emotional development. What may be an urgent concern for one parent may be of little concern to another.

Myrna and her husband, Bob, brought Trey, their 5-month-old, to a local feeding clinic. The young mother discussed the heartache she felt during feeding times with Trey, who was being fed through a gastrointestinal tube. Bob, however, said that feeding times with Trey were enjoyable most of the time. Bob did not appear to experience the same stress that Myrna was feeling. As they discussed the feeding question on ASQ:SE-2 ("Do you and your child enjoy mealtimes together?"), Myrna was able to see Bob's perspective and why he thought Trey was happy. Bob was also able to understand Myrna's fear and anxiety at feeding times.

Multiple Questionnaires Completed by Parents and Other Caregivers

It can be helpful to gather information from more than one person and/or from people who are with the child in different settings (e.g., home, school) when behavioral concerns arise. A child's behavior may vary greatly from setting to setting and/or from caregiver to caregiver. Behaviors that are problematic to one parent or caregiver may not be of concern to another. Behaviors that occur in one setting may not be present in another. This method provides an excellent way to facilitate communication between a parent and another caregiver about a child's behavior. Questionnaires should be independently administered and will result in more than one ASQ:SE-2 score. There may be a discrepancy in ASQ:SE-2 scores because a child's behaviors often differ across settings, and the scores may be significantly different in some cases. Valuable information about the child may surface through discussion of these differences, which may lead to provision of unique supports for the child in a specific setting. More information about the use of ASQ:SE-2 in child care and educational settings can be found in Chapter 9.

Jonah is 20 months old and attends a toddler group 5 mornings a week. In the first few days of Jonah attending school, his toddler teacher expressed concerns about Jonah's aggressive behaviors, including hitting and biting. Jonah's parents were anxious about these reports and worried that Jonah was going to be kicked out of the child care program. Jonah's mother and his teacher both completed ASQ:SE-2 questionnaires for Jonah and compared results. The questionnaire completed by Jonah's mother had a score well below the cutoff, and no concerns were noted. The one completed by Jonah's teacher had a score above the cutoff, indicating the need for a referral. A behavior specialist met with Jonah's teacher and parents, observed Jonah in both settings, and completed a functional behavioral assessment in Jonah's classroom. Because Jonah's behavior was not a problem at home, a behavior plan was developed only for the school setting. The behavior plan will be put into place for 30 days, at which time the teacher, behavior specialist, and Jonah's parents will meet to discuss progress.

MEETING THE NEEDS OF DIVERSE PROGRAMS AND SETTINGS

The ASQ:SE-2 system's great strength is the flexibility it provides in terms of how it can be completed (e.g., mail-out, online, phone interview, home visit, on site/face to face), when it can be used (i.e., with any child from 1 month to 72 months of age), and where it can be used (e.g., at home, in a physician's office). Since publication of the first edition, ASQ:SE has been used by pediatric and family child care practices, well-infant clinics, health care programs, screening clinics, educational intervention programs, research projects, and child welfare programs.

Communities in the United States that provide screening vary considerably in terms of which agencies and professionals have a mission or responsibility to monitor the developmental and behavioral status of young children. The physical facilities, personnel, and resources of these programs require flexibility in screening measures and procedures. Such diversity requires using adaptable measures, such as ASQ:SE-2, which can successfully be used in individual communities employing a wide range of other approaches to collecting questionnaires:

- *Mail-out:* This approach is the first option for ASQ:SE-2 questionnaire completion. This method requires that ASQ:SE-2 be mailed to parents who, in turn, complete questionnaires and return them by mail to a central location, such as the office of the primary health care provider, a clinic, or a screening program.
- *Online:* The ASQ Online Family Access system is the second option for questionnaire completion. The professional directs the caregiver to a secure web site to fill out a questionnaire, and ASQ Family Access ensures that the correct ASQ:SE-2 age interval is selected and that the questionnaire is complete. Data are transmitted to the program's ASQ Online management system account for verification, and the questionnaire is scored and screening results are saved to the child's record. (Personnel using the ASQ Online management system also may enter data from paper questionnaires to be scored and stored in the online management system.)
- *Interview:* The third option involves completing ASQ:SE-2 through an interview over the phone or in person. Using ASQ:SE-2 as an interview tool may be appropriate for programs with limited funds and/or those working with parents with limited reading skills or limited understanding of written questions as a result of language, cognitive, or mental health difficulties.
- *Home visit:* Conducting a home visit is another option for completing ASQ:SE-2. While working with the family in the child's home, the home visitor supports caregivers in completing the questionnaire as necessary.
- *On-site:* ASQ:SE-2 also can be completed on site at a program's physical location, such as in a waiting room or at the preschool on parent night.

Although these are the five primary options typically employed for completing questionnaires, they may be combined or used with other variations as necessary to meet the requirements and resources of programs and their personnel.

Translation Considerations

Translating ASQ:SE-2 may be necessary to adapt the questionnaires for a specific language or culture. (Please see www.agesandstages.com for a list of available ASQ:SE-2 translations.) When translating or adapting ASQ:SE-2, the translator(s) must carefully review all items and come to agreement with the administering program about appropriate translations that fit the intent of the items. See Appendix G: Translation and Adaptation Guidelines for ASQ:SE-2 for more detailed information. Results of questionnaires that are administered in other languages should be interpreted with caution and with consideration to the behavioral norms and expectations of the child and family's culture.

The Steps-Ahead staff decided that their initial contact with parents would be within 1 month of the infant's birth. Based on information on the birth certificate completed in the hospital, the social worker determined whether the child and family met the risk criteria established by the program. The social worker then called the family, explained the purpose of the screening/monitoring program, and asked if the family was interested in participating. When the family expressed interest in participating, an introductory home visit was scheduled. During this visit, the Steps-Ahead social worker obtained the parents' consent to participate, enrolled the family in the program, provided an introduction to ASQ:SE-2, and explained how the tool would gather information that caregivers would use to support their child's development. The social worker answered any questions or concerns the parents had and provided several options for how the family would receive questionnaires, either during home visits, on site, or by mail.

Mail-Out

Mail-out methods generally entail mailing questionnaires to families at set intervals. Parents complete questionnaires and usually return them by mail. Program staff can manually prepare mailings or generate mailings through the ASQ Online management system. Once returned, ASQ:SE-2 is scored, and the results are shared with parents. The mail-out option permits the dynamic monitoring of large populations of infants and children at low cost. The original system was designed as a mail-out system and has consistently been used this way in hundreds, if not thousands, of programs both nationally and internationally.

Mail-Out Considerations

Mailing ASQ:SE-2 for parents or other primary caregivers to complete is appropriate if parents or caregivers are capable of reading the questionnaire items. Prior to mailing a questionnaire, it is important to determine how ASQ:SE-2 will be introduced to parents or caregivers. An initial face-to-face meeting is the preferred way to introduce the screening/monitoring program and ASQ:SE-2. This face-to-face introduction is reassuring and helpful for parental "buy-in," and it may help to maximize ASQ:SE-2 return rates. Chapter 6 offers guidance on introducing ASQ:SE-2 to parents and caregivers. If a face-to-face introduction is not possible, then a letter and the What Is ASQ:SE-2? handout should be sent with the first ASQ:SE-2 questionnaire to introduce the program. (See Chapter 5 for examples of letters; blank letter templates in English and Spanish are available in Appendix D.)

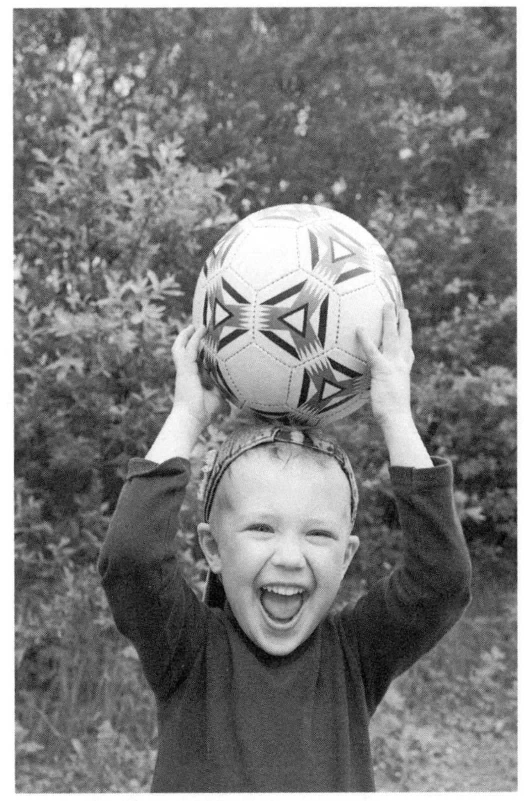

Timely feedback should be given to parents once the completed questionnaires are returned. Sending a properly worded letter is appropriate when the results of the screening indicate a child is developing typically. If the child's performance on ASQ:SE-2 items is above the cutoff score, in the monitoring zone, or if parents indicate any behavioral concerns, then it is important to follow up with a phone call or in-person meeting rather than sending a letter. It is generally recommended that program personnel do not include the Information Summary sheet that shows scoring results when sending parents feedback. This sheet requires explanation by professionals about the scoring cutoffs and results.

Primary health care practices, screening clinics, educational programs, and other types of programs that are monitoring large numbers of children will need a system for keeping track of important dates that include when questionnaires are to be mailed and returned and when feedback needs to be provided to parents. Timely tracking of questionnaire dissemination and feedback requires an electronic or paper-based system. See Appendix 8A for procedures for using a card file tickler system for tracking the mailing of ASQ:SE-2 to families.

Mail-Out Procedures

A master mailing sheet is provided in the ASQ:SE-2 questionnaires box. For programs that use the mail-out completion option, the name of the screening program and its address should be stamped, printed, or typed on a copy of the mailing sheet, and the parent's name and address also should be written or typed on that sheet (see Figure 8.1). A contact phone number, name, and e-mail address should be included on the questionnaire so parents may obtain assistance if necessary. After the child's identifying information is specified on the mailing sheet and the questionnaire is ready to be mailed, the questionnaire and mailing sheet should be folded and taped at the ends and top, with the mailing sheet on the outside of the folded packet. Staff may prefer to use an envelope to mail each ASQ:SE-2. In these cases, a self-addressed stamped envelope should be enclosed to encourage parents to return the completed questionnaire. The return date is a common concern when using the ASQ:SE-2 mail-out method. The following steps are suggested to increase return rates:

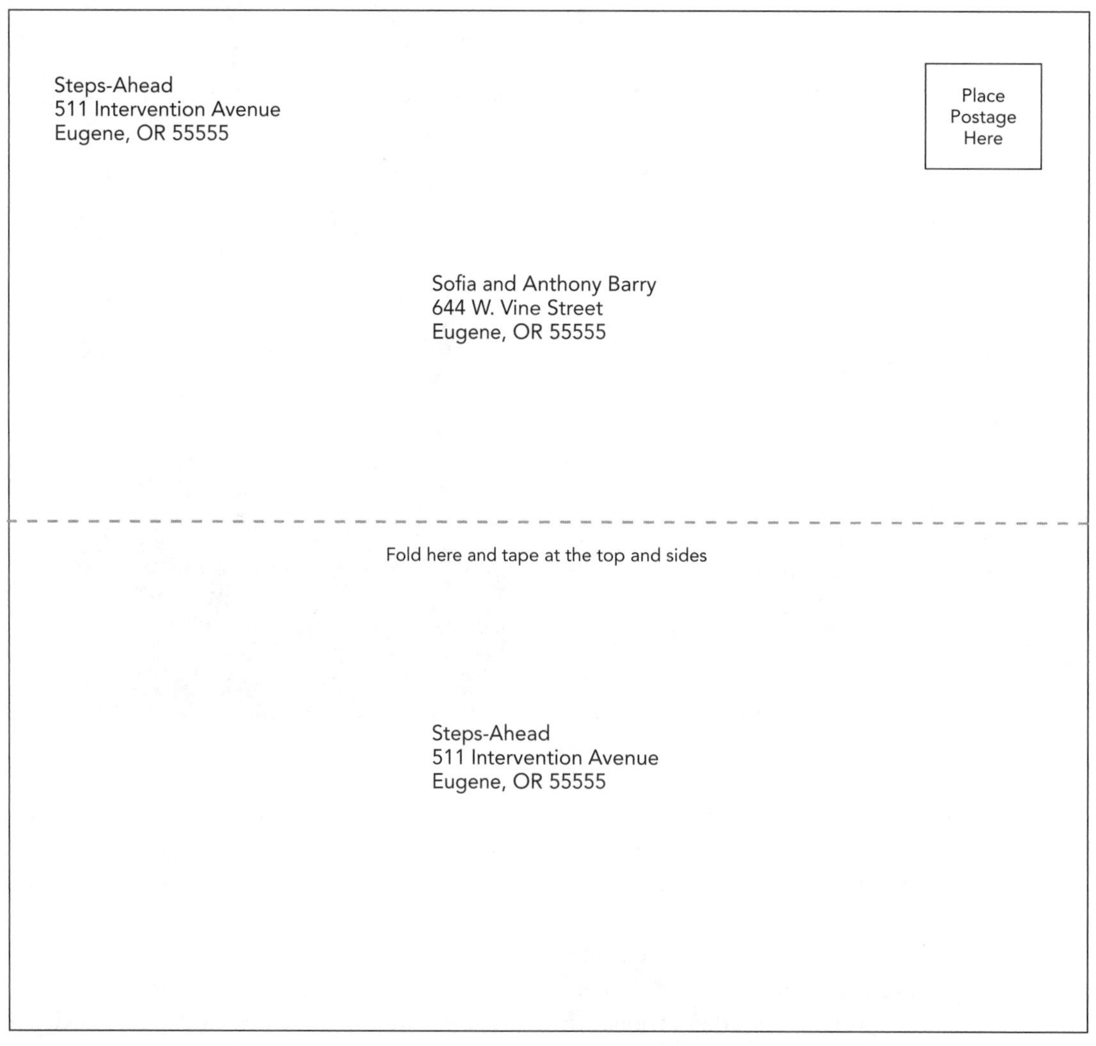

Figure 8.1. Staff who choose the mail-out option can use the master mailing sheet provided with ASQ:SE-2. The example shown here is ready to be mailed to Jackson Barry's family for questionnaire completion.

1. Make a follow-up phone call a few days after ASQ:SE-2 is mailed to ensure receipt and to answer any questions.
2. If the questionnaire is not returned within 2 weeks, then make a second phone call to remind parents to return the questionnaire. A duplicate copy can be mailed at this time if parents cannot be contacted or have not yet responded.

It is important to adhere to the time schedule for sending questionnaires and feedback. Parents should receive the appropriate ASQ:SE-2 interval on time and should receive timely feedback in writing, by phone, or in person. As previously mentioned, it may be important to include an introductory letter to parents in the first questionnaire that explains the screening/monitoring program and purpose of ASQ:SE-2 (see examples of handouts and letters in Chapter 5, Figures 5.6, 5.9, and 5.10).

Examples of Strategies to Improve Return Rates

Some strategies to improve return rates include the following:

- Introduce parents to the screening program and ASQ:SE-2 prior to sending out the first questionnaire. Introductions can be done by letter or ideally through a phone call or face-to-face contact with the family (see Chapter 6 for more information about introductions).
- Provide a contact name, phone number, and e-mail address on the first page of the questionnaire so parents know how to get additional information, if needed.
- Send ASQ:SE-2 in an envelope that will catch a parent's attention or that is personalized in some way (e.g., use a color envelope, stamp "ASQ enclosed" or a due date on the envelope, affix a sticker to help parents keep track).
- Provide a birthday card with the questionnaire on the child's first, second, third, fourth, fifth, and sixth birthdays.

Consider including the following when sending feedback to the families:

- Local restaurant, toy, or book coupons with questionnaire results
- Activity ideas, such as those provided in Appendix E
- A copy of the completed questionnaire for parents

The Follow Along Program is a statewide, Child Find activity in Minnesota that has operated since the late 1980s, supporting young children who are at risk for experiencing developmental delays. Using a mail-out method, parents with children birth to 3 years are given the opportunity to screen their young children using ASQ:SE and ASQ-3. Returned questionnaires are reviewed and scored. If results indicate typical development and parents have not expressed any concerns, then a results letter is sent in the mail along with follow-up activities. If results indicate any red flags or concerns, then parents are contacted by phone to discuss questions and concerns. Resources and local referral options are provided. Counties report different return rates, which range from 30% to 65% and vary based on factors, such as methods for enrolling families, the demographics of the county served, and whether incentives are used to encourage parents to return completed questionnaires (e.g., indicating parents will receive small gifts with results letters). *Visit www.health.state.mn.us/divs/cfh/program/cyshn/follow.cfm for more information on Minnesota's Follow Along Program.*

Online

Online questionnaire completion refers to using ASQ Family Access via the Internet for ASQ-3 or ASQ:SE-2 completion. ASQ Family Access enables programs to set up secure, personalized web sites for parents to complete ASQ:SE-2. The parent enters basic demographic information, is given access to the appropriate ASQ:SE-2 age interval for the child, and may print the ASQ:SE-2 questionnaire and submit responses electronically. Program staff review results transmitted securely from Family Access to the program's ASQ Online management system account (ASQ Pro or ASQ Enterprise).

Staff who use the ASQ Online management system can create and manage child records, screenings, and screening results. The ASQ Online management system scores completed ASQ:SE-2 (and ASQ-3) questionnaires and helps users organize and manage communications with parents, track follow-up and other activities, and run screening program reports.

Online Considerations

The ASQ Online questionnaire completion system is cost effective and can enable programs to reach large numbers of families. Parents have the flexibility to complete a questionnaire online in their home or in another location, such as at a kiosk in a physician's office. Using ASQ Family Access helps address or minimize important issues, such as incomplete questionnaire data, administration of an incorrect age interval or language, and the high cost of mailings. In addition, the ASQ Online management system has some significant advantages over a paper management system in terms of efficiency and accuracy. For instance, the time it takes professionals to score a questionnaire is reduced and scoring errors are eliminated because scoring is automatic.

Parents' level of comfort with this electronic format and their access to the Internet are other important considerations for online questionnaire completion. It is critical that the online method facilitate questionnaire completion without placing a barrier between parent and program, especially for parents who may be uncomfortable in the absence of direct contact with the professional.

Online Procedures

The degree of flexibility afforded by using the ASQ Online questionnaire completion and management systems depends on how the program would like to reach families and whether it has ASQ Pro or ASQ Enterprise as well as ASQ Family Access accounts. Parents are invited to complete a questionnaire online through ASQ Family Access and receive a URL to visit. They set up a user name and password and begin the screening. Staff can direct parents to the URL in the form of a letter, e-mail, or phone call. The program sets up preferences for the web site (e.g., inclusion of logo, welcome message to parents, follow-up note upon completion), and parents simply fill out demographic information and enter responses to the appropriate questionnaire items. Program staff are alerted in the ASQ Pro or ASQ Enterprise management system account when a parent finishes completing a questionnaire, and they can accept the screening for scoring and inclusion in the online management system.

A typical ASQ Online management system user will create and store child records, including results of screenings completed by hand (when parents receive questionnaires in the mail) as well as results collected online via Family Access. The online management system will score the questionnaire, store it, and generate reports and communications as desired by the user. Users can manage general follow-up, subsequent screenings, referrals, and additional communications with parents or caregivers, regardless of the questionnaire delivery and return options.

The online management system does not, however, replace key interaction with a knowledgeable staff person, who should discuss the screening results and next steps with parents or caregivers, respond to questions or concerns, and offer families information for appropriate referrals to local community services if necessary.

Miss Hancock received a 36 month ASQ:SE-2 questionnaire in the mail from her daughter, Rain's, pediatrician. Included with the questionnaire were instructions on completing the questionnaire and bringing it with her to Rain's next scheduled visit. When Miss Hancock arrived, the nurse collected the completed questionnaire and entered it into the computer, generating results that the nurse placed in Rain's file for the doctor to go over with Miss Hancock. ASQ:SE-2 data were added to the program's ASQ Pro account records.

Mrs. Perry took her twin boys, Joe and Jeff, to a primary health care practice that has kiosk-based computer access to ASQ:SE-2 through ASQ Family Access. While waiting in the office for a well-child visit, Mrs. Perry was given directions by office staff on how to access the appropriate ASQ:SE-2 questionnaire for her children. Following the directions, she completed a 36 month ASQ:SE-2 for each boy. She received a reply indicating that the doctor would be discussing the screening results for both children with her shortly. Mrs. Perry then discussed the results with her family physician during the boys' well-child checkup. The physician encouraged Mrs. Perry to contact her local early intervention provider to obtain a more comprehensive assessment for Jeff, who scored above the cutoff on the ASQ:SE-2 questionnaire.

Phone Interview

The interview method often combines the mail-out method with a personal interview over the phone. It is helpful to mail a questionnaire to a parent to review and then follow up by phone to complete the questionnaire. This combination method is effective for families who may not be equipped to independently complete a questionnaire (e.g., parents with limited literacy); however, it is more costly to conduct and therefore most programs may use it only with families who cannot or will not complete the questionnaires without assistance. The interview option can also be used when it is not possible to schedule a visit to a child's home.

Interview Considerations

Programs that have large numbers of children to screen may find that using the mail-out completion option in combination with the phone interview option maximizes effectiveness and resources. The mail-out option was designed for use with parents who can independently complete ASQ:SE-2, whereas the phone interview option can be reserved for the few families who require assistance to complete the questionnaires. The interview option is possible if primary health care practices, screening clinics, or educational programs have personnel who can consistently conduct quality phone interviews.

Interview Procedures

ASQ:SE-2 can be mailed to parents prior to a phone interview, although this step is not critical for accurate completion (unlike for ASQ-3, which requires parents to try items with their child). During the interview, program personnel can follow up with parents regarding questions or concerns and clarify items.

The procedures for implementing phone interview completion closely follow those used for the mail-out system, with a few exceptions. First, the program must dedicate staff time to interview families, and the interviewer must be knowledgeable about child development, local resources, referral agencies, and procedures for completing ASQ:SE-2. Either the interviewer or parents can read items during the interview. Parents and the interviewer can discuss questions and concerns as the items are read; the interviewer must record responses and concerns. Parental concerns and needs can be addressed during the follow-up call.

Luis Mendez was born prematurely and spent 3 weeks in the NICU. The Mendez family members have concerns about Luis's development and behavior and are interested in monitoring using ASQ:SE-2, but they live in a rural area more than 2 hours from the nearest town. Family members indicated that they prefer a home visit rather than receiving the questionnaire by mail, but staff are unable to make home visits at every questionnaire age interval. The questionnaire is mailed prior to a scheduled phone interview when it is not possible for a home visitor to travel to the family. A home visitor then calls or videoconferences with Mrs. Mendez and completes ASQ:SE-2. This approach gives the family some personal contact, and the home visitor can provide immediate feedback if questions arise.

Home Visit

ASQ:SE-2 can be used across a broad range of programs that offer some form of home visitation. The questionnaires are generally incorporated into more comprehensive curricula; for example, ASQ:SE-2 could be used in conjunction with an abuse and neglect prevention program to help parents understand their child's social-emotional development over time. A number of evidence-based home visiting programs—including Nurse–Family Partnerships (NFP), Parents As Teachers, and Healthy Families of America (HFA)—have used ASQ:SE as one component of their evidence-based home visiting services.

Although the home visiting method is the most costly ASQ:SE-2 administrative method, the advantages are numerous. Home visitors, especially if they are working with the family over time, can develop a trusting relationship with families. Parents can ask questions as they complete questionnaires and can discuss behavioral concerns with home visitors. Home visitors can observe if the home environment supports young children's positive behaviors and, if not, provide information and problem solve with parents to create a safe and positive environment. For example, parents who are struggling with their young child's sleeping behaviors may benefit from some information about the importance of routines and how to use routines to support a child's sleep schedule. Home visitors can model positive behavioral strategies with families and use "parent coaching" methods to work with families to incorporate these strategies into day-to-day interactions with their children. Home visitors can also check in frequently with families about behavioral concerns and determine if the parents are feeling more comfortable with their children's behavior and their parenting role.

Home Visit Considerations

It is crucial for home visitors to receive training and guidance on explaining the purpose of social-emotional screening and providing assistance for completing the questionnaire in a home setting. It is important that home visitors understand that ASQ:SE-2 was designed to be completed by parents or other primary caregivers. Home visitors should be nondirective and only offer assistance when requested by parents.

Parents or caregivers should take time to carefully answer each question as well as discuss concerns and results. Parents may become unnecessarily alarmed if results suggest a potential problem when the child's social-emotional development is actually typical for his or her age group.

Home Visit Procedures

The questionnaire ideally should be mailed before the scheduled home visits to give parents the opportunity to review items prior to completing the questionnaire. The home visitor should begin by explaining the screening process and describing his or her role. It is important to explain the purpose of ASQ:SE-2 and provide instructions for completion in language that is easy to understand.

After the questionnaire is completed and reviewed, the home visitor may choose to score the questionnaire with the parents, offering immediate information and feedback and making referrals as appropriate.

There may be times when supervisors choose to have home visitors gather screening information from families but share questionnaire outcomes with supervisors prior to discussing the results with parents. This is particularly important if a home visitor is newly hired or inexperienced or when families have complex needs. When results of ASQ:SE-2 indicate the need for further assessment, it is important for home visitors to be prepared to explain the next steps and to have lists of community resources available. These conversations may be difficult and emotionally charged for family members, and consequentially, home visitors may need to have discussions with supervisors prior to presenting concerning results to parents. Reviewing the discussion in Chapter 6 about communicating results with the family may be helpful.

When discussing results, a home visitor may offer activities that support positive parent–child interactions and encourage children's development. The ASQ:SE-2 Social-Emotional Development Guides and Activities found in Appendix E, or the *ASQ:SE-2™ Learning Activities* handouts can be left with parents. See Appendix 8B at the end of this chapter for specific steps on using ASQ:SE-2 on home visits.

Ginny, a young mother, and her 6-month-old baby were enrolled in Early Head Start soon after her baby was born. Ginny lives with her mother, Pat, and attends a GED program through her local community college. Pat helps take care of the baby while Ginny attends school. The Early Head Start home visitor brings ASQ:SE-2 to complete in the fall and also in the spring. The child's score was in the monitoring zone when Ginny completed ASQ:SE-2 in the fall, and Ginny indicated specific concerns related to sleeping behaviors. Ginny felt exhausted most of the time and was frustrated with how long it took her baby to fall asleep and how often the baby woke up at night. The home visitor provided information and resources on this topic and encouraged Ginny to discuss these concerns with her primary health care provider.

On Site

Questionnaires may be completed on site (e.g., in a doctor's waiting room, at a family center).

On-Site Considerations

It is important to provide an introduction (written or verbally) to the purpose of social-emotional screening. A staff member should be available to support completion of ASQ:SE-2 as needed and discuss concerns and results with parents. Parents may become unnecessarily alarmed if results suggest a potential problem when the child's social-emotional development is actually typical for his or her age group. Scores in the monitoring zone or above the referral cutoffs may require follow-up, so agency staff need to be prepared to provide follow-up and make community referrals for further evaluation or other services as indicated by screening results.

First Place Family Center, a branch of St. Vincent de Paul's in Eugene, Oregon, provides a refuge and place of support for children and their families who are low income, at risk of losing their housing, or already in transition from homelessness and poverty to be safely housed and self-reliant. Center services are comprehensive and include access to a service coordinator for housing and employment assistance, use of on-site facilities for laundry, a kitchen and food bank, clothing, and computer access. Families with children under the age of 5 years are screened with ASQ:SE-2 (and ASQ-3) as part of the intake process. A staff member meets with families in the center and provides an introduction to the purpose of screening and ASQ:SE-2. The family completes ASQ:SE-2 independently or with support as needed. Results and concerns about behavior are discussed with the family at that time. Parents are given information on the social-emotional development of young children and simple strategies for addressing behaviors of concern. Community resources and referral options, as indicated by screening results, are discussed with families. If possible and desired by parents, these referrals are made immediately. In many cases, it is unknown when staff will have another opportunity to meet with the family.

CONCLUSION

ASQ:SE-2 can be administered in many ways. The purpose of this chapter has been to describe five primary ways of completing ASQ:SE-2: mail-out, online, interview, home visit, and on-site completion. Considerations and recommendations for using each option were offered, as well as an example illustrating each method. The ways of administering ASQ:SE-2 described in this chapter can be used separately or combined. It is important for program personnel to examine their screening goals, survey their available resources, and then choose the option that best fits their needs.

8A

Procedures for Using the Card File Tickler System

ASQ:SE-2™

The card file tickler system provides a simple, low-tech approach to tracking all of the activities involved in mailing out ASQ:SE-2. To begin, locate an index card file box. Place dividers for each month (e.g., January, February, March) in the file box. Include subdividers for each month and arrange them by day, week, biweekly interval, or month, depending on the number of children monitored. Complete an individual index card for each child monitored in the program. Figure 8A.1 shows a sample card for Grayson Thomas; a blank sample card is provided as well for program staff to photocopy on an as-needed basis (see Figure 8A.2). The card contains space to record essential identifying information for the child and family, as well as a tracking grid to assist program staff.

The sample grid includes a column listing the program's planned activities in the order the activities are to be administered and columns for each age interval at which a questionnaire is to be completed. Upon completion of each activity in the first column, staff members enter the date in the appropriate column. The activities column contains entries for follow-up, which may not be necessary if the questionnaire is completed and returned to the program on schedule. After a questionnaire is given to the parents, the card is refiled in chronological order under the month and week the questionnaire should be returned. All activities associated with tracking the child's progress are filed by date under the appropriate month and week.

For example, Grayson's card (see Figure 8A.1) is filed under the week of June 1 because that date is 1 week before Grayson will become 12 months old. The card is reviewed when June 1 arrives, and Grayson's parents are sent a 12 month ASQ:SE-2. A notation is made on the card indicating that a reminder call should be made to the parents on June 5, approximately 4 days after the questionnaire was mailed, and the questionnaire should be returned by June 19. The card is filed under the week of June 5 until the call is made and the questionnaire is returned.

Child's name *Grayson Thomas*

Parent's or guardian's name *Ryan & Lindsay Thomas*

Address *1172 Riviera Drive, Chicago, IL*

Telephone *541-555-0149* Message *None*

Corrected date of birth *None*

Child's gender *M*

Date of birth *June 8, 2015*

Activity	2 MO	6 MO	12 MO	18 MO	24 MO	30 MO	36 MO	48 MO	60 MO
Send questionnaire			6-1-16	12-1-16					
Sent questionnaire			6-1-16						
Call—instructions			6-5-16						
Called			6-5-16						
Expected return			6-19-16						
Returned			6-13-16						
If not, called									
Results			OK						
Feedback sent			6-19-16						
Parent called with concern			—						
Physician notified			—						
Referral			—						
Refile card (y/n)			Y						

Comments:

Figure 8A.1. The card file tickler system includes a card for each child participating in the program. As shown on this sample card completed for Grayson Thomas, essential identifying information is recorded, and staff use the grid to track the distribution and return of questionnaires. Basic results are also recorded.

If the questionnaire were to be returned before June 19, then this would be indicated on the card. In addition, other important information should be recorded on the card when possible (e.g., feedback from the family, results, whether child was referred for services). A space also is provided at the bottom of the card to record any additional comments or information relevant to the child. The date for mailing the next questionnaire is recorded, and the card is refiled under the appropriate month and day.

Grayson's parents returned the questionnaire on June 13; the results indicated typical development, and staff sent the family feedback on June 19. Grayson's parents are scheduled to receive the 18 month questionnaire next; thus, the card is refiled under the week of December 1, approximately 6 months after the last questionnaire was completed. If Grayson's parents had not returned the questionnaire by June 19, then they would have been called and a new return date would have been recorded on the card.

SPECIFIC STEPS FOR USING A TICKLER SYSTEM

Careful adherence to the following steps is the first guideline for ensuring a high return rate. In all steps, *target* refers to the assigned date for completing the questionnaire; for infants who were born 3 or more weeks premature and who are less than 24 months of age, this target date corresponds with the corrected age rather than the date of birth.

1. Pull the child's card from the tickler file box.
2. Complete the identifying information on the first page of the appropriate ASQ:SE-2 interval.
3. Record the questionnaire target date (e.g., the date the child will be 18 months) under *Expected return* on the tickler file card.
4. Prepare the questionnaire for mailing, either by folding in half and stapling or taping the ends or by putting it in an envelope. If stapled or taped, then the program's return address and a stamp should be added to the mailing sheet. If mailed in an envelope, then a program-addressed, stamped return envelope should be included.
5. Record the date the questionnaire is mailed on the child's tickler file card under *Sent questionnaire.*
6. Record a date 3 or 4 days after mailing in the *Call—instructions* row.
7. Refile the card under the date marked in the *Call—instructions* row.
8. Check the tickler file and call parents on the date marked for *Call—instructions* to ensure that the questionnaire was received and to answer any questions the parents may have about completing the questionnaire.
9. Record the date the parents were contacted in the *Called* row.
10. Refile the tickler file card in the file box under the date in the *Expected return* row.
11. If the questionnaire is returned before the expected return date, then record the date returned under the *Returned* row.
12. If the questionnaire is not returned by the expected return date, then call the child's parents and record the date in the *If not, called* row.
13. Score the questionnaire according to the instructions in Chapter 6 and record the results on the Information Summary sheet.
14. If the questionnaire results indicate the child is developing typically, then send a feedback letter (see Chapter 5 for examples of feedback letters; see Appendix D for blank letter templates in English and Spanish) and Social-Emotional Development Guides and Activities

Child's name ______________________ Corrected date of birth ______________________

Parent's or guardian's name ______________________ Child's gender ______________________

Address ______________________ Date of birth ______________________

Telephone ______________ Message ______________

Activity	2 MO	6 MO	12 MO	18 MO	24 MO	30 MO	36 MO	48 MO	60 MO
Send questionnaire									
Sent questionnaire									
Call—instructions									
Called									
Expected return									
Returned									
If not, called									
Results									
Feedback sent									
Parent called with concern									
Physician notified									
Referral									
Refile card (y/n)									

Comments:

Figure 8A.2. This blank sample card for the card file tickler system may be photocopied for program use. (Please see the conditions of the Photocopying Release on p. xx.)

(see Appendix E). If program resources permit, then send parents additional incentives that may increase return rate (see discussion in this chapter about mail-out incentives).

15. If the questionnaire results indicate that a child is identified as needing an in-depth assessment, then call the child's parents to discuss options. Refer the child for further assessment, if indicated.
16. Ask the parents if they want the questionnaire results sent to the child's physician. Obtain the parents' written consent to share questionnaire results with other agencies and the child's physician.
17. Determine whether the child will continue to be monitored using the questionnaires. Monitoring would be discontinued for three reasons: 1) at the parent's request, 2) if the child is older than 6 years, or 3) if developmental delays are identified on the follow-up assessment and the child then begins receiving early intervention services.
18. Refile the child's tickler file card under the date that corresponds to 1 week before the target date for the next questionnaire age interval.

8B

Using ASQ:SE-2 on Home Visits

ASQ:SE-2™

This appendix describes the steps and decisions involved in implementing the ASQ:SE-2 system while on a home visit.

Prepare for the Home Visit

- Obtain consent from the parent(s) to participate in the screening/monitoring program (this step can also be done at the home visit).
- Schedule a home visit date and time.
- Photocopy the language-appropriate (English or Spanish) and age-appropriate questionnaire.
- Arrange for an interpreter if necessary.
- *(Optional)* Mail the age-appropriate questionnaire to the child's home before the visit so the family can review items.

Begin the Home Visit

- Determine whether the parents are capable of understanding and completing ASQ:SE-2 independently. If they are, then be available to answer questions. If not, then provide assistance with reading, or interpret items as needed.
- Introduce the purpose of screening and ASQ:SE-2. For example, the home visitor may say, "The purpose of this questionnaire is to check your child's social-emotional development. Your answers will help me know what type of information I may be able to gather for you. Some of the questions are not very specific, but answer based on your knowledge of your child's behavior."

Explain the Scoring System

Discuss how to score the questionnaire before parents begin. Ensure parents know how to mark concerns and understand the different scoring options:

- *Often or always:* Child is performing the behavior often or always.
- *Sometimes:* Child is performing behavior occasionally but not consistently.
- *Rarely or never:* Child rarely or never performs the behavior.

Administer ASQ:SE-2

Have parents complete the questionnaire as independently as possible:

- When necessary, read each item aloud to parents.
- When necessary, paraphrase items for parents who seem to need clarification.
- When appropriate, rephrase questions in terms of the family's values or cultural orientation.
- *Note:* Be careful not to lead the parent in choosing a response. ASQ:SE-2 should be completed based on the parent's experience with their child, their observations of the child's behaviors, and their opinion or interpretation of those behaviors. For example, if a parent wants clarification about an item asking about the child liking to be around other children, reword the item (e.g., "Does Albert enjoy visiting cousins and playing with them or having them visit your apartment?"). Don't offer your opinion based on what he does in the classroom; encourage Albert's mother to think about her experiences and base her answers on these examples.

Score ASQ:SE-2

Compare the child's results to the cutoff score indicated on the Information Summary sheet.

Discuss Results of ASQ:SE-2 with the Family

- Discuss the child's strengths, and reinforce positive parent–child interactions.
- Discuss items that individually score 10 or 15 points.
- Discuss parents' answers to open-ended questions.
- Review the child's score and compare it with the cutoff.

Discuss Referral Considerations when the Total Score Is Above the Cutoff or in the Monitoring Zone

For scores in the monitoring zone or above the cutoff, the next steps will depend on several factors, including time/setting, the child's developmental level, health factors, and culture/family factors. These factors should be discussed with the parents and supports and/or referral options should be given based on child and family strengths and needs. These factors are described in more detail in Chapter 6.

Review These General Guidelines for Decision Making with ASQ:SE-2

Below Cutoff

- Provide ASQ:SE-2 activities.
- Follow up on any items of concern.
- Share results with the child's primary health care provider.
- Monitor (readminister ASQ:SE-2).

Monitoring Zone (Close to Cutoff)

- Follow up on any items of concern.
- Provide ASQ:SE-2 development guides and activities.
- Provide information, education, and support to the family.
- Monitor the child using ASQ:SE-2.
- Share results with the child's primary health care provider.
- Make referrals as appropriate; if child is a girl, consider referral for further evaluation.

Above Cutoff

- Make referrals. Examples:
    - Early intervention/early childhood special education
    - Primary health care provider
    - Mental health services (adult, parent–child, or play therapy)
    - Local community agencies
    - Feeding and/or sleeping clinics
    - Community groups: YMCA, Birth to Three, church groups
    - Parenting groups
    - Behavior management classes for parents
    - Healthy Start, Early Head Start, Head Start
- Share results with the child's primary health care provider.

9

ASQ:SE-2 Settings

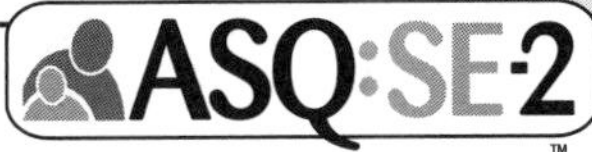

The ASQ:SE-2 system's flexibility in terms of how and in what settings it can be used is a great strength of the tool. As indicated in Chapter 8, the mail-out, online, phone interview, home visit, and on-site options for ASQ:SE-2 completion can be used across a variety of programs that may wish to conduct social-emotional screening (Johnson-Staub, 2014). Any program or setting that interfaces with parents who have young children has the potential to offer social-emotional screening as a service. This chapter highlights the variety of settings that provide opportunities for social-emotional screening, including screening clinics, child care and center-based educational programs (e.g., preschools, Head Start programs), health and primary care practices, early intervention/early childhood special education (EI/ECSE) programs, and child welfare programs. Some programs may administer the screening test and refer families to other community agencies for follow-up, as indicated by screening results (e.g., a screening clinic); other programs may administer the tool and provide the majority of follow-up within their agencies (e.g., a Head Start center). The following sections offer information and recommendations for social-emotional screening across diverse settings.

SCREENING CLINICS

Screening clinics (also known as roundups) usually are joint community efforts held annually to provide screenings to a large number of children related to general development, social-emotional development, hearing, and vision, as well as medical and dental evaluations. Recommendations and referrals are made to EI/ECSE programs, hospitals, and other community resources as appropriate. Screening clinics usually are sponsored by a network of providers who combine their agencies' efforts to provide communitywide early childhood assessments.

ASQ:SE-2 is a good measure of choice for many screening clinics conducted throughout the United States for several reasons. First, because a child's behavior often varies in different settings or with different people, it is difficult during the short duration of a screening clinic for professionals to observe a child long enough to get an accurate picture of his or her social-emotional development. Gathering information from parents is imperative when assessing behavioral or social-emotional development. Second, ASQ:SE-2 is economical to use because questionnaires can be completed by parents rather than professional staff. Third, most parents and other caregivers find the questionnaires to be user friendly, easy to complete, and a reasonable time investment. Fourth, parents comment on the value of completing an ASQ:SE-2 questionnaire because it gives them a better understanding of their child's social-emotional development. Finally, the extensive data backing the reliability and validity of ASQ:SE-2 permit professional staff to be confident that ASQ:SE-2 results will be accurate in most cases.

Parents can complete ASQ:SE-2 independently or with support from staff. Information on community resources and referrals can be given to families when necessary.

Pretend City is a children's museum designed to meet the developmental needs of children younger than 5 years located in Orange County, California. Pretend City's mission is to create a "community which builds better brains through fun, whole body learning experiences and empowers children and their grown-ups to meaningfully connect with and expand their world" (Pretend City, 2013). In addition to offering developmental screenings, health screenings, and follow-up, Pretend City provides opportunities for parents to screen their child's social-emotional development with ASQ:SE. Pretend City holds special social-emotional screening events, with a behavior specialist on site to answer questions regarding children's social-emotional and behavioral concerns. *Visit http://pretendcity.org for more information.*

Three human services agencies in a small rural county offer an annual screening clinic to all interested parents of children birth to 5 years of age. Maria, a single mother, brought her infant Santiago to the screening clinic, where she completed a 6 month ASQ:SE-2 questionnaire. Upon completion, a staff member reviewed and scored the questionnaire. The total score was in the monitoring zone, and Maria had indicated two concerns related to feeding and sleeping items on the questionnaire. Maria also completed an ASQ-3 questionnaire, with results indicating that Santiago's development was on schedule. Maria was able to meet with a nurse who determined that Santiago's height and weight were in good proportion and that he was in good physical health. A staff person talked with Maria about her concerns and shared resources for parents in their community. Maria liked the idea of going to a parent support group, so together they contacted a local birth-to-3 parenting group. With Maria's permission, the staff member arranged to share the ASQ:SE-2 results with her infant's health care provider and developed a plan to monitor Santiago's social-emotional development by rescreening him at 12 months of age.

CHILD CARE AND CENTER-BASED EDUCATIONAL SETTINGS

Communities offer a wide variety of child care options for families, and most communities offer center-based educational programs for young children. Many of these programs, such as Head Start, target preschool-age children, whereas other programs, such as Early Head Start, focus on infants and toddlers. Some child care programs offer developmental and social-emotional screenings for children as part of their services, and more providers are offering screening as part of their involvement in state or national programs. Programs such as Head Start and Early Head Start are required to provide developmental and social-emotional screening to all children. The quality rating and improvement system (QRIS) uses rating and improvement strategies to elevate the quality of care in state early care and education systems. In some states, the QRIS requires programs to provide developmental and social-emotional screening to children as part of the quality ratings approach.

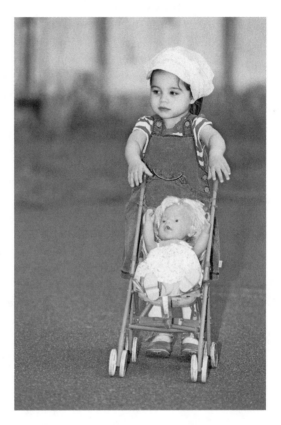

In addition to identifying children in need of additional behavioral support services, using ASQ:SE-2 universally in child care and educational settings helps to facilitate discussions between parents and child care providers about children's behavior across settings. A child may be exhibiting positive social-emotional behaviors at home while exhibiting negative social-emotional behaviors in the school setting—or vice versa. ASQ:SE-2 provides an excellent springboard for a child's caregivers to compare notes and ensure that a child and/or a child's caregiver is receiving adequate support to ensure the child's optimum social-emotional development. As previously mentioned, if someone other than a parent completes ASQ:SE-2, he or she should know the child well and have at least 15–20 hours per week of contact with the child. Enrollment in a child care program or a center-based educational program is an excellent time to introduce the purpose of screening and ASQ:SE-2 to parents. Parent meetings are a second opportunity to discuss screening. Including screening as one of the program's activities makes it a universal process and therefore does not stigmatize any child or family. Parents can be given the age-appropriate ASQ:SE-2 questionnaire for their children during enrollment. A meeting or home visit can be arranged between the parent and teacher or child care provider to review the results of the questionnaire. Both the parent and the provider can independently complete an ASQ:SE-2 questionnaire, and differences in observations of the child's behavior can be discussed. If the parent does not bring the questionnaire to the meeting, then the parent can complete ASQ:SE-2 before the meeting begins.

Although there is some flexibility in ASQ:SE-2 administration procedures, providers need to keep in mind the three main options for completing ASQ:SE-2: 1) the parent completes ASQ:SE-2 independently, 2) the teacher completes ASQ:SE-2 independently, or 3) both teacher and parent complete ASQ:SE-2 questionnaires independently and compare results.

Especially when the preschool teacher or child care provider completes ASQ:SE-2 for a child, parents should be provided the opportunity to complete the questionnaire for two important reasons. First, many parents learn what to expect at different ages and benefit by acquiring information about their child's social-emotional development. This information may help to lessen a parent's concerns about their child's behavior, "normalize" behaviors of concern, and facilitate conversations about age-appropriate strategies for implementing positive behavioral support in the home. Second, parents usually know more about their children than anyone else; certainly parents know more about their children's behavior at home than anyone else. Because a child will spend the majority of his or her time in the home environment, it is important to problem-solve behaviors of concern with parents and facilitate positive parent–child relationships in the home.

Having a child care provider or teacher work in partnership with a parent and compare the child's behaviors at home with behaviors in child care settings also follows the 2009 position statement *Developmentally Appropriate Practice in Early Childhood Programs Serving Children from Birth Through Age 8* by the National Association for the Education of Young Children (NAEYC). In this position statement, NAEYC recommended that important decisions about a child always be made on the basis of results from more than one developmental assessment or screening instrument and that families are involved as important sources of information when screening indicates the need for a referral. Meeting together to compare observations and discuss a child's social-emotional development provides the opportunity to discuss the child's strengths and, if necessary, discuss any behavioral concerns.

Albina Head Start is the largest Head Start in the Portland metro area and serves children in 32 classrooms across north and northeast Portland. Albina Head Start uses ASQ:SE during the initial parent–teacher meeting each fall. Each family has an individual meeting with an assigned teacher prior to the first day of school. During this meeting, the parent and child visit the classroom, set goals for the year, and complete ASQ-3 and ASQ:SE. Results are immediately discussed with the family, and parents are informed of support services available if needed. Any family whose child scores above the ASQ:SE cutoff is given the opportunity to be referred to a mental health consultant for further screening and observation, consultation to the classroom and possibly referral, or ongoing individual treatment. In Multnomah County, where Albina Head Start is located, early childhood mental health consultation is provided to Head Start programs and child care agencies at a rate subsidized by the county. This allows the Portland metro area Head Start programs additional access to mental health staff than other programs have in many different parts of the state. When a child is referred to the mental health consultant, the consultant, teacher, and family work collaboratively to meet the child's needs both at home and at school. Children scoring near the cutoff are rescreened in 3 months.

HEALTH AND PRIMARY CARE PRACTICES

A child's development and health go hand-in-hand. Good overall health provides an important foundation for a child's early brain development and a child's ability to achieve new skills and develop to his or her fullest potential. A child's health is influenced by early events, such as a mother's health before and during pregnancy as well as positive early experiences after birth and throughout childhood (National Scientific Council on the Developing Child & National Forum on Early Childhood Policy and Programs, 2010). A number of evidence-based home visiting programs that are part of health initiatives, such as NFP and HFA, have used ASQ:SE-2 as one component of their evidence-based home visiting services. See Chapter 8 for more information on using ASQ:SE-2 in home visiting programs. Any health initiative that interfaces with families who have young children provides a potential setting for developmental and behavioral screening. For example, the Special Supplemental Nutrition Program for Women, Infants, and Children (WIC) provides federal grants to states to provide supplemental foods, health care referrals, and nutrition education to families with infants and children up to age 5 years who are found to be at nutritional risk. WIC programs have used this touch point with families as a way to provide information on developmental milestones, introduce the purpose of screening in early childhood, and share information on community resources that are available if families have concerns about their children's development or behaviors (e.g., EI/ECSE). Programs can either administer screenings on site and/or enroll children in other community screening/monitoring programs. The remainder of this section provides considerations and recommendations for conducting screening during primary health care well-child checkups, an excellent opportunity to provide universal screening of all young children.

Primary health care providers can use ASQ:SE-2 questionnaires to gather information on children prior to physical examinations. Although the American Academy of Pediatrics (AAP) recommendations call for using a standardized developmental screening of young children at regular intervals (and autism screening at 18 and 24 months), research also points to the importance of social-emotional development on general well-being versus risk (Briggs et al., 2012). Health care providers may save time by sending questionnaires to parents prior to their children's appointments, directing parents to an online method of completing questionnaires, or having parents complete questionnaires while in the waiting room just before their appointments. These methods help parents identify concerns prior to the appointment with their primary health care provider and provide a focus for the examination and subsequent discussion.

When parents contact their children's pediatric offices to schedule well-child visits, office staff may ask if parents have Internet access at home. If parents say yes, then office staff may direct them to complete ASQ:SE-2 prior to the well-child visit via the ASQ Family Access online questionnaire completion system. If a parent does not have Internet access, then the office staff can mail the age-appropriate questionnaire with an explanation about the screening/monitoring program. When parents receive appointment reminder calls prior to well-child visits, the messaging system may also include a prompt for parents to go to the web site to complete ASQ:SE-2 or a reminder to complete their paper questionnaire and bring it to their appointments. Results from ASQ:SE-2 questionnaires completed online through ASQ Family Access are transmitted to the ASQ Online management system for scoring, and results can be placed in the child's physical file.

If parents have not completed ASQ:SE-2 prior to the well-child visit, then they should be given the appropriate questionnaire to complete once they arrive in the waiting room. Offices may provide paper copies of questionnaires or set up a computer station or kiosk with ASQ Family Access.

A staff member should be appointed to assist parents as necessary while they complete ASQ:SE-2. One of the advantages of the ASQ:SE-2 system is that paraprofessionals, office staff, and assistant medical health professionals (e.g., a certified nurse assistant) can receive training and provide excellent support to parents. Support may range from directing caregivers to the ASQ:SE-2 station to helping them complete the questionnaire by reading or clarifying the intent of items.

Before meeting with the primary health care provider, trained support staff can meet with parents to remind them about the purpose of social-emotional screening, discuss the results of the completed ASQ:SE-2, and share local community resource information related to parenting and child development. This meeting is intended to be a brief conversation (i.e., 5–10 minutes) to help parents become better informed about social-emotional development and resources in their community. Information about immediate concerns as well as referrals to community agencies for more in-depth assistance may be given to parents at this time. This touch point is a critical one for parents, particularly for those whose children will require a referral for EI/ECSE or behavioral support agencies. The designated ASQ:SE-2 staff person should receive extensive training on how to introduce ASQ:SE-2, support parents in completing ASQ:SE-2, and score and interpret results, as well as training on how to communicate results to parents in a sensitive, supportive, and nonthreatening manner (see Chapter 6 for more information on how to talk to parents).

Screening a child with ASQ:SE-2 will result in one of three findings: 1) the child appears to be developing typically at the time of administration, and there are no behavioral concerns; 2) the child may need follow-up because results are in the monitoring zone; or 3) the child should be referred for an in-depth behavioral assessment because the child's score is above the established cutoff.

If the child is developing typically (i.e., the score is below the established cutoff point) and the parent has no specific concerns, then the designated ASQ:SE-2 staff will discuss and emphasize these results with parents and provide them with a general information packet. This packet can include age-appropriate activities as well as general community resources for families and young children.

If the child's score is close to the cutoff (in the monitoring zone), or if the parent has any specific concerns or questions, then staff should reinforce the child's strengths and provide information that is tailored to the parents' concerns. For example, if a parent is struggling with behaviors related to feeding, then staff can provide information about feeding relevant to the child's age. If a parent wants information about community child care options, then staff can refer the parent to the local child care resource and referral agency.

If a child's score is above the cutoff, then staff will discuss behaviors of concern with the parent. Staff will note any of these discussions or considerations and alert the primary health care provider to these considerations when sharing the ASQ:SE-2 Information Summary sheet. Parents should be encouraged to discuss their concerns with the child's primary care provider during the next visit. Initial information about local referral agencies and the services offered to children and families should also be provided.

The ASQ:SE-2 Information Summary sheet, with any additional information noted by the staff member, should be placed in the child's file for the primary health care provider to review. In the majority of cases, primary health care providers can simply comment on social-emotional strengths that children exhibit and celebrate these accomplishments with families. When referrals are warranted, the primary care provider should discuss this with the parents and obtain consent if necessary to refer the child to the local EI/ECSE agency or other agencies that assess children's behavioral/social-emotional development. It is assumed that the majority of these screenings will indicate typical development, and in most cases, there will be minimal time necessary for discussing behavioral concerns with a child's primary health care provider.

Results from the child's social-emotional screening, including any referrals made based on screening results, should be entered into the child's medical record so that social-emotional progress can be monitored over time. See Appendix D for blank templates of letters and forms that can be used in medical settings.

Montefiore Medical Group, located in the Bronx, New York City, uses ASQ:SE in 13 of its medical clinics to identify children at risk for social-emotional difficulties. Clinics offer monitoring and referral services, and some employ infant/toddler specialists (ITS), who offer on-site clinical evaluations and intervention. During a child's visit, nursing staff give the appropriate ASQ:SE while the family waits for the provider. Families are also given a letter of explanation (in English or Spanish) that reviews the purpose of the screening. Parents can complete ASQ:SE during the visit, ask staff for help with completion, or decline to complete ASQ:SE. The ITS reviews and scores the questionnaire, and keeps the ASQ:SE Information Summary sheet for the child's records. If a child's score is above the ASQ:SE cutoff, then the ITS offers to complete a more comprehensive assessment. The ITS makes treatment and referral decisions from ASQ:SE results and, in consultation with the pediatric provider, either delivers the treatment or closely follows all referrals made.

Source: Briggs, Stettler, Johnson Silver, Schrag, Nayak, Chinitz, and Racine (2012); see http://pediatrics.aappublications.org/content/129/2/e377.full for more information.

EARLY INTERVENTION AND EARLY CHILDHOOD SPECIAL EDUCATION SETTINGS

The Individuals with Disabilities Education Improvement Act (IDEA) of 2004 (PL 108-446) guarantees infants and toddlers (under Part C) and preschool and school-age children (under Part B) with disabilities the right to a free appropriate public education in the least restrictive environment. ASQ:SE-2 can be used in a variety of different ways as part of Part C early intervention and Part B, Section 619, early childhood special education services. Although some children enter or become eligible for services based on social-emotional delays, many children are referred to or become eligible for these services based on general developmental delays (e.g., motor, cognitive) and may have undetected behavioral or social-emotional delays. The incidence of social-emotional delays in children with disabilities is estimated at 40%, much higher than the 16%–20% estimated in the general population (Clifford, Squires, Twombly, Bricker, & Yockelson, 2012). Therefore, it is critical to identify early indicators of social-emotional delays in this population and address parent concerns as early as possible. *Note:* ASQ:SE-2 may not be necessary or appropriate if a child is eligible for services based on behavioral or social-emotional delays and is receiving comprehensive behavioral or mental health supports.

Early intervention programs have successfully used ASQ:SE-2 as part of the intake/eligibility evaluation (see the program profile that follows), providing an opportunity for parents to share and discuss behavioral concerns during this process. Service providers have used ASQ:SE as a way to establish a relationship early on with a family, regardless of the child's disability. In future work with a family, the service provider considers a parent's behavioral concerns when planning interventions to support the child's development. ASQ:SE questionnaires have also been included as part of a child's transition between Part C and Part B services to ensure that social-emotional development is evaluated when behavioral concerns are present. Finally, if early childhood special education services are being provided in a preschool setting, with a minimal parent involvement, then ASQ:SE-2 can be given to parents as a way to facilitate the home–school connection and address behaviors that may be of concern at home but are not present in the school environment.

Early intervention programs in Illinois are using a relationship-based model for promoting social-emotional development in Part C early intervention. The goal is to support social-emotional development for all children in early intervention and to more effectively serve children who demonstrate social-emotional difficulties and their families. Providing the opportunity for parents who have not yet completed ASQ:SE to do so during the initial intake process is one component of this comprehensive approach. Completing ASQ:SE allows parents to share their concerns and start conversations about the social-emotional needs of their children. This process helps the service coordinator feel more knowledgeable and connected to the family, and sets parents' expectations for what is to come. After the initial intake, the service coordinator consults with a social-emotional specialist to determine what follow-up may be needed to address the parents' questions and concerns. Decisions are made regarding what types of expertise are needed to address the parents' questions and concerns, what disciplines are needed to conduct further assessment, and how to involve the family in this process. The service coordinator benefits from these consultations by better understanding families' concerns and learning effective strategies to address the social-emotional needs of very young children in early intervention.

Source: Gilkerson and Kopel (2004); see https://www.erikson.edu/wp-content/uploads/OPgilkerson.pdf for more information.

CHILD WELFARE SETTINGS

The Child Abuse Prevention and Treatment Act (CAPTA) of 1974 (PL 93-247) requires that states have provisions and procedures for the referral to early intervention services funded by Part C of IDEA for children younger than 3 years who are involved in substantiated cases of child abuse or neglect. Part C of IDEA was reauthorized in 2004 and contains a provision very similar to the one in CAPTA. These laws were put into place to ensure that the developmental and social-emotional needs of very young children are being met. Twenty percent of children in foster care are younger than 3 years (U.S. Department of Health and Human Services, 2010). A study indicated that 42.3% of children ranging in age from 1 year to 5 years involved in child welfare investigations had some social-emotional or developmental need that may have qualified them for services under Part C (Casanueva et al., 2012). States have the discretion whether to refer such children under the age of 3 to early intervention or to first employ a screening process to determine whether a referral is needed.

Using ASQ:SE-2 in child welfare settings requires some important considerations. If the child has been placed in a new setting (e.g., a foster home), then the child should be given some time to adjust to this new setting prior to administering ASQ:SE-2. Children who have undergone a recent change in placement may undergo a "honeymoon" period in which they do not exhibit problem behaviors for some time, or they may exhibit problem behaviors that lessen as they adjust to their new environment. Providing a minimum of 30 days for a child to adjust to his or her new setting (and more time if possible) is recommended prior to administering ASQ:SE-2 with a new caregiver. In addition, sometimes parents who are involved with child welfare may not be accurate reporters because of their lack of trust in the child protection system. Caseworkers will need to have developed a positive and trusting relationship with these parents prior to administering ASQ:SE-2. Caseworkers should be clear with parents about why the tool is being administered, how results will be used, and with whom results will be shared.

Children who have been abused or neglected have a high incidence of behavioral and social-emotional delays. Caregivers of these children, including biological, adoptive, and foster parents, require education and support on the potential behaviors they will encounter as well as positive behavioral strategies for responding to behaviors of concern. Using ASQ:SE-2 with caregivers provides an opportunity to open dialogue about what type of social-emotional behaviors are typical and what behaviors are cause for concern. Using ASQ:SE-2 in the child welfare system also necessitates the development of a process for referring children as indicated by ASQ:SE-2 results and for supporting caregivers in gaining access to services in the community. Monitoring with ASQ:SE-2 can help determine if education and supports provided are making a difference for caregivers and children. Although ASQ:SE-2 is not an evaluative measure, looking at trends in ASQ:SE-2 scores does provide information on a child's behavior over time.

The state of Pennsylvania implemented a law in September 2008 to meet the CAPTA and IDEA mandate requiring that all children younger than 3 years with substantiated cases of child abuse or neglect be referred or screened for possible referral for Part C early intervention services. Pennsylvania's policy goes beyond the federal requirements by also encouraging screening for all children younger than 5 years who are receiving child welfare services. The state selected ASQ:SE and ASQ-3 as screening tools. Training was provided to staff from public and private children and youth social services agencies. Caseworkers reported that the screening process helped them engage parents and better understand children's development. Research indicated that more children are being screened and receiving services for developmental and social-emotional problems as a result of the state's early intervention referral policy for infants and toddlers involved with child welfare. *See the University of Pittsburgh's web site at www.pacwrc.pitt.edu/ASQ.htm for more information on the referral policy and the University of Pittsburgh's evaluation of it.*

CONCLUSION

The purpose of this chapter has been to describe specific settings for using ASQ:SE-2. Screening clinics, child care and center-based educational programs, health and primary care practices, early intervention settings, and child welfare are some examples of the variety of environments where ASQ:SE-2 can be used. The flexibility of ASQ:SE-2 and the numerous completion methods make it possible for programs to use the questionnaires in a variety of ways, including ongoing monitoring of a child's social-emotional status, one-time screening to identify delays or concerns, and as a platform to gather information from parents about their children's social-emotional strengths as well as areas of concern. Those working with families in these diverse settings will need to be trained on how to administer ASQ:SE-2, including describing the purpose of screening, offering assistance without being directive, discussing results with families, and offering services and supports as a follow-up to questionnaire results. Using ASQ:SE-2 may assist parents, teachers, and care providers in identifying and discussing children's strengths and concerns as well as in providing parents with needed resources for supporting their young children's optimal development.

10

ASQ:SE-2 Family Studies

ASQ:SE-2™

This chapter comprises a series of scenarios designed to illustrate the use of ASQ:SE-2 across various programs and settings. They are intended to help users consider how ASQ:SE-2 results are interpreted and to support work with families. These examples may be a useful training tool for program staff new to ASQ:SE-2. The following case studies include examples of screening through the foster care system, clinic-based screening, center-based educational screening, and screening through a home visiting program. The following brief descriptions may be used as a guide to locate the examples that will be most relevant based on the user's needs.

1. *Lilah:* The first case study is about 3-year-old Lilah, whose foster mother works with a caseworker to screen Lilah.
2. *Adrian:* The second case study is about Adrian, a 10½-month-old whose questionnaires were administered through a clinic-based program for a well-child visit.
3. *Marcus:* The third case study is about 3-year-old Marcus, whose family experienced on-and-off homelessness. Marcus received screening through an early childhood program run through a day center's services for families in transition.
4. *Celia:* The last case study is about Celia, who is 14 weeks old, with an adjusted age of 10 weeks. Celia was screened through a home visiting program that is designed to support families as they make the transition from the NICU to home.

LILAH

Lilah is 3 years 2 months old and lives in a foster home with her 18-month-old brother Sam. Lilah and Sam entered protective custody after witnessing domestic violence between their mother and her boyfriend. Lilah's mother is receiving supervised visitation with Lilah and Sam for 1 hour a week. Lilah's biological father's rights were terminated soon after Sam's birth.

Denise, the protective services caseworker, brought ASQ:SE-2 for Lilah's foster mother to complete 5 weeks after Lilah was placed in her home (see Figure 10.1). Every child who is brought into protective custody younger than age 5 is administered a developmental and a social-emotional screening within the first 45 days of placement. Lilah's total score on ASQ:SE-2 is 80 points, which is in the monitoring zone (the cutoff score for her ASQ:SE-2 age interval is 105). Lilah's foster mother indicated specific concerns about sleeping, nightmares, and Lilah's general mood.

Setting/Time Factors

Lilah's foster mother reported that Lilah is happiest when she is with her brother. She also reported that Lilah is upset when she returns from visits with her mother. Lilah cries and says she wants to go home.

Developmental Factors

Lilah's ASQ-3 scores indicate that her communication, gross motor, and fine motor skills are in the monitoring zone (see Figure 10.2). Lilah's problem-solving and personal-social skills are above the cutoff, however, indicating those skills appear to be on schedule. Lilah's foster mother indicated that Lilah is "a really quiet kid" who only talks to adults and peers when asked direct questions. She does hear Lilah talking to her brother, although Lilah stops if anyone gets too close.

Health Factors

Lilah was born 4 weeks premature. She has not been to regular well-child checkups. She had an overall health evaluation when she entered foster care and her general health is good, although she is underweight for her age. Hearing and vision screenings indicated no concerns.

Family/Cultural Factors

In her foster home, Lilah lives with her brother Sam and two teenagers who are the foster family's biological children. The foster parents are experienced caregivers, and Denise considers the home a good placement for the children.

ASQ:SE-2 Interpretation and Follow-Up

Denise discussed the results of Lilah's ASQ:SE-2 with her foster mother. In reviewing the responses, Denise noticed that the items on ASQ:SE-2 that Lilah received points on are all considered internalizing behaviors (e.g., fearfulness, nightmares, lack of interest in things in her environment) versus externalizing behaviors (e.g., aggression, dangerous behaviors, not following rules).

- Although Lilah's ASQ:SE-2 score is only in the monitoring zone, Denise wants to refer Lilah to an early childhood mental health therapist for a mental health evaluation. She based this decision on the fact that Lilah is a girl (and girls' total scores are generally lower than boys' scores on ASQ:SE-2), as well as the knowledge that the internalizing behaviors Lilah demonstrates may be a result of witnessing domestic violence.

36 Month Information Summary

33 months 0 days through 41 months 30 days — ASQ:SE-2

Child's name: Lilah — Date ASQ:SE-2 completed: 3/17/15

Child's ID #: 0084 — Child's date of birth: 1/12/12

Person who completed ASQ:SE-2: Amanda — Child's age in months and days: 38 months 5 days

Administering program/provider: Early Check — Child's gender: ○ Male ● Female

1. **ASQ:SE-2 SCORING CHART:**
   - Score items (*Z* = 0, *V* = 5, *X* = 10, *Concern* = 5).
   - Transfer the page totals and add them for the total score.
   - Record the child's total score next to the cutoff.

		Cutoff	Total score
TOTAL POINTS ON PAGE 1			
TOTAL POINTS ON PAGE 2		105	80
TOTAL POINTS ON PAGE 3			
TOTAL POINTS ON PAGE 4			
Total score			

2. **ASQ:SE-2 SCORE INTERPRETATION:** Review the approximate location of the child's total score on the scoring graphic. Then, check off the area for the score results below.

no or low risk — 75 — monitor — 105 — refer → 155+ (90%ile)

___ The child's total score is in the ☐ area. It is below the cutoff. Social-emotional development appears to be on schedule.
✓ The child's total score is in the ▒ area. It is close to the cutoff. Review behaviors of concern and monitor.
___ The child's total score is in the ■ area. It is above the cutoff. Further assessment with a professional may be needed.

3. **OVERALL RESPONSES AND CONCERNS:** Record responses and transfer parent/caregiver comments. YES responses require follow-up.

1–35. Any Concerns marked on scored items? (YES) no — Comments: Lilah doesn't talk much & seems fearful.

36. Eating/sleeping/toileting concerns? (YES) no — Comments: She doesn't sleep well & sometimes has nightmares.

37. Other worries? YES (no) — Comments:

4. **FOLLOW-UP REFERRAL CONSIDERATIONS:** Mark all as Yes, No, or Unsure (Y, N, U). See pages 98–103 in the *ASQ:SE-2 User's Guide.*

Y **Setting/time factors** (e.g., Is the child's behavior the same at home as at school?)
U **Developmental factors** (e.g., Is the child's behavior related to a developmental stage or delay?)
N **Health factors** (e.g., Is the child's behavior related to health or biological factors?)
Y **Family/cultural factors** (e.g., Is the child's behavior acceptable given the child's cultural or family context? Have there been any stressful events in the child's life recently?)
Y **Parent concerns** (e.g., Did the parent/caregiver express any concerns about the child's behavior?)

5. **FOLLOW-UP ACTION:** Check all that apply.

✓ Provide activities and rescreen in 3 months.
✓ Share results with primary health care provider.
___ Provide parent education materials.
___ Provide information about available parenting classes or support groups.
___ Have another caregiver complete ASQ:SE-2. List caregiver here (e.g., grandparent, teacher): ______
___ Administer developmental screening (e.g., ASQ-3).
___ Refer to early intervention/early childhood special education.
✓ Refer for social-emotional, behavioral, or mental health evaluation.
___ Follow up with items of concern.
✓ Other: Refer to Head Start

P201360600

Figure 10.1. Lilah's ASQ:SE-2 Information Summary sheet.

ASQ-3 — 36 Month ASQ-3 Information Summary

34 months 16 days through 38 months 30 days

Child's name: Lilah — Date ASQ completed: 3/17/15

Child's ID #: 0084 — Date of birth: 1/12/12

Administering program/provider: Early Check

1. **SCORE AND TRANSFER TOTALS TO CHART BELOW:** See *ASQ-3 User's Guide* for details, including how to adjust scores if item responses are missing. Score each item (YES = 10, SOMETIMES = 5, NOT YET = 0). Add item scores, and record each area total. In the chart below, transfer the total scores, and fill in the circles corresponding with the total scores.

Area	Cutoff	Total Score	0	5	10	15	20	25	30	35	40	45	50	55	60
Communication	30.99	40	●	●	●	●	●	●	●	○	●	○	○	○	○
Gross Motor	36.99	45	●	●	●	●	●	●	●	●	○	●	○	○	○
Fine Motor	18.07	25	●	●	●	●	○	●	○	○	○	○	○	○	○
Problem Solving	30.29	45	●	●	●	●	●	●	●	○	○	●	○	○	○
Personal-Social	35.33	60	●	●	●	●	●	●	●	○	○	○	○	○	●

2. **TRANSFER OVERALL RESPONSES:** Bolded uppercase responses require follow-up. See *ASQ-3 User's Guide,* Chapter 6.

1. Hears well? (Yes) NO — Comments:
2. Talks like other children his age? Yes (NO) — Comments: She doesn't talk very much.
3. Understand most of what your child says? (Yes) NO — Comments:
4. Others understand most of what your child says? (Yes) NO — Comments:
5. Walks, runs, and climbs like other children? (Yes) NO — Comments:
6. Family history of hearing impairment? YES (No) — Comments:
7. Concerns about vision? YES (No) — Comments:
8. Any medical problems? YES (No) — Comments:
9. Concerns about behavior? YES (No) — Comments:
10. Other concerns? (YES) No — Comments: She is underweight.

3. **ASQ SCORE INTERPRETATION AND RECOMMENDATION FOR FOLLOW-UP:** You must consider total area scores, overall responses, and other considerations, such as opportunities to practice skills, to determine appropriate follow-up.

If the child's total score is in the ☐ area, it is above the cutoff, and the child's development appears to be on schedule.
If the child's total score is in the ▒ area, it is close to the cutoff. Provide learning activities and monitor.
If the child's total score is in the ■ area, it is below the cutoff. Further assessment with a professional may be needed.

4. **FOLLOW-UP ACTION TAKEN:** Check all that apply.

✓ Provide activities and rescreen in 3 months.
✓ Share results with primary health care provider.
___ Refer for (circle all that apply) hearing, vision, and/or behavioral screening.
___ Refer to primary health care provider or other community agency (specify reason): ______.
___ Refer to early intervention/early childhood special education.
___ No further action taken at this time
✓ Other (specify): Refer to Head Start.

5. **OPTIONAL:** Transfer item responses (Y = YES, S = SOMETIMES, N = NOT YET, X = response missing).

	1	2	3	4	5	6
Communication						
Gross Motor						
Fine Motor						
Problem Solving						
Personal-Social						

P101360800

Figure 10.2. Lilah's ASQ-3 Information Summary sheet.

- When Denise makes the referral, she plans to ask the therapist to help the foster mother learn strategies for supporting Lilah at home. Denise asks Lilah's foster mother to talk to the therapist about her concerns about nightmares and Lilah's distress after visiting her mother.
- The protective service plan is to work with Lilah's biological mother with the end goal of returning Lilah and Sam to her care. Lilah's ASQ:SE-2 and ASQ-3 results will be shared with Lilah's biological mother so that she can stay informed about Lilah's development and how she is adjusting to foster care.
- Denise is going to refer Lilah to Head Start so that she can interact with peers and participate in activities to support her overall development.
- Denise shares the ASQ:SE-2 guide to social-emotional development at 36 months with Lilah's foster mother and her biological mother, as well as ideas about social-emotional activities that can be done together in the foster home or during visitation times.
- Denise is planning to rescreen Lilah in 3 months using ASQ:SE-2 and ASQ-3 because the results of both screening tools indicated the need to monitor.
- ASQ:SE-2 and ASQ-3 results will be shared with Lilah's health care provider by Denise, with the foster mother's permission. Lilah's general health and weight gain will be monitored by her primary health care provider.

ADRIAN

Adrian is 10½ months old and lives with his big sister and his mother and father. Adrian's mother describes Adrian as a "good baby," who eats and sleeps well overall and is generally easy to care for.

Adrian's mother completed ASQ:SE-2 and ASQ-3 online using Family Access before attending a well-child checkup at her children's primary health care provider's office. Adrian's total score on ASQ:SE-2 is 70 points, above the cutoff score of 50 points for his ASQ:SE-2 age interval (see Figure 10.3). His mother did not indicate any concerns on scored questions or Overall questions.

Setting/Time Factors

Adrian's mother, Jessica, is Adrian's primary caregiver. Adrian has been cared for by babysitters and his grandmother but has not been in an out-of-home caregiving setting. Jessica reported on ASQ:SE-2 that no one had expressed concerns about Adrian's behavior.

Developmental Factors

Adrian's scores on ASQ-3 indicate his development is on schedule in the areas of fine motor and problem-solving skills (see Figure 10.4). His scores for communication and personal-social skills are in the monitoring zone. His score in the gross motor area is below, but close to, the cutoff at 30 points (the referral cutoff is below 30.6). Jessica did not report any concerns on any of the Overall questions.

Health Factors

Adrian was born full term at 7½ pounds. Jessica received prenatal care throughout her pregnancy, and there were no complications at birth. Adrian's health has been very good in his first year, and he is on track for his height and weight for his age.

12 Month Information Summary *9 months 0 days through 14 months 30 days* — ASQ:SE-2

Baby's name: Adrian Date ASQ:SE-2 completed: 6/15/15

Baby's ID #: 22784 Baby's date of birth: 7/21/14

Person who completed ASQ:SE-2: Jessica Baby's age/adjusted age in months and days: 10 months 25 days

Administering program/provider: Johnson Family Medicine Baby's gender: ● Male ○ Female

1. ASQ:SE-2 SCORING CHART:

- Score items (*Z* = 0, *V* = 5, *X* = 10, *Concern* = 5).
- Transfer the page totals and add them for the total score.
- Record the baby's total score next to the cutoff.

TOTAL POINTS ON PAGE 1	
TOTAL POINTS ON PAGE 2	
TOTAL POINTS ON PAGE 3	
Total score	

Cutoff	Total score
50	70

2. ASQ:SE-2 SCORE INTERPRETATION: Review the approximate location of the baby's total score on the scoring graphic. Then, check off the area for the score results below.

no or low risk — 40 — monitor — 50 — refer → 75+ (90%ile)

___ The baby's total score is in the ☐ area. It is below the cutoff. Social-emotional development appears to be on schedule.
___ The baby's total score is in the ▒ area. It is close to the cutoff. Review behaviors of concern and monitor.
✓ The baby's total score is in the ■ area. It is above the cutoff. Further assessment with a professional may be needed.

3. OVERALL RESPONSES AND CONCERNS: Record responses and transfer parent/caregiver comments. YES responses require follow-up.

1–27. Any Concerns marked on scored items? YES (no) Comments:

28. Eating/sleeping concerns? YES (no) Comments:

29. Other worries? YES (no) Comments:

4. FOLLOW-UP REFERRAL CONSIDERATIONS: Mark all as Yes, No, or Unsure (Y, N, U). See pages 98–103 in the *ASQ:SE-2 User's Guide.*

N **Setting/time factors** (e.g., Is the baby's behavior the same at home as at school?)
U **Developmental factors** (e.g., Is the baby's behavior related to a developmental stage or delay?)
U **Health factors** (e.g., Is the baby's behavior related to health or biological factors?)
N **Family/cultural factors** (e.g., Is the baby's behavior acceptable given the baby's cultural or family context? Have there been any stressful events in the baby's life recently?)
N **Parent concerns** (e.g., Did the parent/caregiver express any concerns about the baby's behavior?)

5. FOLLOW-UP ACTION: Check all that apply.

✓ Provide activities and rescreen in 2 months.
___ Share results with primary health care provider.
✓ Provide parent education materials.
___ Provide information about available parenting classes or support groups.
___ Have another caregiver complete ASQ:SE-2. List caregiver here (e.g., grandparent, teacher): ______
___ Administer developmental screening (e.g., ASQ-3).
✓ Refer to early intervention/early childhood special education.
___ Refer for social-emotional, behavioral, or mental health evaluation.
✓ Other: See ASQ-3 (hearing screening)

P201120500

Figure 10.3. Adrian's ASQ:SE-2 Information Summary sheet.

ASQ-3 — 10 Month ASQ-3 Information Summary *9 months 0 days through 10 months 30 days*

Baby's name: Adrian Date ASQ completed: 6/15/15

Baby's ID #: 22784 Date of birth: 7/21/14

Administering program/provider: Johnson Family Medicine Was age adjusted for prematurity when selecting questionnaire? ○ Yes ● No

1. SCORE AND TRANSFER TOTALS TO CHART BELOW: See *ASQ-3 User's Guide* for details, including how to adjust scores if item responses are missing. Score each item (YES = 10, SOMETIMES = 5, NOT YET = 0). Add item scores, and record each area total. In the chart below, transfer the total scores, and fill in the circles corresponding with the total scores.

Area	Cutoff	Total Score
Communication	22.87	25
Gross Motor	30.07	30
Fine Motor	37.97	50
Problem Solving	32.51	45
Personal-Social	27.25	35

2. TRANSFER OVERALL RESPONSES: Bolded uppercase responses require follow-up. See *ASQ-3 User's Guide,* Chapter 6.

1. Uses both hands and both legs equally well? (Yes) **NO** Comments:
2. Feet are flat on the surface most of the time? (Yes) **NO** Comments:
3. Concerns about not making sounds? **YES** (No) Comments:
4. Family history of hearing impairment? **YES** (No) Comments:
5. Concerns about vision? **YES** (No) Comments:
6. Any medical problems? **YES** (No) Comments:
7. Concerns about behavior? **YES** (No) Comments:
8. Other concerns? **YES** (No) Comments:

3. ASQ SCORE INTERPRETATION AND RECOMMENDATION FOR FOLLOW-UP: You must consider total area scores, overall responses, and other considerations, such as opportunities to practice skills, to determine appropriate follow-up.

If the baby's total score is in the ☐ area, it is above the cutoff, and the baby's development appears to be on schedule.
If the baby's total score is in the ▒ area, it is close to the cutoff. Provide learning activities and monitor.
If the baby's total score is in the ■ area, it is below the cutoff. Further assessment with a professional may be needed.

4. FOLLOW-UP ACTION TAKEN: Check all that apply.

✓ Provide activities and rescreen in 2 months.
___ Share results with primary health care provider.
✓ Refer for (circle all that apply) (hearing), vision, and/or behavioral screening.
___ Refer to primary health care provider or other community agency (specify reason): ______
✓ Refer to early intervention/early childhood special education.
___ No further action taken at this time
___ Other (specify): ______

5. OPTIONAL: Transfer item responses (Y = YES, S = SOMETIMES, N = NOT YET, X = response missing).

	1	2	3	4	5	6
Communication						
Gross Motor						
Fine Motor						
Problem Solving						
Personal-Social						

P101100700

Figure 10.4. Adrian's ASQ-3 Information Summary sheet.

Family/Cultural Factors

Adrian's middle class family lives in a large home in a suburban neighborhood outside a major city. Adrian's father works full time and earns a living wage. The family is very close, and everyone was excited about Adrian's arrival. Adrian's mother is a loving and responsive parent who works part time from home.

ASQ:SE-2 Interpretation and Follow-Up

Adrian's pediatrician, Dr. Marks, reviewed Adrian's ASQ:SE-2 and ASQ-3 results and discussed them with Adrian's mother. Jessica indicated on ASQ:SE-2 that Adrian "rarely or never" demonstrates the ability to calm himself down when he becomes upset, nor does he turn his head when someone calls his name. She did not note concerns for any of the items. Jessica also indicated a number of items that "sometimes" occur—it takes more than 30 minutes to feed Adrian, he only asks for things he wants, and he only communicates back and forth with sounds. Adrian received scores in the monitoring zone in three ASQ-3 areas, and he is at the upper age level for the administration window for that tool (Adrian's age at administration was 10 months 25 days, and the 10 month ASQ-3 can be administered up to 10 months 29 days). Dr. Marks discussed the following with Jessica.

- Although Adrian's newborn hearing screening does not indicate any concerns, Dr. Marks advises that Adrian undergo a hearing evaluation. This advice is based on Adrian's ASQ-3 communication area score in the monitoring zone. It is also based on his mother's responses to specific ASQ:SE-2 items, such as Adrian's lack of response to his name and inconsistencies in repeating sounds back to his mother.
- In addition to this referral for hearing testing, Dr. Marks talks to Jessica about making a referral to early intervention for a full developmental evaluation. He feels the result above the cutoff score on ASQ:SE-2, combined with results in the monitoring zone and below the cutoff on ASQ-3, indicate the need for further evaluation. Adrian's mother is reluctant to refer Adrian and questions the need for involving early intervention if the problem is Adrian's hearing. She wants to wait until the results of the hearing evaluation come back. Dr. Marks lets her know that early intervention is a free, confidential service that is intended to support her infant's development. Dr. Marks shares that early intervention specialists can take a closer look across all areas of Adrian's development and provide services and strategies that will support Adrian's development. Dr. Marks stresses the importance of a child's development in the first 5 years and that it is better not to wait. He shares that, in his experience, it is best to make the referral and get the early intervention system process started. Adrian's mother agrees to the referral, and Dr. Marks says she should expect a call soon from the local provider.
- Dr. Marks shares social-emotional development information with Jessica along with activities that would be fun for the whole family to do together with Adrian.
- Dr. Marks wants to see Adrian again soon. His medical practice has developed a process with the local early intervention provider to stay updated on the results of the early intervention evaluation and obtain a copy of Adrian's individualized family service plan if he becomes eligible for services.

MARCUS

Marcus is 3 years 11 months old and lives with his mother Tessa, twin brothers who are 28 months old, and a baby sister who is 9 months old. Marcus's family moved to a low-income apartment complex right before Marcus's baby sister was born. Prior to this, the family had experienced on and off homelessness since Marcus was born.

Marcus's mother has access to a day center's services for families in transition. Family Place's services include washer/dryer facilities, a clothing closet, a food bank, showers, and kitchen facilities. In addition, families with children younger than 5 years of age can participate in an early childhood program that includes drop-in therapeutic child care as well as developmental and social-emotional screening and referral services.

Ellen, the lead teacher at Family Place, worked with Tessa to screen Marcus with both ASQ:SE-2 and ASQ-3 (see Figures 10.5 and 10.6). Marcus's 48 month ASQ:SE-2 total score is 120 points (above the cutoff score for referral, which is 85 points). Tessa reported concerns about Marcus's behaviors, such as destroying and damaging things, not being able to calm down, throwing tantrums, hurting himself, and eating problems.

Setting/Time Factors

Tessa noted on ASQ:SE-2 that Marcus's grandmother has expressed concerns about Marcus's "angry behaviors." In addition, Tessa's boyfriend, who lives with Tessa and her children, has gotten angry at Marcus and has spanked him. Ellen has observed that Marcus is interested in playing with other children and often follows rules at playgroup, which he loves to attend. She is concerned that Marcus gets frustrated sometimes. For example, he once grabbed a toy from another child and also kicked a chair when it was time to clean up and move to a new activity. Marcus only attends playgroup a few times a month, so Ellen has not had the opportunity to spend the 15–20 hours per week minimum time she would need to complete ASQ:SE-2 for him.

Developmental Factors

Marcus was screened with ASQ-3 at 27 months, and at that time, his scores in all areas were well above cutoffs. At this screening, Marcus's ASQ-3 results indicate his development is on schedule in the gross motor, fine motor, and personal-social areas, and in the monitoring zone in the communication and problem-solving areas. Tessa reported in the Overall section on ASQ-3 that other people have a hard time understanding Marcus, although she can understand what he is saying most of the time.

Health Factors

Marcus was born 2 weeks early at 6 pounds, 7 ounces. Tessa did not receive prenatal care while she was pregnant with Marcus, but there were no complications at delivery. Although Tessa reported smoking marijuana when she was pregnant with her twins, she stated that she did not use any drugs or alcohol when she was pregnant with Marcus, who has been generally healthy, aside from some colds. Tessa reported she could not remember the last time she brought Marcus to the doctor.

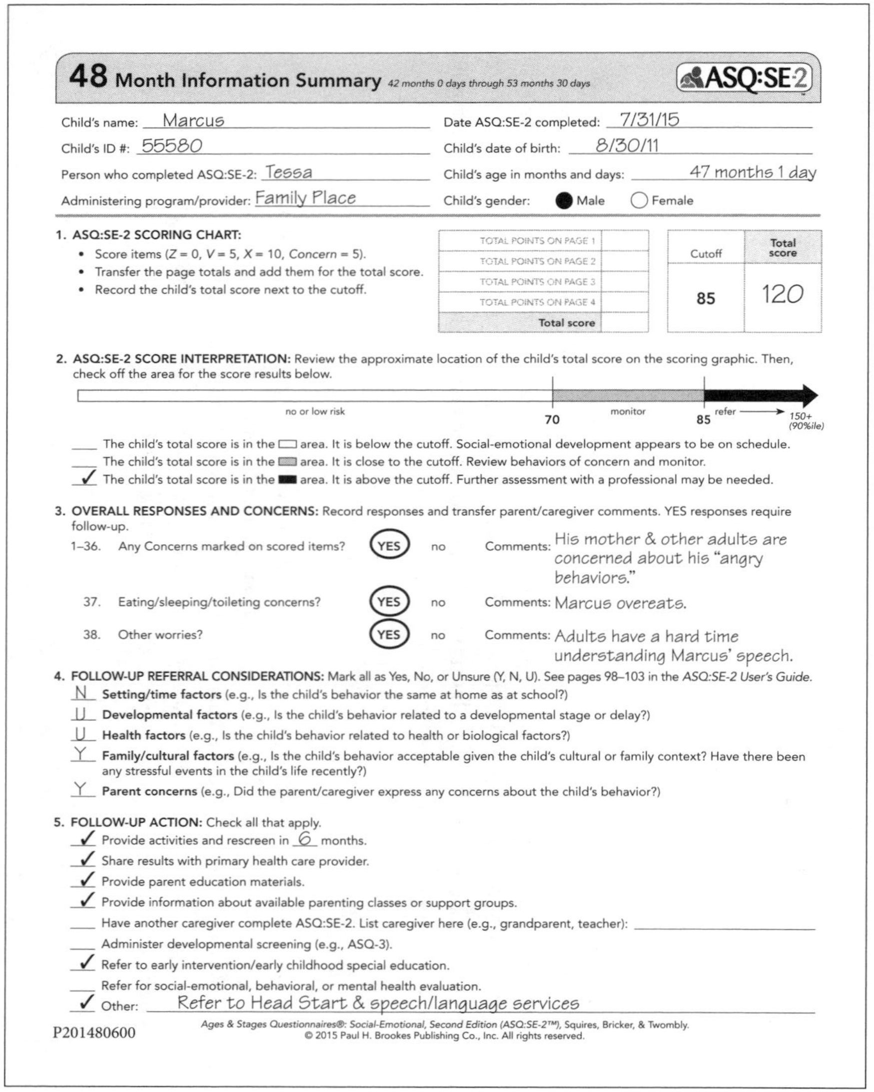

48 Month Information Summary *42 months 0 days through 53 months 30 days* — ASQ:SE-2

Child's name: Marcus — Date ASQ:SE-2 completed: 7/31/15

Child's ID #: 55580 — Child's date of birth: 8/30/11

Person who completed ASQ:SE-2: Tessa — Child's age in months and days: 47 months 1 day

Administering program/provider: Family Place — Child's gender: ● Male ○ Female

1. ASQ:SE-2 SCORING CHART:

- Score items (*Z* = 0, *V* = 5, *X* = 10, *Concern* = 5).
- Transfer the page totals and add them for the total score.
- Record the child's total score next to the cutoff.

TOTAL POINTS ON PAGE 1	
TOTAL POINTS ON PAGE 2	
TOTAL POINTS ON PAGE 3	
TOTAL POINTS ON PAGE 4	
Total score	

Cutoff	Total score
85	120

2. ASQ:SE-2 SCORE INTERPRETATION: Review the approximate location of the child's total score on the scoring graphic. Then, check off the area for the score results below.

no or low risk — 70 — monitor — 85 — refer → 150+ (90%ile)

___ The child's total score is in the ☐ area. It is below the cutoff. Social-emotional development appears to be on schedule.
___ The child's total score is in the ▒ area. It is close to the cutoff. Review behaviors of concern and monitor.
✓ The child's total score is in the ■ area. It is above the cutoff. Further assessment with a professional may be needed.

3. OVERALL RESPONSES AND CONCERNS: Record responses and transfer parent/caregiver comments. YES responses require follow-up.

1–36. Any Concerns marked on scored items? (YES) no — Comments: His mother & other adults are concerned about his "angry behaviors."

37. Eating/sleeping/toileting concerns? (YES) no — Comments: Marcus overeats.

38. Other worries? (YES) no — Comments: Adults have a hard time understanding Marcus' speech.

4. FOLLOW-UP REFERRAL CONSIDERATIONS: Mark all as Yes, No, or Unsure (Y, N, U). See pages 98–103 in the *ASQ:SE-2 User's Guide*.

N **Setting/time factors** (e.g., Is the child's behavior the same at home as at school?)
U **Developmental factors** (e.g., Is the child's behavior related to a developmental stage or delay?)
U **Health factors** (e.g., Is the child's behavior related to health or biological factors?)
Y **Family/cultural factors** (e.g., Is the child's behavior acceptable given the child's cultural or family context? Have there been any stressful events in the child's life recently?)
Y **Parent concerns** (e.g., Did the parent/caregiver express any concerns about the child's behavior?)

5. FOLLOW-UP ACTION: Check all that apply.

✓ Provide activities and rescreen in 6 months.
✓ Share results with primary health care provider.
✓ Provide parent education materials.
✓ Provide information about available parenting classes or support groups.
___ Have another caregiver complete ASQ:SE-2. List caregiver here (e.g., grandparent, teacher): ______
___ Administer developmental screening (e.g., ASQ-3).
✓ Refer to early intervention/early childhood special education.
___ Refer for social-emotional, behavioral, or mental health evaluation.
✓ Other: Refer to Head Start & speech/language services

P201480600

Figure 10.5. Marcus's ASQ:SE-2 Information Summary sheet.

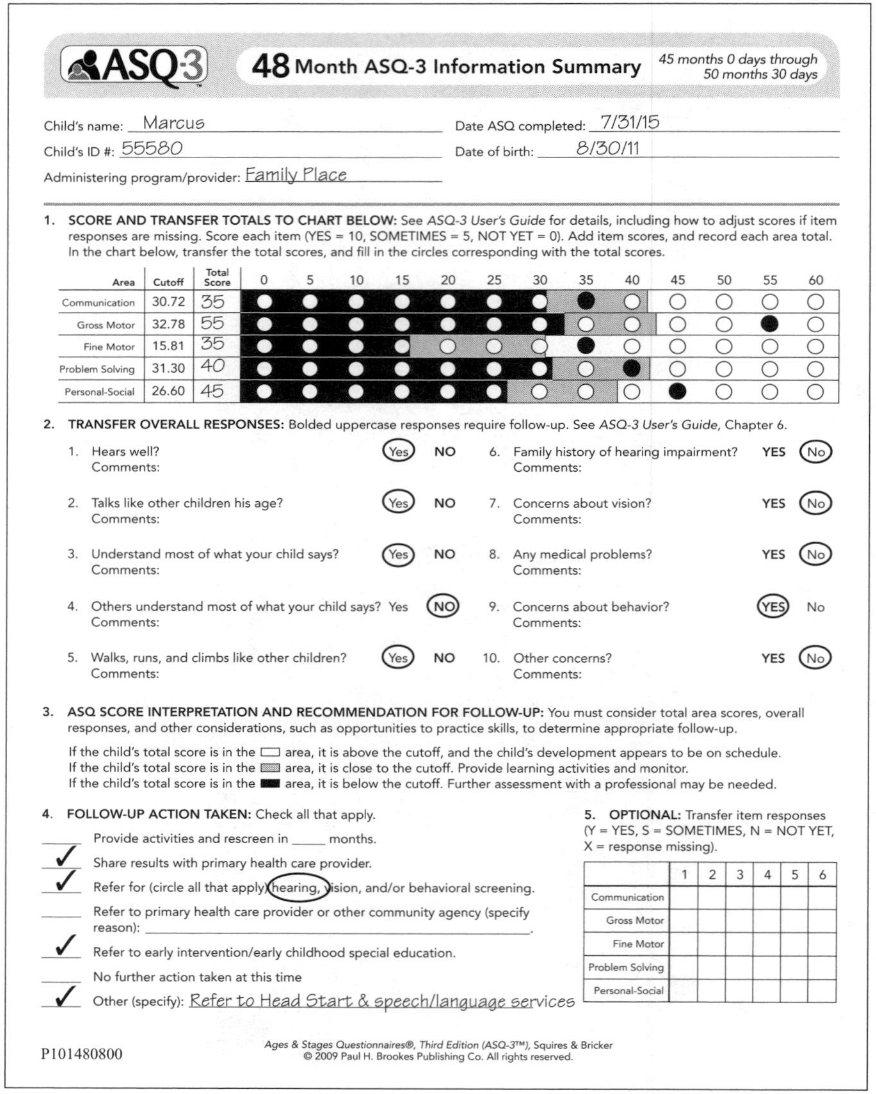

ASQ-3 — 48 Month ASQ-3 Information Summary *45 months 0 days through 50 months 30 days*

Child's name: Marcus — Date ASQ completed: 7/31/15

Child's ID #: 55580 — Date of birth: 8/30/11

Administering program/provider: Family Place

1. SCORE AND TRANSFER TOTALS TO CHART BELOW: See *ASQ-3 User's Guide* for details, including how to adjust scores if item responses are missing. Score each item (YES = 10, SOMETIMES = 5, NOT YET = 0). Add item scores, and record each area total. In the chart below, transfer the total scores, and fill in the circles corresponding with the total scores.

Area	Cutoff	Total Score	0	5	10	15	20	25	30	35	40	45	50	55	60
Communication	30.72	35								●					
Gross Motor	32.78	55												●	
Fine Motor	15.81	35								●					
Problem Solving	31.30	40									●				
Personal-Social	26.60	45										●			

2. TRANSFER OVERALL RESPONSES: Bolded uppercase responses require follow-up. See *ASQ-3 User's Guide*, Chapter 6.

1. Hears well? (Yes) **NO** — Comments:
2. Talks like other children his age? (Yes) **NO** — Comments:
3. Understand most of what your child says? (Yes) **NO** — Comments:
4. Others understand most of what your child says? Yes (**NO**) — Comments:
5. Walks, runs, and climbs like other children? (Yes) **NO** — Comments:
6. Family history of hearing impairment? **YES** (No) — Comments:
7. Concerns about vision? **YES** (No) — Comments:
8. Any medical problems? **YES** (No) — Comments:
9. Concerns about behavior? (**YES**) No — Comments:
10. Other concerns? **YES** (No) — Comments:

3. ASQ SCORE INTERPRETATION AND RECOMMENDATION FOR FOLLOW-UP: You must consider total area scores, overall responses, and other considerations, such as opportunities to practice skills, to determine appropriate follow-up.

If the child's total score is in the ☐ area, it is above the cutoff, and the child's development appears to be on schedule.
If the child's total score is in the ▒ area, it is close to the cutoff. Provide learning activities and monitor.
If the child's total score is in the ■ area, it is below the cutoff. Further assessment with a professional may be needed.

4. FOLLOW-UP ACTION TAKEN: Check all that apply.

___ Provide activities and rescreen in ___ months.
✓ Share results with primary health care provider.
✓ Refer for (circle all that apply) (hearing,) vision, and/or behavioral screening.
___ Refer to primary health care provider or other community agency (specify reason): ______
✓ Refer to early intervention/early childhood special education.
___ No further action taken at this time
✓ Other (specify): Refer to Head Start & speech/language services

5. OPTIONAL: Transfer item responses (Y = YES, S = SOMETIMES, N = NOT YET, X = response missing).

	1	2	3	4	5	6
Communication						
Gross Motor						
Fine Motor						
Problem Solving						
Personal-Social						

P101480800

Figure 10.6. Marcus's ASQ-3 Information Summary sheet.

Family/Cultural Factors

Tessa was 18 years old when she had Marcus, and she is now 23 years old and the primary caregiver to her children. Tessa's mother provides child care because Tessa recently got a part-time job at a department store. This has been a big adjustment for all of the children. Tessa's mother has told Tessa it is too much for her to watch all of the kids. Marcus's father is not involved in his life. The father of Marcus's baby sister lives with them in their apartment.

ASQ:SE-2 Interpretation and Follow-Up

Ellen discussed the results of ASQ:SE-2 with Tessa. Marcus's ASQ:SE-2 total score of 120 points is well above the cutoff of 85. Although Marcus's ASQ-3 does not indicate the need for a referral, Tessa indicated that other people have a hard time understanding Marcus. Ellen also has a difficult time understanding Marcus, as do other volunteers and children in that setting. Based on ASQ:SE-2 results, Tessa's concerns, and her own observations, Ellen discussed the following with Tessa.

- Ellen suggests that Marcus be referred to his primary health care provider. Ellen encourages Tessa to have the doctor check Marcus's hearing because of concerns about Marcus's articulation. Tessa is open to bringing Marcus to the doctor because it has been a long time since his last visit. Ellen works with Tessa to find a primary health care provider so that all of Tessa's children can attend well-child checkups.
- Ellen encourages Tessa to enroll Marcus in the Head Start extended day program. Tessa reported that she and Marcus participated in Early Head Start for a few months when Marcus was an infant, but they stopped participating when she had to move. Tessa feels embarrassed about how she left the program and is reluctant to get back in touch with the program. Ellen reassures her that program staff will understand and says they could call together. In addition to Marcus attending Head Start, Ellen hopes that the twins can be enrolled in Early Head Start extended day program also to relieve Tessa's mother of child care responsibilities.
- Ellen talks to Tessa about Marcus's general development and emphasizes the areas of strength for Marcus (gross motor, fine motor, and personal-social skills). She talks to Tessa about her report that it is hard for other caregivers to understand Marcus. Ellen discusses how this might lead to frustration for Marcus and contribute to some of his problem behaviors. Tessa is reluctant to refer Marcus because her boyfriend "didn't want anyone coming around the house." Ellen lets Tessa know that the local Part B early childhood special education program could send someone to Family Place to meet with her and Marcus. She also shares that Marcus could receive speech-language services when he is placed in a Head Start classroom. Tessa feels it will be okay as long as providers do not have to come to their apartment. She and Ellen make a referral together to early childhood special education to look at Marcus's articulation.
- Ellen discusses the results of Marcus's ASQ:SE-2 and Tessa's concerns about Marcus's behavior. Ellen comments that the combination of Head Start's comprehensive services and speech-language therapy could really decrease Marcus's problem behaviors. Because it may take a few weeks to get enrolled into services, Ellen talks to Tessa about the behaviors that were of concern, and together they come up with some ideas to try with Marcus. Ellen also talks to Tessa about a parenting class through Family Place that is starting in a week, asking if Tessa and her boyfriend would like to attend. Tessa is interested but is not sure her boyfriend will be willing to go. She agrees to ask him and get back to Ellen.

- Ellen shares a social-emotional development guide and ideas about social-emotional activities that would be fun for the whole family to do together.
- Ellen plans to check in with Tessa in a few days to invite her again to the parenting class. She is hopeful that Tessa's boyfriend also will attend because it sounds like he has gotten frustrated with Marcus and uses spanking as a punishment. She wants to stay in close touch and provide emotional support to Tessa and continue to provide information and talk to her about Marcus's behaviors. She also plans on checking with Head Start and the early childhood special education referral to make sure Marcus gets services as soon as possible.

CELIA

Celia is 14 weeks old, with an adjusted age of 10 weeks. She lives with her mother, Donna, her father, James, and her 2-year-old sister in a large city. The family was looking forward to Celia's birth, which did not go as planned. Donna is a strong proponent of natural childbirth and breast feeding and was saddened by complications at birth that lead to a caesarian section as well as by subsequent health and feeding difficulties for her infant.

Donna has been bringing Celia to a high-risk infant follow-up clinic at the hospital for health and feeding difficulties. Celia's health has been improving in the last few weeks, and she has started to gain weight. When Celia was first discharged from the NICU, Donna was told she could receive home visits from a nurse through a program called Baby Steps. This program is designed to help support families while they make the transition from the NICU to home. At first, Donna did not think she needed or wanted to be part of the program. She only wanted to take her infant home and be her mother. When this was brought up again, however, Donna agreed that it might be a good idea to receive some support from someone more familiar with premature infants.

Genine, a home visitor with Baby Steps, had Donna complete ASQ:SE-2 on her first home visit (see Figure 10.7). She wanted to learn more about Donna's concerns about Celia's behavior. Celia's ASQ:SE-2 score of 65 points was well above the cutoff of 35 points.

Setting/Time Factors

Celia has been taken care of almost exclusively by her mother. Celia's father does not feel comfortable feeding her and stated that she's "always crying and fussy." He has also expressed concerns about Celia's health and weight.

Developmental Factors

The doctors and nurses who work with Celia at the high-risk follow-up clinic report that Celia seems to be meeting milestones. Celia has not been assessed with a formal tool.

Health Factors

Celia was delivered by caesarian section, 4 weeks premature and weighing 5 pounds. She developed gastroesophageal reflux (milk would not stay down after feedings) and was not gaining weight as expected. She was often very uncomfortable and fussy. Donna was given strategies for feeding Celia, and recently the doctor prescribed medication for Celia, which Donna has been giving her. Celia is keeping down more milk and seems to be less fussy, except during feedings.

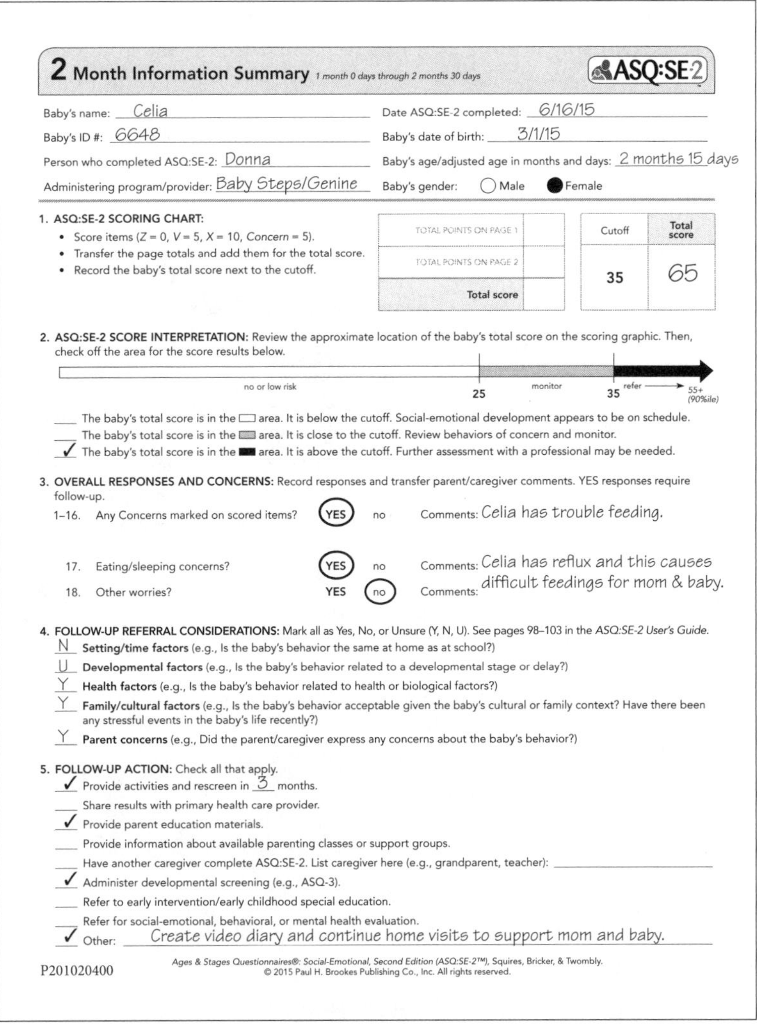

2 Month Information Summary 1 month 0 days through 2 months 30 days — ASQ:SE-2

Baby's name: Celia — Date ASQ:SE-2 completed: 6/16/15

Baby's ID #: 6648 — Baby's date of birth: 3/1/15

Person who completed ASQ:SE-2: Donna — Baby's age/adjusted age in months and days: 2 months 15 days

Administering program/provider: Baby Steps/Genine — Baby's gender: ◯ Male ● Female

1. ASQ:SE-2 SCORING CHART:

- Score items (Z = 0, V = 5, X = 10, Concern = 5).
- Transfer the page totals and add them for the total score.
- Record the baby's total score next to the cutoff.

TOTAL POINTS ON PAGE 1	
TOTAL POINTS ON PAGE 2	
Total score	

Cutoff	Total score
35	65

2. ASQ:SE-2 SCORE INTERPRETATION: Review the approximate location of the baby's total score on the scoring graphic. Then, check off the area for the score results below.

no or low risk — 25 — monitor — 35 — refer — 55+ (90%ile)

___ The baby's total score is in the ☐ area. It is below the cutoff. Social-emotional development appears to be on schedule.
___ The baby's total score is in the ▒ area. It is close to the cutoff. Review behaviors of concern and monitor.
✓ The baby's total score is in the ■ area. It is above the cutoff. Further assessment with a professional may be needed.

3. OVERALL RESPONSES AND CONCERNS: Record responses and transfer parent/caregiver comments. YES responses require follow-up.

1–16. Any Concerns marked on scored items? (YES) no — Comments: Celia has trouble feeding.

17. Eating/sleeping concerns? (YES) no — Comments: Celia has reflux and this causes difficult feedings for mom & baby.

18. Other worries? YES (no) — Comments:

4. FOLLOW-UP REFERRAL CONSIDERATIONS: Mark all as Yes, No, or Unsure (Y, N, U). See pages 98–103 in the *ASQ:SE-2 User's Guide.*

N **Setting/time factors** (e.g., Is the baby's behavior the same at home as at school?)
U **Developmental factors** (e.g., Is the baby's behavior related to a developmental stage or delay?)
Y **Health factors** (e.g., Is the baby's behavior related to health or biological factors?)
Y **Family/cultural factors** (e.g., Is the baby's behavior acceptable given the baby's cultural or family context? Have there been any stressful events in the baby's life recently?)
Y **Parent concerns** (e.g., Did the parent/caregiver express any concerns about the baby's behavior?)

5. FOLLOW-UP ACTION: Check all that apply.

✓ Provide activities and rescreen in 3 months.
___ Share results with primary health care provider.
✓ Provide parent education materials.
___ Provide information about available parenting classes or support groups.
___ Have another caregiver complete ASQ:SE-2. List caregiver here (e.g., grandparent, teacher): ___
✓ Administer developmental screening (e.g., ASQ-3).
___ Refer to early intervention/early childhood special education.
___ Refer for social-emotional, behavioral, or mental health evaluation.
✓ Other: Create video diary and continue home visits to support mom and baby.

P201020400

Ages & Stages Questionnaires®: Social-Emotional, Second Edition (ASQ:SE-2™), Squires, Bricker, & Twombly.

Figure 10.7. Celia's ASQ:SE-2 Information Summary sheet.

Family/Cultural Factors

Celia's mother and father are highly educated professionals who work at a city university. Both of them were working full time when Celia's was born, but Donna has been on leave since Celia's birth. Celia's early arrival was stressful for the entire family. Celia had to be in the NICU for 5 days, and Donna described this as "traumatic." James supported Donna as much as possible but worked a lot during this time. Donna had to begin pumping breast milk to feed Celia from a bottle because of Celia's feeding difficulties. Donna has been troubled by this and says she is sad she cannot breast-feed her baby like she did her older daughter. She is also feeling guilty about the lack of attention she has been giving her 2-year-old, who has been going to child care full time since the birth of her sister and is very clingy and fussy when she comes home.

ASQ:SE-2 Interpretation and Follow-Up

Genine has concerns about Donna's wellness and whether she might be experiencing postpartum depression. Donna seems exhausted and shows little emotion or joy in her interactions with

Celia and tears up at times during their conversation. Genine observed that neither Donna nor Celia seems relaxed during feedings. Donna has to swaddle Celia, and feedings take a very long time. Genine and Donna reviewed the ASQ:SE-2 results together and talked about next steps.

- Genine starts the follow-up conversation about ASQ:SE-2 results by focusing on Celia's strengths. There are behaviors that Genine highlights for Donna and celebrates, including liking to be picked up and held, enjoying watching and listening to people in her environment, and sometimes beginning to calm herself. Genine talks to Donna about how difficult the experience of having a premature baby is for parents and that it is not uncommon for parents to feel overwhelmed by the experience.

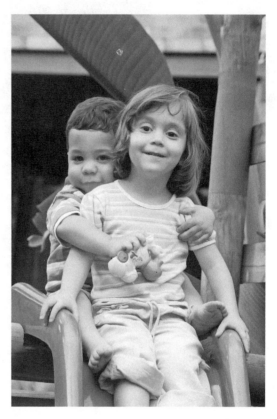

- Donna spends time talking about her concerns about feeding and her sadness about not being able to breast-feed Celia. During this conversation, Donna shares how much time feeding takes—every 2 hours, she needs to give Celia medicine, wait 30 minutes, feed Celia 3 ounces, keep her quiet and upright for 30 minutes, and then start pumping breast milk again for the next round of feeding. She shares that Celia's pediatrician said she could try formula, but she wanted to do the right thing and give Celia breast milk. Genine asks Donna if she would like to explore the possibility of formula further. Donna says she will think about it because she "is so tired all the time and really wants to have some energy to be a good mother to Celia." Genine agrees to bring more information to the next home visit but encourages Donna to discuss this issue with Celia's pediatrician.
- Genine talks to Donna about whether she is willing to let her create a video diary of Celia. Genine explains that at each home visit she will take a short video with her phone and then string the clips together for the family to keep. She suggests watching the videos together to talk about Celia's development. Donna thinks that would be okay. Genine receives training through Baby Steps in how to support parent–child relationships using a video feedback process. In particular, she hopes to focus on Donna and Celia's feeding times and build on Donna and Celia's strengths during this interaction.
- Genine talks to Donna about what support she is receiving and how she can get some breaks for herself. Donna says that Celia's father is very supportive and helps with her older daughter, but Donna is reluctant to let him help with Celia. Genine encourages her to let her husband learn to feed Celia so that Donna can take some breaks.
- Genine is planning on bringing ASQ-3 for Donna to complete in a couple of weeks. For the next visit, she wants to focus on Donna and Celia's feeding relationship and continue to address Donna's concerns.

- Genine shares a social-emotional development guide and activities that would be fun for the family.
- Although Celia's results on ASQ:SE-2 indicate the need for a referral, the home visits Donna is receiving are comprehensive and include services to support Donna, her relationship with her infant, and Celia's social-emotional development. The clinic also is closely monitoring Celia's health. Genine plans to monitor Celia's social-emotional development with the 6 month ASQ:SE-2 when Celia is a few months older.

References

ASQ:SE-2™

Achenbach, T.M., & Rescorla, L.A. (2001). *Manual for the ASEBA School-Age Forms & Profiles.* Burlington: University of Vermont, Research Center for Children, Youth, & Families.

American Academy of Pediatrics. (2001). Developmental surveillance and screening of infants and young children. *Pediatrics, 108*(1), 192–196.

American Academy of Pediatrics. (2006). Identifying infants and young children with developmental disorders in the medical home: An algorithm for developmental surveillance and screening. *Pediatrics, 118*(1), 405–420.

American Academy of Pediatrics. (2014). *Bright Futures guidelines package.* Elk Grove Village, IL: Author.

Bandura, A. (1997). *Self-efficacy: The exercise of control.* New York, NY: Freeman.

Boyd, B.A., Odom, S.L., Humphreys, B.P., & Sam, A.M. (2010). Infants and toddlers with autism spectrum disorder: Early identification and early intervention. *Journal of Early Intervention, 32,* 73–96.

Bricker, D., Macy, M., Squires, J., & Marks, K. (2013). *Developmental screening in your community: An integrated approach for connecting children with services.* Baltimore, MD: Paul H. Brookes Publishing Co.

Bricker, D., Squires, J., Kaminski, R., & Mounts, L. (1988). The validity, reliability and cost of a parent completed questionnaire system to evaluate their at-risk infants. *Journal of Pediatric Psychology, 13*(1), 55–68.

Briggs, R.D., Stettler, E.M., Silver, E.J., Schrag, R.D.A., Nayak, M., Chinitz, S., Racine, A.D. (2012). Social-emotional screening for infants and toddlers in primary care. *Pediatrics, 129*(2), e377–e384.

Bureau of the Census. (2011, March). *Overview of race and Hispanic origin: 2010 census briefs.* Retrieved from http://www.census.gov/2010census/data

Cambell, F., Conti, G., Heckman, J., Moon, S., Pinto, R., Pungello, E., & Pan, Y. (2014). Early childhood investments substantially boost adult health. *Science, 343*(6178), 1478–1485.

Campos, J., Mumme, D., Kermoina, R., & Campos, R. (1994). A functional perspective on the nature of emotion. *Monographs of the Society for Research in Child Development, 59*(2–3), Serial No. 240, 284–303.

Casanueva, C., Wilson, E., Smith, K., Dolan, M., Ringeisen, H., & Horne, B. (2012). *NSCAW II wave 2 report: Child well-being.* Retrieved from www.acf.hhs.gov/programs/opre/resource/nscaw-ii-wave-2-report-child-well-being

Casey, P.H., Whiteside-Mansell, L., Barrett, K., Bradley, R., & Gargus, R. (2006). Impact of prenatal and/or postnatal growth problems in low birth weight preterm infants on school-age outcomes: An 8-year longitudinal evaluation. *Pediatrics, 118*(3), 1078–1086.

Centers for Disease Control and Prevention. (2007). *CDC releases new data on autism spectrum disorders from multiple communities in the United States* [Press release]. Retrieved from http://www.cdc.gov/media/pressrel/2007/r070208.htm?s_cid=mediarel_r070208_x

Centers for Disease Control and Prevention. (2014, May 13). *Injury prevention & control: Division of Violence Prevention.* Retrieved from http://www.cdc.gov/violenceprevention/acestudy

Chen, X., & Rubin, K. (2011). *Social emotional development in cultural context.* New York, NY: Guilford.

Child Abuse Prevention and Treatment Act (CAPTA) of 1974 (PL 93-247), 42 U.S.C. §§ 5101 *et seq.*

Cicchetti, D. (1993). Developmental psychopathology. *Developmental Review, 13,* 471–502.

Cicchetti, D., Ackerman, B.P., & Izard, C.E. (1995). Emotions and emotion regulation in developmental psychopathology [Special issue]. *Development and Psychopathology, 7,* 1–10.

Cicchetti, D., & Toth, S.L. (2000). Child maltreatment in the early years of life. In J.D. Osofsky & H.E. Fitzgerald (Eds.), *WAIMH handbook of infant mental health: Infant mental health in groups at high risk* (Vol. 4, pp. 255–294). New York, NY: Wiley.

Clifford, J., Squires, J., Twombly, E., Bricker, D., & Yockelson, S. (2012). Developmental screening in early childhood: Past trends, current practices, and recommendations for future navigation. In *Gathering information to make informed decisions: Contemporary perspectives about assessment in early intervention and early childhood special education: Young exceptional children monograph 13* (pp. 16–42). Missoula, MT: Division for Early Childhood.

Diamond, A., Barnett, W.S., Thomas, J., & Munro, S. (2007). Preschool program improves cognitive control. *Science, 317* (1387). doi:10.1126/science.1151148

Dieterich, S., Landry, S., Smith, K., Swank, P., & Hebert, H. (2006). Impact of community mentors on maternal behaviors and child outcomes. *Journal of Early Intervention, 28*(2), 111–124.

Dishion, T., French, D., & Patterson, G. (1995). The development and ecology of antisocial behavior. In D. Cicchetti & D. Cohen (Eds.), *Developmental psychology: Risk, disorder, and adaptation* (Vol. 2). New York, NY: Wiley.

Drotar, D., Stancin, T., & Dworkin, P. (2008, February 26). *Part 1: Defining Your Practice's Screening Needs.* Retrieved from http://www.commonwealthfund.org/General/General_show.htm?doc_id=622420

Duncan, G., & Brooks-Gunn, J. (2000). Family, poverty, welfare reform, and child development. *Child Development, 71*(1), 188–196.

Durlak, J., Weissberg, R., Dymnicki, A., Taylor, R., & Schellinger, K. (2011). The impact of enhancing students' social and emotional learning: A meta-analysis of school-based universal interventions. *Child Development, 82*(1), 405–432.

Dunlap, G., Smith, B.J., Fox, L., & Blase, K. (2014). *Road map to statewide implementation of the pyramid model* (Roadmap to Effective Intervention Practices No. 6). Tampa: University of South Florida, Technical Assistance Center on Social Emotional Intervention for Young Children. Retrieved from http://challengingbehavior.fmhi.usf.edu/do/resources/documents/roadmap_6.pdf

Education of the Handicapped Act Amendments of 1983, PL 98-199, 20 U.S.C. §§ 1400 *et seq.,* 97 Stat. 1357.

Education of the Handicapped Act Amendments of 1986, PL 99-457, 20 U.S.C. §§ 1400 *et seq.*

Emde, R., Korfmacher, J., & Kubicek, L. (2000). Toward a theory of early relationship-based interventions. In J. Osofsky & H. Fitzgerald (Eds.), *WAIMH handbook of mental health: Early intervention, evaluation, and assessment* (Vol. 2). New York, NY: Wiley.

Feil, E., Frey, A., Walker, H., Small, J., Seeley, J., Golly, A., & Forness, S. (2014). The efficacy of a home–school intervention for preschoolers with challenging behaviors: A randomized controlled trial of preschool first step to success. *Journal of Early Intervention, 36*(3), 151–170.

Fenson, L., Marchman, V., Thal, D., Dale, P., Reznick, S., & Bates, E. (2007). *MacArthur Communicative Developmental Inventories: User's guide and technical manual.* Baltimore, MD: Paul H. Brookes Publishing Co.

Fernald, L., Kariger, K., Engle, E., & Raikes, A. (2009). *Examining early childhood development in low-income countries: A toolkit for the assessment of children in the first five years of life.* Washington, DC: World Bank.

Frankenburg, W.K., & Bresnick, B. (1998). *Denver Prescreening Developmental Questionnaire II (PDQ II).* Denver, CO: Denver Developmental Materials.

Frankenburg, W., Dodds, J., Archer, P., Bresnick, B., Maschka, P., Edelman, N., & Shapiro, H. (1996). *The Denver II technical manual.* Denver, CO: Denver Developmental Materials.

Freeman, P.C. (2014). Prevalence and relationship between adverse childhood experiences and child behavior among young children. *Infant Mental Health Journal, 35*(6), 544–554.

Garbarino, J., & Ganzel, B. (2000). The human ecology of early risk. In J.P. Shonkoff & S.J. Meisels (Eds.), *Handbook of early childhood intervention* (2nd ed., pp. 76–93). New York, NY: Cambridge University Press.

Giannoni, P., & Kass, P. (2012). Predictors of developmental outcomes of high risk and developmentally delayed infants and children enrolled in a state early childhood intervention program. *Infants & Young Children, 25*(3), 244–264.

Glascoe, F.P. (2001). Can teachers' global ratings identify children with academic problems? *Journal of Developmental and Behavioral Pediatrics, 22*(3), 163–168.

Glascoe, F.P., & Robertshaw, N.S. (2007). *PEDS: Developmental milestones* (assessment version). Nolensville, TN: Ellsworth & Vandermeer Press.

Guralnick, M.J. (1997). Second-generation research in the field of early intervention. In M.J. Guralnick (Ed.), *The effectiveness of early intervention* (pp. 3–22). Baltimore, MD: Paul H. Brookes Publishing Co.

Guralnick, M.J. (2011). Why early intervention works: A systems perspective. *Infants & Young Children, 24,* 6–28.

Guralnick, M.J. (2013). Developmental science and preventive interventions for children at environmental risk. *Infants and Young Children, 26,* 270–285.

Hack, M., Taylor, H.G., Drotar, D., Schluchter, M., Cartar, L., Wilson-Costello, D., . . . Morrow, M. (2005). Poor predictive validity of the Bayley scales of infant development for cognitive function of extremely low birth weight children at school age. *Pediatrics, 116*(2), 333–341.

Halfon, N., Regalado, M., Sareen, H., Inkelas, M., Peck Reuland, C., Glascoe F., & Olson, L. (2004). Assessing development in the pediatric office. *Pediatrics, 113*(6), 1926–1933.

Heo, K., & Squires, J. (2012). Adaptation of a parent-completed social emotional screening instrument for young children: Ages and Stages Questionnaires-Social Emotional. *Early Human Development, 88*(3), 151–158.

Heo, G., Squires, J., Yovanoff, P., & Lee, H. (2006). Psychometric study on a parent-completed screening instrument for Korean infants and preschoolers. *Journal of Korean Special Education, 8*(3), 261.

Individuals with Disabilities Education Act (IDEA) of 1990, PL 101-476, 20 U.S.C. §§ 1400 *et seq.*

Individuals with Disabilities Education Act Amendments (IDEA) of 1997, PL 105-17, 20 U.S.C. §§ 1400 *et seq.*

Individuals with Disabilities Education Improvement Act (IDEA) of 2004, PL 108-446, 20 U.S.C. §§ 1400 *et seq.*

Jellinek, M., Murphy, J., Little, M., Pagano, M., Comer, D., & Kelleher, K. (1999). Use of pediatric symptom checklist to screen for psychosocial problems in pediatric primary care: A national feasibility study. *Archives of Pediatrics and Adolescent Medicine, 153*(3), 254–260.

Johnson, C.P., & Myers, S.M. (2007). American Academy of Pediatrics, Council on Children with Disabilities: Identification and evaluation of children with autism spectrum disorders. *Pediatrics, 120*(5), 1183–1215.

Johnson, C., Myers, S., & Council on Children with Disabilities. (2005). Identification and evaluation of children with autism spectrum disorders. *Pediatrics, 120*(5), 1183–1215.

Johnson, C., Myers, S., & Council on Children with Disabilities. (2007). Identification and evaluation of children with autism spectrum disorders. AAP Clinical Report. *Pediatrics, 120*(5), 1183–1215.

Johnson-Staub, C. (2014, October). *First steps for early success: State strategies to support developmental screening in early childhood settings.* Retrieved from www.clasp.org/resources-and-publications/publication-1/State-Strategies-to-Support-Developmental-Screening-in-Early-Childhood-Settings.pdf

Jones, S., & Bouffard, S. (2012). Social and emotional learning in schools: From programs to strategies. *Social Policy Report, 26*(4), 1–32.

Keeping Children and Families Safe Act of 2003, PL 108-36, 21 U.S.C. §§ 802 *et seq.*

Kim, Y.S., Leventhal, B.L., Koh, Y.J., Fombonne, E., Laska, E., Lim, E.C., . . . Richard, R. (2011). Prevalence of autism spectrum disorders in a total population sample. *American Journal of Psychiatry, 168*(9), 904–912.

Knitzer, J. (2000). Early childhood mental health services: A policy and systems development perspective. In J.P. Shonkoff & S.J. Meisels (Eds.), *Handbook of early childhood intervention* (2nd ed., pp. 416–438). New York, NY: Cambridge University Press.

Knitzer, J., & Perry, D. (2009). Poverty and infant and toddler development facing the complex challenges. In C. Zeanah (Ed.), *Handbook of infant mental health* (pp. 135–152). New York, NY: Guilford Press.

Knitzer, J., Theberge, S., & Johnson, K. (2008, January). *Reducing maternal depression and its impact on young children: Toward a responsive early childhood policy framework.* New York, NY: National Center for Children in Poverty. Retrieved from http://www.nccp.org/publications/pub_791.html

Knobloch, H., Stevens, F., Malone, A., Ellison, P., & Risemburg, H. (1979). The validity of parental reporting of infant development. *Pediatrics, 63*(6), 872–878.

Landy, S. (2009). *Pathways to competence: Encouraging healthy social and emotional development in young children* (2nd ed.). Baltimore, MD: Paul H. Brookes Publishing Co.

Lyman, D., Njoroge, W., & Willis, D. (2007). Early childhood psychosocial screening in culturally diverse populations: A survey of clinical experience with the Ages & Stages Questionnaires: Social-Emotional. *Zero to Three, 27*(5), 46–54.

Macy, M. (2012). The evidence behind developmental screening instruments. *Infants and Young Children: An Interdisciplinary Journal of Special Care Practices, 25*(1), 19–61.

Mardell, C., & Goldenberg, D.S. (2011). *Developmental Indicators for the Assessment of Learning–Fourth (DIAL-4).* New York, NY: Pearson.

Marks, K.P., & Glascoe, F. (2010). Helping parents understand developmental-behavioral screening. *Contemporary Pediatrics, 27,* 54–61.

Marks, K., & LaRosa, A. (2012). Understanding developmental-behavioral screening measures. *Pediatrics in Review, 33*(10), 448–458.

Martoccio, T., Brophy-Herb, H., & Onaga, E. (2014). Road to readiness: Pathways from low-income children's early interactions to school readiness skills. *Infants & Young Children, 27*(3), 193–206.

McKinney-Vento Homeless Assistance Act of 1987, PL 100-77, 42 U.S.C. §§ 11301 *et seq.*

Meisels, S., Marsden, D., Wiske, M., & Henderson, L. (2008). *The Early Screening Inventory–Revised, 2008 Edition.* Ann Arbor, MI: Rebus.

Merrell, K., & Holland, M. (1997). Social-emotional behavior of preschool-age children with and without developmental delays. *Research in Developmental Disabilities, 18*(6), 393–405.

Mitchell, A.W. (2005). *Stair steps to quality: A guide for states and communities developing quality rating systems for early care and education.* Retrieved from United Way web site: http://www.earlychildhoodfinance.org/downloads/2005/MitchStairSteps_2005.pdf

National Scientific Council on the Developing Child. (2007). *A science-based framework for early childhood policy: Using evidence to improve outcomes in learning, behavior, and health for vulnerable children.* Retrieved from http://www.developingchild.harvard.edu

National Scientific Council on the Developing Child & National Forum on Early Childhood Policy and Programs. (2010). *The foundations of lifelong health are built in early childhood.* Retrieved from http://developingchild.harvard.edu/resources/reports_and_working_papers/foundations-of-lifelong-health/

O'Neill, L. (2007). Embodied hermeneutics: Gadamer meets Woolf in a room of one's own. *Educational Theory, 57*(3), 325–337.

Osofsky, J.D., & Thompson, M.D. (2000). Adaptive and maladaptive parenting: Perspectives on risk and protective factors. In J.P. Shonkoff & S.J. Meisels (Eds.), *Handbook of early childhood intervention* (2nd ed., pp. 55–73). New York, NY: Cambridge University Press.

Ostrov, J., & Keating, C. (2004). Gender differences in preschool aggression during freeplay and structured interactions: An observational study. *Social Development, 1312,* 255–276.

Owens, R. (2010). *Language development: An introduction.* Boston, MA: Pearson.

Patterson, G.R., Reid, J.B., & Dishion, T.J. (1992). *Antisocial boys.* Eugene, OR: Castalia.

Pizur-Barnekow, K., Erickson, S., Johnston, M., Bass, T., Lucinski, L., & Bleuel, D. (2010). Early identification of developmental delays through surveillance, screening, and diagnostic evaluation. *Infants and Young Children, 23*(4), 323–330.

Radecki, L., Sand-Loud, N., O'Connor, K.G., Sharp, S., & Olson, L.M. (2011). Trends in the use of standardized tools for developmental screening in early childhood: 2002-2009. *Pediatrics, 128,* 14–19.

Raver, C., & Zigler, E. (1997). Social competence: An untapped dimension in evaluating Head Start's success. *Early Childhood Research Quarterly, 12,* 363–385.

Reid, J. (1993). Prevention of conduct disorder before and after school entry: Relating intervention to developmental findings. *Development and Psychology, 5,* 243–262.

Sameroff, A.J. (Ed.). (2009). *The transactional model of development: How children and contexts shape each other.* Washington, DC: American Psychological Association.

Sameroff, A.J. (2010). A unified theory of development: A dialectic integration of nature and nurture. *Child Development, 81*(1), 6–22.

Sameroff, A.J., & Chandler, M.J. (1975). Reproductive risk and the continuum of caretaking casualty. In F. Horowitz, M. Hetherington, S. Scarr-Salapatek, & G. Siegel (Eds.), *Review of child development research* (pp. 187–244). Chicago, IL: University of Chicago Press.

Sameroff, A.J., & Fiese, B.H. (2000). Transactional regulation: The developmental ecology of early intervention. In J.P. Shonkoff & S.J. Meisels (Eds.), *Handbook of early childhood intervention* (2nd ed., pp. 135–139). New York, NY: Cambridge University Press.

Sameroff, A., Seifer, R., & McDonough, S. (2004). Contextual contributors to the assessment of infant mental health. In R. DelCarmen-Wiggins & A. Carter (Eds.), *Handbook of infant, toddler, and preschool mental health assessment* (pp. 61–78). New York, NY: Oxford University Press.

Sandall, S., Hemmeter, M.L., Smith, B., & McLean, M. (2005). *DEC recommended practices: A comprehensive guide for practical application in early intervention/early childhood special education.* Longmont, CO: Sopris West Educational Services.

Serenius, F., Kallen, K., Blennow, M., Ewald, U., Fellman, V., Holmstrom, G., . . . Stromberg, B. (2013). Neurodevelopmental outcome in extremely preterm infants at 2.5 years after active perinatal care in Sweden. *Journal of the American Medical Association, 309*(17), 1810–1820.

Sheldrick, R.C., & Perrin, E.C. (2013). Evidence-based milestones for surveillance of cognitive, language and motor development. *Academic Pediatrics, 13*(6), 577–586. doi:10.1016/j.acap.2013.07.001.

Simard, M.N., Luu, T.M., & Gosselin, J. (2012). Concurrent validity of Ages & Stages Questionnaires in preterm infants. *Pediatrics, 130*(1), 108–114.

Sontag-Padilla, L., Schultz, D., Reynolds, K., Lovejoy, S., & Firth, R. (2013). *Maternal depression: Implications for systems serving mother and child.* Retrieved from http://www.rand.org/content/dam/rand/pubs/research_reports/RR400/RR404/RAND_RR404.pdf

Squires, J. (2012). Assessing young children's social emotional development. In S. Summers & R. Chazen-Cohen (Eds.), *Understanding early childhood mental health: A practical guide for professionals.* Baltimore, MD: Paul H. Brookes Publishing Co.

Squires, J., & Bricker, D. (2007). *An activity-based approach to developing young children's social emotional competence.* Baltimore, MD: Paul H. Brookes Publishing Co.

Squires, J., Bricker, D., & Clifford, J. (2010). Developmental screening measures: Stretching the use of the ASQ for other assessment purposes. *Infants & Young Children, 23*(1), 14–22.

Squires, J., Bricker, D., Heo, K., & Twombly, E. (2001). Identification of social-emotional problems in young children using a parent-complete screening measure. *Early Childhood Research Quarterly, 16,* 405–419.

Squires, J., Bricker, D., & Potter, L. (1995). *Ages & Stages Questionnaires® user's guide.* Baltimore, MD: Paul H. Brookes Publishing Co.

Squires, J., Bricker, D., & Potter, L. (1997). Revision of a parent-completed developmental screening tool: Ages & Stages Questionnaires. *Journal of Pediatric Psychology, 22*(3), 313–328.

Squires, J., Bricker, D., & Twombly, E. (2002). *Ages & Stages Questionnaires®: Social-Emotional (ASQ:SE): A parent-completed child-monitoring system for social-emotional behaviors.* Baltimore, MD: Paul H. Brookes Publishing Co.

Squires, J., Bricker, D., & Twombly, E. (2004). Parent-completed screening for social emotional problems in young children: Effects of risk/disability status and gender on performance. *Infant Mental Health, 25*(1), 62–73.

Squires, J., Bricker, D., Waddell, M., Funk, K., Clifford, J., & Hoselton, R. (2014). *Social-Emotional Assessment/Evaluation Measure (SEAM™), Research Edition.* Baltimore, MD: Paul H. Brookes Publishing Co.

Squires, J., Nickel, R., & Bricker, D. (1990). Use of parent-completed developmental questionnaires for child-find and screening. *Infants & Young Children, 3*(2), 46-57.

Squires, J., Nickel, R.E., & Eisert, D. (1996). Early detection of developmental problems: Strategies for monitoring young children in the practice setting. *Journal of Developmental and Behavioral Pediatrics, 17*(6), 410–427.

Summers, S., & Chazen-Cohen, R. (2012). (Eds.). *Understanding early childhood mental health: A practical guide for professionals.* Baltimore, MD: Paul H. Brookes Publishing Co.

Thomas, S.A., Cotton, W., Pan, X., & Ratliff-Schaub, K. (2012). Comparison of systematic developmental surveillance with standardized developmental screening in primary care. *Clinical Pediatrics, 51*(2), 154–159.

U.S. Department of Health and Human Services. (2010). *The Abuse and Prevention Act of 2010.* Retrieved from http://www.acf.hhs.gov/programs/cb/resource/capta2010

Wade, M., Moore, C., Astington, J.W., Frampton, K., & Jenkins, J.M. (2015). Cumulative contextual risk, maternal responsivity, and social cognition at 18 months. *Development and Psychopathology, 27*(1), 189–203. doi: 10.1017/S0954579414000674

Walker, H., & Shinn, M. (2010). Systematic, evidence-based approaches for promoting positive student outcomes using a multi-tier framework: Moving from efficacy to effectiveness. In M. Shinn & H. Walker (Eds.), *Interventions for achievement and behavior problems in a three-tier model including RTI* (pp. 1–26). Bethesda, MD: National Association of School Psychologists.

Wallace, K., & Rogers, S. (2010). Intervening in infancy: Implications for autism spectrum disorders. *Journal of Child Psychology and Psychiatry, 51*(12), 1300–1320.

Waters, E., & Sroufe, L.A. (1983). Social competence as a developmental construct. *Developmental Review, 3,* 79–87.

Weissbourd, R., Bouffard, S.M., & Jones, S.M. (2013). School climate, moral and social development. In T. Dary & T. Pickeral (Eds.), *School climate: Practices for implementation and sustainability. A school climate.* (Practice Brief, Number 1). New York, NY: National School Climate Center.

Yoshikawa, H., Weiland, C., Brooks-Gunn, J., Burchinal, M., Espinosa, L., . . . Zaslow, M.J. (2013). *Investing in our future: The evidence base on preschool education.* New York, NY: Society for Research in Child Development & Foundation for Child Development.

Zeanah, C. (Ed.). (2009). *Handbook of infant mental health* (3rd ed.). New York, NY: Guilford Press.

Zeanah, C., & Zeanah, P. (2009). The scope of infant mental health. In C. Zeanah (Ed.), *Handbook of infant mental health* (pp. 5–21). New York, NY: Guilford Press.

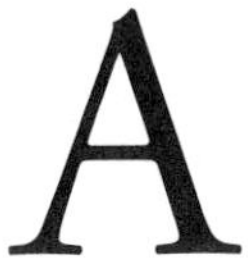

Suggested Readings

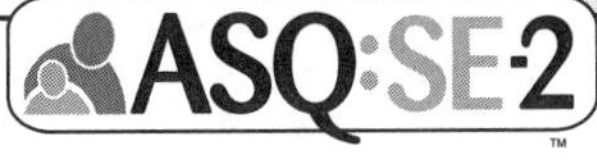

American Academy of Pediatrics. (2006). Identifying infants and young children with developmental disorders in the medical home: An algorithm for developmental surveillance and screening. *Pediatrics, 118*(1), 405–420.

Baggett, K., Warlen, L., Hamilton, J., Roberts, J., & Staker, M. (2007). Screening infant mental health indicators: An Early Head Start initiative. *Infants and Young Children, 20*(4), 300–310.

Beeber, L.S., Holditch-Davis, D., Perreira, K., Schwartz, T., Lewis, V., Blanchard, H., . . . Goldman, B. (2010). Short-term, in-home intervention reduces depressive symptoms in Early Head Start Latina mothers of infants and toddlers. *Research in Nursing and Health, 33*(1), 60–76.

Bennett, F., Nickel, R., Squires, J., & Woodward, B. (1997). Developmental screening/surveillance. In H. Wallace, R. Biehl, R. MacQueen, & J. Blackman (Eds.), *Children with disabilities and chronic illnesses* (pp. 236–247). St. Louis, MO: Mosby.

Bricker, D., Shoen Davis, M., & Squires, J. (2004). Mental health screening in young children. *Infants and Young Children, 17*(2), 129–144.

Briggs, R., Stettler, E., Silver, E., Schrag, M., Chinitz, S., & Racine, A. (2012). Social-emotional screening for infants and toddlers in primary care. *Pediatrics, 129*(2), e377–e384.

Brown, M., Copeland, K., Sucharew, H., & Kahn, R. (2012). Social-emotional problems in preschool-aged children: Opportunities for prevention and early intervention. *Archives of Pediatric and Adolescent Medicine, 166*(10), 926–932.

Chan, B., & Taylor, N. (1998). The follow along program cost analysis in southwest Minnesota. *Infants and Young Children, 10*(4), 71–79.

Committee on Children with Disabilities. (2006, July). Developmental surveillance and screening of infants and young children. *Pediatrics, 108*(1), 192–196.

D'Aprano, A., Silburn, S., Johnston, V., Roboinson, G., Oberklaid, F., & Squires, J. (2014). Adaptation of the Ages & Stages Questionnaires for remote aboriginal Australia. *Qualitative Health Research,* doi: 10.177/10497323/456289

Dobrez, D., Sasso, A.L., Holl, J., Shalowitz, M., Leon, S., & Budetti, P. (2001). Estimating the cost of developmental and behavioral screening of preschool children in general pediatric practice. *Pediatrics, 108*(4), 913–922.

Drotar, D., Stancin, T., & Dworkin, P. (2008). *Pediatric developmental screening: Understanding and selecting screening instruments.* New York, NY: The Commonwealth Fund.

Earls, M., & Hay, S. (2006). Setting the stage for success: Implementation of developmental and behavioral screening and surveillance in primary care practice—The North Carolina Assuring Better Child Health and Development (ABCD) project. *Pediatrics, 118*(1), 183–188.

Feeney-Kettler, K., Kratochwill, T., Kaiser, A., Hemmeter, M., & Kettler, R. (2015). Screening young children's risk for mental health problems: A review of four measures. *Assessment for Effective Intervention, 35*(4), 218–230.

Filipek, P., Accardo, P., Ashwal, S., Baranek, G.T., Cook, E.H., Jr., Dawson, G., . . . Volkmar, F.R. (2000). Practice parameter: Screening and diagnosis of autism. A report of the quality standards subcommittee of American Academy of Neurology and the Child Neurology Society. *Neurology, 55*(4), 468–479.

Frisk, V., Lee, E., Green, P., & Whyte, H. (2004). Deciding on a screening test for medically-at-risk children: An evidence-based approach. *IMPrint: Newsletter of the Infant Mental Health Promotion Project, 40,* 16.

Gilkerson, L., & Kopel, C. (2005). Relationship-based systems change: Illinois model for promoting social-emotional development in Part C early intervention. *Infants and Young Children, 18*(4), 349–365.

Glascoe, F.P. (2000). Evidence-based approach to developmental and behavioral surveillance using parents' concerns. *Child: Care, Health and Development, 26*(2), 137–149.

Handal, A., Lozoff, B., Breilh, J., & Harlow, S. (2007). Effects of community residence on neurobehavioral development in infants and young children in a flower-growing region of Ecuador. *Environmental Health Perspectives, 115*(1), 128–133.

Heo, K., & Squires, J. (2012). Adaptation of a parent-completed social emotional screening instrument for young children: Ages & Stages Questionnaires: Social-Emotional. *Early Human Development, 88*(3), 151–158.

Hillen, T., Gafson, L., Drage, L., & Conlan, L. (2012). Assessing the prevalence of mental health disorders and mental health needs among preschool children in care in England. *Infant Mental Health Journal,* doi: 10.1002/imhj.21327

Hix-Small, H., Marks, K., Squires, J., & Nickel, R. (2007). Implementing developmental screening at 12 and 24 months in a primary care pediatric office. *Pediatrics, 120*(2), 1–9.

James Bell Associates. (2009). *Early Head Start/Child Welfare Services Initiative: Final synthesis report: Volume II. Compendium of grantee-specific findings.* Washington, DC: Office on Child Abuse and Neglect, Children's Bureau.

Jee, S., Conn, M., Szilagyi, P., Blumkin, A., Baldwin, C., & Szilagyi, M. (2010). Identification of social-emotional problems among young children in foster care. *Journal of Child Psychology and Psychiatry, 51*(12), 1351–1358.

Jeon, L., Buettner, C., & Hur, E. (2014). Family and neighborhood disadvantage, home environment, and children's school readiness. *Journal of Family Psychology, 28*(5), 718–727.

Klamer, A., Lando, A., Pinborg, A., & Greisen, G. (2005, May). Ages & Stages Questionnaire used to measure cognitive deficit in children born extremely preterm. *Acta Paediatrica, 94*(9), 1327–1329.

Kucuker, S., Kupci, E., & Uslu, R. (2011). Evaluation of the Turkish version of the Ages & Stages Questionnaires: Social-Emotional in identifying children with social-emotional problems. *Infants and Young Children,* 24(2), 207–220.

Lando, A., Klamer, A., Jonsbo, J., Weiss, J., & Greisen, G. (2005, May). Developmental delay at 12 months in children born extremely preterm. *Acta Paediatrica, 94*(11), 1604–1607.

Lipkin, P. (2006). Moving forward in development screening. *Pediatric News, 40*(9), 34.

Lyman, D.R., Njoroge, W., & Willis, D. (2007). Early childhood psychosocial screening in culturally diverse populations: Survey of clinical experience with Ages & Stages Questionnaires: Social-Emotional. *Zero to Three, 27*(5), 46–54.

Marks, K., & LaRosa, A. (2012). Understanding developmental-behavioral screening measures. *Pediatrics in Review, 33*(10), 448–458.

Maternal and Child Health Bureau. (n.d.). *Developmental and behavioral pediatrics* (2nd ed.). Retrieved from http://mchb.hrsa.gov/training/projects.asp?program=6

Meisels, S., & Shonkoff, J. (Eds.). (2000). *Handbook of early childhood intervention* (2nd ed.). New York, NY: Cambridge University Press.

Nicol, P. (2006). Using the Ages & Stages Questionnaires to teach medical students developmental assessment: A descriptive analysis. *BMC Medical Education, 6,* 29. Retrieved from http://biomedcentral.com/1472-6920/6/29

Pinto-Martin, J., Dunkle, M., Earls, M., Fliedner, D., & Landes, C. (2004). Developmental stages of developmental screening: Steps to implementation of a successful program. *American Journal of Public Health, 95*(11), 6–10.

Printz, P.H., Borg, A., & Demarree, M.A. (2003). *A look at social, emotional, and behavioral screening tools for Head Start and Early Head Start.* Newton, MA: Education Development Center, Center for Children & Families.

Radecki, L., Sand-Loud, N., O'Connor, K.G., Sharp, S., & Olson, L.M. (2011). Trends in the use of standardized tools for developmental screening in early childhood: 2002–2009. *Pediatrics, 128,* 14–19.

Rais-Bahrami, K., & Short, B.L. (2013). Premature and small-for-dates infants. In M.L. Batshaw, N.J. Roizen, & G.R. Lotrecchiano (Eds.), *Children with disabilities* (7th ed., pp. 87–104). Baltimore, MD: Paul H. Brookes Publishing Co.

Ringwalt, S. (2008). *Developmental screening and assessment instruments with an emphasis on social and emotional development for young children ages birth through five.* Retrieved from http://www.nectac.org/-pdfs/pubs/screening.pdf

Roan, B., Valleley, R., & Allen, K. (2012). Impact of Ages & Stages Questionnaires scores on pediatrician referral patterns. *Infants and Young Children, 25*(2), 149–157.

Salomonsson, M., Sorjonen, K., & Salomonsson, B. (2015). A long-term follow-up of a randomized controlled trial of mother-infant psychoanalytic treatment: Outcomes on the child. *Infant Mental Health Journal,* 36(1), 12–29.

Squires, J. (2000, June/August). Early detection of development delays: Parents as first-level screeners. *Journal of Intellectual Disability Research, 44*(3–4), 471.

Squires, J., Bricker, D., Heo, K., & Twombly, E. (2001). Identification of social-emotional problems in young children using a parent-complete screening measure. *Early Childhood Research Quarterly, 16,* 405–419.

Squires, J., Bricker, D., & Twombly, E. (2004). Parent-completed screening for social emotional problems in young children: Effects of risk/disability status and gender on performance. *Infant Mental Health, 25*(1), 62–73.

Squires, J., Carter, A., & Kaplan, P. (2003). Developmental monitoring of children conceived by intracytoplasmic sperm injection and in vitro fertilization. *Fertility and Sterility, 79*(2), 453–454.

Squires, J., Katzev, A., & Jenkins, F. (2002, June). Early screening for developmental delays: Use of parent completed questionnaires in Oregon's Healthy Start program. *Early Child Development and Care, 172*(3), 275–282.

Squires, J., Nickel, R., & Eisert, E. (1996). Early detection of developmental problems: Strategies for monitoring young children in the practice setting. *Journal of Developmental and Behavioral Pediatrics, 17*(6), 410–427.

Squires, J., Potter, L., Bricker, D., & Lamorey, S. (1998). Parent-completed developmental questionnaires: Effectiveness with low and middle income parents. *Early Childhood Research Quarterly, 13*(2), 347–356.

Squires, J., Twombly, E., Bricker, D., & Potter, L. (2009). *ASQ-3™ user's guide.* Baltimore, MD: Paul H. Brookes Publishing Co. (*Note:* Includes technical report with research data on ASQ-3.)

U.S. Department of Health and Human Services (2014, March). *Birth to 5: Watch me thrive! A compendium of screening measures for young children.* Washington, DC: Author.

Vacca, J.J. (2005). Review of the Ages & Stages Questionnaires: Social-Emotional. In B.S. Plake & J.C. Impara (Eds.), *The sixteenth mental measurements yearbook.* Lincoln, NE: Buros Institute of Mental Measurements.

Werner, E.E., & Smith, R.S. (2004). Journeys from childhood to midlife: Risk, resilience, and recovery. *Pediatrics, 114*(2), 492.

Worcester, S. (2007, September). Ages & Stages' screen improves referral rates. *Pediatric News, 41*(9), 24–25

Wright, C., & Holm-Hansen, C. (2010). Mental health concerns in young children: Developing a comprehensive early identification and referral system. *Zero to Three, 31*(1), 48–53.

Yovanoff, P., & Squires, J. (2006). Determining cut-off scores on a developmental screening measure: Comparison of receiver operating characteristics and item response theory approaches. *Journal of Early Intervention, 29*(1), 48–62.

B

Glossary

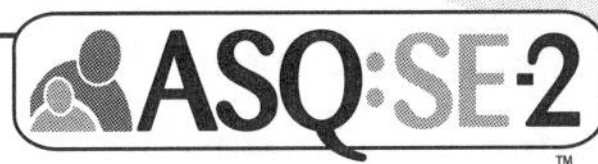

above the cutoff An ASQ:SE-2 total score that is above the statistically derived referral cutoff point. A score above the cutoff indicates a need for further evaluation and/or additional follow-up actions.

adaptive functioning A child's success or ability to cope with physiological needs (e.g., sleeping, eating, elimination, safety).

adjusted age An age correction for weeks of prematurity when the actual date of birth is 3 or more weeks earlier than the expected birth date. To calculate a corrected age, the weeks of prematurity are subtracted from the child's chronological age.

chronological age – number of weeks premature = corrected age

For example, a child who was born 8 weeks prematurely and whose chronological age is 14 weeks will be given a corrected age of 6 weeks. The authors recommend that the corrected age be used until the child reaches 24 months of age.

adjusted total score An average item score obtained by adding scores on ASQ:SE-2 items for a total score and then dividing by the number of questions answered. Average score is used in calculating the child's final total score when parents leave up to three items unanswered:

total score + (average score × number of questions not answered) = final total score

affect A child's ability or willingness to demonstrate his or her own feelings and empathy for others.

ASQ Abbreviation for *Ages & Stages Questionnaires®, Third Edition (ASQ-3™)*, which is a developmental screening tool that examines milestones in five domains. ASQ:SE-2™ refers specifically to *Ages & Stages Questionnaires®: Social-Emotional, Second Edition.*

ASQ:SE-2 Abbreviation for the *Ages & Stages Questionnaires®: Social-Emotional, Second Edition,* which is a screening tool that examines social-emotional behaviors in young children.

autonomy A child's ability or willingness to self-initiate or respond without guidance (i.e., moving to independence).

below the cutoff An ASQ:SE-2 score that is below the statistically derived referral cutoff point and is below the monitoring zone. If there are no concerns about the child's behavior, then a total score in this area indicates that the child's social-emotional development appears to be on schedule at the time of administration.

CAPTA *See* Child Abuse Prevention and Treatment Act.

CBA *See* curriculum-based assessment.

CDOB *See* corrected date of birth.

Child Abuse Prevention and Treatment Act (CAPTA) of 1974 (PL 93-247) A law providing federal funding to states in support of prevention, assessment, investigation, prosecution, and treatment of child abuse. It specifically directs states to provide developmental screening to all children placed in foster care.

Child Find A component of the Individuals with Disabilities Education Improvement Act (IDEA) of 2004 (PL 108-446) that requires states to identify, locate, and evaluate all children with disabilities from birth to age 21, who are in need of early intervention or special education services.

compliance A child's ability or willingness to conform to the direction of others and follow rules.

corrected date of birth (CDOB) A chronological date correction for weeks of prematurity when the actual date of birth is 3 or more weeks earlier than the expected birth date. To calculate CDOB, add the weeks of prematurity to the child's date of birth. (The CDOB is essentially the same as the child's original due date.)

curriculum-based assessment (CBA) Measurement that uses direct observation and recording of a child's performance as a basis for gathering information to make instructional decisions and develop intervention goals.

cutoff point Also known as *referral cutoff point.* Empirically derived score that indicates when a child's performance is suspect and referral for further assessment is appropriate.

developmental assessment An assessment that establishes baseline, or entry level of measurement, of a child's skills across developmental areas.

developmental surveillance An important technique used by pediatricians that includes a flexible, continual process whereby knowledgeable professionals perform skilled observations of children during the provision of health care. The components of developmental surveillance include eliciting and attending to parental concerns, obtaining a relevant developmental history, making accurate and informative observations of children, and sharing opinions and concerns with other relevant professionals. Pediatricians often use age-appropriate developmental checklists to record milestones during preventive care visits as part of developmental surveillance.

early intervention/early childhood special education (EI/ECSE) Supports offered to children with developmental delays.

emotional competence The ability to effectively regulate emotions to accomplish one's goals (Campos et al., 1994; Squires et al., 2014; Summers & Chazen-Cohen, 2012).

false positive Those who test positive but are negative (i.e., do not have the condition).

IDEA *See* Individuals with Disabilities Education Act.

identified Also known as *screened.* Descriptive of children whose scores on a screening tool, such as ASQ:SE-2, are above the cutoff score and who are identified as needing further assessment.

Individuals with Disabilities Education Act (IDEA) IDEA was originally enacted by the U.S. Congress as the Education for All Handicapped Children Act of 1975 (PL 94-142) to make sure that children with disabilities have the opportunity to receive a free appropriate public education. IDEA guides how states and school districts provide special education and related services to more than 6 million eligible children with disabilities. IDEA was reauthorized in 2004 as Individuals with Disabilities Education Improvement Act (PL 108-446).

interaction A child's ability or willingness to respond to or initiate social responses to parents, other adults, and peers.

interobserver reliability Also known as *interrater reliability.* The degree of agreement among raters. It gives a score of how much homogeneity, or consensus, there is in the ratings given by judges.

Local Early Intervention Interagency Coordinating Council (LICC) An interagency group that operates in most communities to coordinate services under IDEA.

mean (*M*) The arithmetic average of a set of values, or distribution.

median Fiftieth percentile of a distribution; point below which half of the observations fall.

monitoring Periodic developmental screening of young children.

monitoring zone An empirically derived range of scores that indicate that a child's development should be monitored further over time. A child's ASQ:SE-2 total score that is in this area indicates a need for monitoring and may require follow-up actions. The monitoring zone begins at the 65th percentile of ASQ:SE-2 score distribution gathered in the normative sample and ends at the established cutoff score.

multidisciplinary team A group of people from different disciplines and professions who work together as equal stakeholders in addressing a common challenge.

multidisciplinary team approach A screening approach that involves highly trained professionals representing a range of disciplines assessing specific groups of young children at risk for developmental disabilities at designated intervals, such as screening groups of premature infants with low birth weights who meet specific criteria.

Overall question Last section of ASQ:SE-2, which asks questions about a child's overall social-emotional development and about any concerns that a parent may have about his or her child's development.

overidentification Also known as *overreferral* or *overscreening.* The proportion of children incorrectly identified as in need of further assessment by the screening tool.

paraprofessional Job title for certain people working in education, health care, and related fields. These individuals have obtained the necessary knowledge and experience that enables them to perform tasks requiring significant expertise but do not have the occupational licenses to perform at professional levels in the field.

parent monitoring approach A screening approach whereby parents monitor their children's development. Measures suitable for a parent monitoring approach require minimal professional input, such as ASQ:SE-2 and ASQ-3.

Part B, Section 619, IDEA Early childhood special education program for children ages 3–21 years with disabilities.

Part C, IDEA Early intervention program for infants and toddlers with disabilities.

percent agreement The proportion of agreement between the screening tool and standardized assessments.

percent screened The percentage of children who are identified as needing further assessment by a screening tool.

positive predictive value The probability that a child identified by the screening tool as needing further assessment will have intervention needs.

psychometric study Research examining the validity, reliability, and utility of an assessment instrument.

quality rating and improvement system (QRIS) "A method to assess, improve, and communicate the level of quality in early care and education settings" (Mitchell, 2005, p. 4). The QRIS in some states requires programs to provide developmental and social-emotional screening to children.

receiver operating characteristic (ROC) curve Procedure to determine optimal cutoff points on a screening tool. Curves are generated (using a computer program) from potential cutoff points. These cutoff points are then selected that maximize sensitivity (true positives) and specificity (true negatives).

roundup approach A screening approach, also called *screening clinics,* that involves parents bringing their young children to a community-based event or evaluation center that offers screening. Roundups are typically scheduled one to four times per year and are staffed by professionals and volunteers.

referral The outcome when parent concerns and/or a child's score on a screening measure, such as ASQ:SE-2, indicate that follow up to a community agency for further assessment is warranted.

reliability Consistency of test scores over time and between testers; the extent to which it is possible to generalize from one test result conducted by one person to test results conducted at different times or by different observers.

screening A brief procedure to determine whether a child requires further and more comprehensive assessment.

SD *See* standard deviation.

self-regulation A child's ability or willingness to calm or settle down or adjust to physiological or environmental conditions or stimulation.

semi-interquartile range One half of the distance between the first quartile of scores (25% of distribution) and the third quartile (75% of distribution): (Quartile 3 – Quartile 1) ÷ 2.

skewed curve Asymmetrical distribution in which the majority is very high or very low. ASQ:SE-2 scores are positively skewed, with the majority of scores between 0 and 25.

sensitivity The proportion of children correctly identified as needing further assessment by the screening tool and who perform below the expected level on a standardized assessment or assessment battery.

social competence An array of behaviors that permits one to develop and engage in positive interactions with peers, siblings, parents, and other adults (Chen & Rubin, 2011; Raver & Zigler, 1997; Squires, 2012).

social-communication A child's ability or willingness to interact with others by responding to or initiating verbal or nonverbal signals to indicate interests or needs, feelings, affective, or internal states.

specificity The proportion of children correctly excluded as developing typically by the screening tool and who perform at the expected level on a standardized assessment.

standard deviation (SD) A measure of the dispersion of a set of values or data points.

standardized test A test that is administered and scored in a consistent manner so that the questions and conditions for administering, scoring, and interpreting results are performed in a predetermined, standard manner.

test–retest reliability The consistency of a measure from one time to another.

tickler system A method of keeping track of the steps involved in ASQ:SE-2. A file box of index cards is sorted by weeks or months in a year, and as cards get pulled and refiled, they alert program staff as to when certain activities need to occur.

tracking Periodic and sequential developmental screening and referral of young children for intervention services.

true positive Those who test positive for a condition and are positive (i.e., have the condition).

utility Usefulness; ease of use of the screening tool or procedure.

underidentification Also known as *underreferral* or *underscreening.* The proportion of children incorrectly identified as developing typically by the screening tool.

universal screening approach A screening approach whereby all children have access to developmental and social-emotional screening at regular intervals. This approach is characterized by the quick, low-cost, and repeatable testing of age-appropriate skills and requires large-scale coordination and collaboration between agencies that provide services to children and families.

validity Extent to which a test measures what its authors claim it measures; appropriateness of the inferences that can be made from test results.

well below the cutoff *See* below the cutoff.

well-child checkup approach A screening and monitoring approach to identify infants and young children who are at risk for developmental delays at well-child checkups in physicians' offices or in public health facilities.

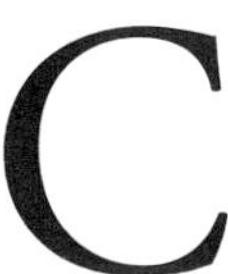

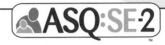

ASQ:SE-2 Technical Report

ASQ:SE-2™

Jane Squires, Diane Bricker, Elizabeth Twombly,
Kimberly Murphy, and Rob Hoselton,
with contributions from Jill Dolata and Chieh-Yu Chen

This technical report focuses on the development and study of the psychometric properties of the *Ages & Stages Questionnaires®: Social-Emotional, Second Edition* (*ASQ:SE-2*™), including revisions and additions to the first edition of ASQ:SE. Psychometric studies completed on ASQ:SE-2 are also described in detail, including results across the nine questionnaire intervals.

The first section addresses the development of the first edition, including item selection and revision, and is followed by a description of the iterative process used for developing, revising, and studying ASQ:SE-2. The next section describes ASQ:SE-2 data collection procedures, including participant recruitment, as well as procedures for the validity and reliability studies. Next, this technical report offers an overview of the demographic characteristics of the ASQ:SE-2 normative sample. The following section reports psychometric findings, including internal consistency, test–retest reliability, and convergent and known group validity. Finally, findings on the utility of ASQ:SE-2 are reported.

DEVELOPMENT OF ASQ:SE

This section briefly describes the development of the first edition of ASQ:SE.

Item Selection

A developmental and behavioral lens was used to select items for ASQ:SE. The tool includes items that focus on acceptable, prosocial behaviors as well as problem behaviors, with attention paid to developmentally appropriate expectations for children. The knowledge that cultural and family factors as well as situational circumstances affect appropriateness of behaviors also guided our item selection.

ASQ:SE items initially were developed using a variety of sources, including standardized social-emotional and developmental assessments, research studies, textbooks and other resources in developmental and abnormal psychology, education and intervention resources, and language and communication materials. We ensured that items are as follows:

1. Representative of critical adaptive and maladaptive behaviors at targeted age intervals
2. Easy for parents/caregivers to understand and recognize
3. Appropriate for a variety of cultural groups and families

Each item was written using common words that did not exceed a sixth-grade reading level. When possible, quantitative descriptors (e.g., 15 minutes, within 24 hours) and concrete examples (e.g., smiles, kicks, bites other children) were provided to assist with interpretation of the item meanings.

Iterative Item Development and Testing

Items were assembled into a field test version, which was titled the Behavior-Ages & Stages Questionnaires (B-ASQ; Bricker, Squires, Twombly, Yockelson, & Kim, 1996). The field test version contained seven age intervals. The number of items per interval varied from 21 items at 6 months to 33 items at 48 months. The items in this field test version were reviewed by experts in psychology, psychiatry, education, early childhood development, pediatrics, nursing, and mental health. Experts provided feedback on the items regarding their appropriateness, ease of understanding, scoring format, and content validity.

Concurrently, practitioners in approximately 50 programs across the United States used the B-ASQ with a diverse population of young children and parents, including families served by Healthy Start in Hawaii and Oregon; inner-city families in Cincinnati, Ohio, Portland, Oregon, and San Francisco, California; Head Start and Migrant Head Start families in California, Texas, and Washington; Child Development and Rehabilitation Center professors in Eugene, Oregon; and families with young children identified with social-emotional delays in Arizona, California, Oregon, Utah, and Washington. Utility surveys completed by service providers and parents offered feedback on the clarity of item meaning, appropriateness of items, missing content, and suggestions for revisions or additional items.

The B-ASQ was revised and renamed the Ages & Stages Questionnaires: Social-Emotional (ASQ:SE) based on the input gathered from experts, parents, and practitioners and on preliminary data analyses. Revisions included eliminating or combining items with overlapping and similar content; rewording items that were difficult to understand; adding items to fill content gaps (e.g., items were added to target so-called "red flags" for autism and adding a questionnaire for 60 months).

DEVELOPMENT OF ASQ:SE-2

Beginning in late 2009, we began the process of revising and updating ASQ:SE based on data and comments from professionals and parents who had used the tool for more than 6 years. Early intervention program faculty, staff, and doctoral students again delved into an updated literature base on social-emotional development, including studies documenting the rise in the awareness and prevalence of autism spectrum and related disorders in young children, as well as the continuing and persistent problem with late identification of social-emotional delays and disabilities in the preschool population. We began to develop and revise items for the second edition of ASQ:SE with a focus on capturing symptoms related to autism and communication disorders and developing additional items to identify competence and problem behaviors in infants and toddlers. Our main goals for the second edition revisions included the following:

1. Extend the age range of ASQ:SE in both directions—to include infants from 1 month to facilitate enrolling and monitoring children from birth, and to expand items to cover children's behavioral repertoire to age 6 (i.e., 72 months) when children generally enter school settings
2. Develop new questionnaire items that directly target social-emotional, early communication, regulatory, and autism spectrum disorder (ASD) behaviors, and do so for children at a younger age
3. Update the format, including response options, to enhance the user friendliness of ASQ:SE
4. Update the normative sample to reflect the current, more diverse population of young children in in the United States
5. Incorporate the addition of a monitoring zone similar to that used in ASQ-3 to aid in score interpretation and follow-up decision making

Extended Age Range

Extending the ASQ:SE-2 age windows included testing and modifying the 6 month interval to include infants as young as 1 month of age, as well as expanding the upper age range of the 60 month interval to include children to age 6 years.

Development of the 2 Month Age Interval

The 2 month questionnaire was developed in response to requests from program personnel monitoring the development of newborns and older infants, who wanted an initial ASQ:SE to give parents soon after the birth of their children. With a 2 month questionnaire, professionals would be able to screen those infants whose parents had great concerns shortly after birth.

Analyses indicated that infants 1–2 months of age were inconsistently performing several items on the ASQ:SE-2 6 month questionnaire. A 2 month questionnaire for children from 1 to 3 months was developed and was composed of 16 scored items from the 6 month questionnaire, which were revised to be more developmentally appropriate. For example, "Does your baby let you know when she is hungry or sick?" was revised to "Does your baby let you know when she is hungry, tired, or uncomfortable? For example, does she fuss or cry?"

Extension of the Upper Age Range to 72 Months

The ASQ:SE-2 60 month questionnaire (with no additional items) was given to children 60–72 months of age to assist with screening children during kindergarten and entry to school. Analyses suggested that mean scores did not significantly differ between children 60–65 and 66–72 months of age. By extending the upper age range to 72 months, programs will be better able to continuously monitor children until their entry into first grade in public or private school settings, thus improving efforts to identify social-emotional and behavioral issues during children's early school years.

Item Additions

Additional ASQ:SE-2 items were formulated and field-tested in a series of eight iterative versions between 2010 and 2013. Items were added primarily to target early communication and behaviors associated with ASD, as well as internalizing behaviors in young children that might go undetected, such as excessive shyness and lack of reciprocity in social situations. We identified internalizing and communication behaviors and other more subtle behaviors associated with ASD in children 14 months of age and older, as these behaviors become easier to identify at this time. For infants, we looked at what behaviors parents would notice that are indicative of the communication, social, cognitive, and behavioral impairments at young ages (e.g., no back-and-forth sharing of sounds, no or few social smiles, no babbling or gesturing by 12 months) that might lead to early identification and improved outcomes.

Between three and seven additional items were added to each of the previously existing age intervals, and minor wording changes were made to existing ASQ:SE items. We made minor edits to existing ASQ:SE items based on item response modeling analyses and feedback from users. Examples of new items include the following:

- "Does your baby make sounds and look at you while playing with you?" (6 months)
- "When you copy sounds your baby makes, does your baby repeat the same sounds back to you?" (12 months)
- "Does your child play with objects by pretending? For example, does your child pretend to talk on the phone, feed a doll, or fly a toy airplane?" (18–30 months)
- "Is your child too worried or fearful?" (24–60 months)

New items are listed in Chapter 1, Table 1.1.

Format Changes

Three major format changes were made to ASQ:SE-2—response options, scoring indicators, and the Information Summary sheet. First, we modified response options to make items easier for parents to interpret and respond. The previous response options of *most of the time, sometimes,* and *rarely or never* were changed to *often or always, sometimes,* and *rarely or never.* Both practitioners and parents felt that using *often or always* would assist in responding to items such as "Does your child cry, scream, or have tantrums for long periods of time?" The previous option (*most of the time*) was confusing for some parents, and focus groups of parents and practitioners felt that *often or always* was easier to understand.

Scoring Indicators

Changes to streamline the scoring procedure were made to assist professionals in adding individual items' scores (i.e., 15, 10, 5, 0) page by page before transferring the scores to the Information Summary sheet. Scoring lines were added in the right margin for each ASQ:SE-2 item as well as at the bottom of each page for total points per page, which can then be transferred to the Information Summary for calculating the child's total score. In addition, a "V" was added next to each item concern circle to prompt professionals to add 5 points to any item score marked by the parent as a concern.

Information Summary Sheet

The third format change was to revise the Information Summary sheet of each ASQ:SE-2 questionnaire so that it contains more information to summarize a child's score, interpret results, and indicate next steps for referral and evaluation. The Information Summary revisions were based on feedback from five focus groups with students, four focus groups with ASQ:SE users, as well as a final design review with professionals representing six programs with extensive experience using ASQ:SE. The revised Information Summary includes a scoring graphic illustrating the range of normative scores from 0% to 90% (the range of children's scores is too wide to accurately illustrate in the space on each questionnaire—often up to 350 points—so the 90th percentile score is indicated). The child's total score can be reviewed on the scoring graphic to get a visual representation of where the score falls on the distribution.

Monitoring Zone

We developed a monitoring zone, or "questionable" area, just under the empirically derived cutoff score for each of the nine age intervals. The monitoring zone cutoff for each interval was set above the median at the 65th percentile, and each monitoring zone includes a range of 10–30 points below the at-risk cutoff score, depending on the specific age interval. The monitoring zone will identify an additional 14% of children across the ASQ:SE-2 intervals. It is depicted on the Information Summary sheet as a light gray area on the scoring graphic, as it is on ASQ-3.

This monitoring zone was included to assist programs in talking to parents about results and the relationship between the child's score and normative data, and to assist with decisions regarding referral options. Significant parent concerns paired with a child's total score in the monitoring zone may indicate a need for immediate referral to a mental health agency. See Chapter 6, Table 6.3, for additional information to guide professionals on aspects to consider regarding referral, including parent concerns.

ASQ:SE-2 Pilot Version

Once initial content revisions were finalized in 2010, we began piloting an expanded version of ASQ:SE-2 to investigate 1) potential cutoff scores and psychometric properties with a new and larger normative population; 2) the accuracy of items extending the age range of ASQ:SE down to 1 month (from the original 3 months) and up to 72 months, or 6 years (from the original 66 months); and 3) how this expanded version identified children with and without ASD diagnoses. Parents of children from 1 month to 72 months of age were invited to complete the ASQ:SE-2 expanded pilot version, in both paper and electronic formats.

DATA COLLECTION PROCEDURES

This section describes data collection procedures and iterative analyses and revisions.

Participant Recruitment

Children between the ages of 1 and 72 months and their parents were recruited for the normative study. Approximately 10% were recruited through newspaper and magazine advertisements; 25% through agency personnel who attended national conferences and agreed to field-test ASQ:SE-2; and 65% through recruiting efforts via electronic bulletin boards and parenting web sites. Additional recruiting methods included posting advertisements on other web sites (e.g., Craigslist), social media, and in parenting resource guides; sending recruitment letters to child care providers in Oregon and California; and contacting personnel in agencies serving high-risk families and young children with disabilities in several states (including California, Connecticut, Florida, Hawaii, Michigan, North Carolina, Ohio, Oregon, and Washington).

An attempt was made to stratify the normative sample so that children/families would be representative of the U.S. population in terms of race/ethnicity, geographic region, parent education and income, and gender of children. Recruitment letters and research protocols were approved by the University of Oregon Human Subjects Compliance Committee prior to beginning data collection. Data from the normative sample were first collected, followed by recruitment of samples for assessing convergent validity—the agreement of the classification outcomes of ASQ:SE-2 (i.e., risk, okay) with other screening and evaluation measures—and ASQ:SE-2's internal consistency, test–retest reliability, and interrater reliability.

Measures

ASQ:SE-2 and a demographic form were the primary measures that were completed by parents. ASQ:SE-2 is a series of questionnaires at nine age intervals from 1 month to 72 months, as described previously. The questionnaires are designed to be completed by parents or other caregivers who can provide information on a child's social-emotional competence across situations.

The demographic form asked parents to provide information on the child's age, date of birth, gender, and race/ethnicity. Information about mother's age at child's birth, mother's education level, and family income also were requested.

Convergent Validity

Several measures were used as comparators for ASQ:SE-2 outcomes to measure convergent validity. Due to the lack of "gold standard" assessments for the evaluation of general social-emotional difficulties in children from birth to 6 years (DelCarmen-Wiggins & Carter, 2004), we chose to compare ASQ:SE-2 outcomes with several evidence-based measures that focus on social-emotional outcomes in one or more age groups within the 1- to 72-month age range. We chose the term *convergent validity* to suggest that we were investigating the correspondence between ASQ:SE-2 and these measures rather than comparing ASQ:SE-2 with one gold standard of diagnosis. Convergent measures included the Devereux Early Childhood Assessment for Infants and Toddlers (DECA-IT; Mackrain, LeBuffe, & Powell, 2007), the Infant Toddler Social Emotional Assessment (ITSEA; Carter & Briggs-Gowan, 2006), and the Child Behavior Checklist (CBCL; Achenbach & Rescorla, 2000).

DECA-IT (Mackrain et al., 2007) is an assessment designed for parent or teacher completion and measures protective and risk factors for children's social-emotional development. Reliability studies by the DECA-IT authors indicated internal consistency ranged from .90 to .94, test–retest reliability from .83 to .94, and interrater reliability from .68 to .72. The Infant Interval, designed for children from birth to 18 months, was used with a subset of infants and toddlers in the ASQ:SE-2 normative sample between 1 and 13 months of age.

ITSEA (Carter & Briggs-Gowan, 2006), a standardized norm-referenced assessment with solid psychometric properties that evaluates social-emotional competence in young children from 1 year to 3 years of age (Printz, Borg, & Demaree, 2003), was used with a subset of children between 12 and 36 months in the ASQ:SE-2 normative sample. National standardization data suggested high internal consistency (the majority of Cronbach's alphas are above .70), acceptable test–retest reliability (intraclass correlations = .61–.91), evidence for concurrent validity (problem scores correlated significantly with Child Behavior Checklist 2/3; r = .28–.78), and acceptable factor loading on the designated subscales (Carter & Brigg-Gowan, 2006).

Three subscales (i.e., Compliance, Negative Emotionality, and Prosocial Peer Relations) were used as comparators for ASQ:SE-2, based on recommendations from the ITSEA first author (Carter) as measures critical for social-emotional assessment (Beeber et al., 2007).

The CBCL (Achenbach & Rescola, 2000) was used as a convergent measure for a subset of children whose ages were in the 18 months to 5 years range in the ASQ:SE-2 normative sample. CBCL is a well-standardized and validated checklist that has been used widely with diverse populations. CBCL is completed by parents and/or teachers, has solid psychometric evidence, and contains approximately 100 items targeting problem behaviors in young children (Whitcomb & Merrell, 2013).

Diagnostic Status

Additional children with a formal diagnosis of social-emotional disability, developmental disability, or ASD were recruited. Multidisciplinary teams in both educational and medical settings evaluated these children who received a diagnosis for eligibility for specialized early intervention/early childhood special education services. The disability status of these children was then compared with their overall classification on ASQ:SE-2 (at risk/okay) as a measure of convergent validity.

Procedures with Parents

Parents willing to participate in the study were presented with a packet of materials containing a consent form, ASQ:SE-2 questionnaire, demographic form, and one or more convergent validity measures, depending on the child's age and the research phase. Packets were distributed in one of three ways: by mailing packets to parents (e.g., those who were contacted through advertisements, social network sites, online parenting sites) who agreed to participate; by preschool teachers directly to parents; and via the Internet through a research web portal. The forms were automatically scored for those using the portal, and the parents immediately received results online after completion. Parents were asked to complete paper research forms within 1 week and return them by mail to the researchers.

Iterative Questionnaire Development

In order to develop ASQ:SE-2, an initial version was developed and distributed to parents during a 2-year period, between 2009 and 2011. Between 1 and 7 items were initially added to each ASQ:SE interval to test the ability of these new items to differentiate between children with social-emotional difficulties and those without. Data were collected in an ongoing fashion and analyzed every 2–3 months to test item functioning, utility, and agreement with convergent measures. Item response modeling and correlational and chi-square analyses were performed to test the functioning of the new items and their agreement with other measures and clusters of items. Every 5–6 months, focus groups of students, researchers, practitioners, and parents were assembled to review the ASQ:SE-2 questionnaires, make comments, suggest revisions, and evaluate utility. Eight different field test versions with differing numbers of new items were tested and analyzed; items that did not differentiate children with social-emotional difficulties were deleted from subsequent data analyses.

Out of the 20 new items tested, a total of 16 were added to ASQ:SE-2 across the 9 intervals. The final item set was developed in late 2012, at which time investigation of convergent validity and test–retest reliability outcomes were instigated.

DEMOGRAPHIC CHARACTERISTICS OF NORMATIVE SAMPLE

Children between the ages of 1 month and 72 months were recruited to examine the psychometric properties of ASQ:SE-2. Data for demographic variables such as race/ethnicity, family income, and mother's education level were not always provided by parents or primary caregivers for a variety of reasons (e.g., privacy, information unknown). The number of questionnaires completed without corresponding demographic information is noted for each analysis.

The ASQ:SE-2 total sample included 14,074 children. The total number of ASQ:SE-2 assessments completed on these children was 16,424. The distribution of these questionnaires by age interval and gender is shown in Table C.1. The majority of parents completed one ASQ:SE-2 interval; however, some parents completed more than one ASQ:SE-2 as their child aged (e.g., contributing questionnaires for the same child at 12, 24, and 36 months).

For those children born 3 or more weeks premature, an adjusted age was used to correct for prematurity up to 24 months of age. This adjusted age corresponded to the expected due date. Note that ASQ-3 uses the same procedure for determining which questionnaire a caregiver should complete for the child.

Table C.2 contains a comparison of U.S. Census Bureau estimates of the race/ethnicity distribution with those of the ASQ:SE-2 normative sample. This comparison is not straightforward, given that the U.S. Census did not use the category of "mixed" race/ethnicities on the 2010 Census and used a two-part question that separated categories of race from ethnicity (e.g., Hispanic or Latino/White not Hispanic or Latino).

According to data provided by the U.S. Census, the ASQ:SE-2 normative sample had a higher percentage of well-educated mothers than found generally in the United States (see Table C.3). Comparisons are not straightforward, however, given differing categories of analysis. A comparison between the U.S. Census data and the ASQ:SE-2 sample on annual family income level indicates the ASQ:SE-2 sample was composed of a similar percentage of families across the income levels (see Table C.4).

Data taken from the demographic form permitted dividing the ASQ:SE-2 normative sample into four groups according to the children's developmental status in order to compare

Table C.1. Number of questionnaires and gender distribution by ASQ:SE-2 age interval[a]

	Number of questionnaires		
ASQ:SE-2 age interval	Total	Males	Females
2 month	287	148	139
6 month	2,042	1,066	976
12 month	2,274	1,278	996
18 month	2,214	1,329	885
24 month	1,808	1,101	707
30 month	1,509	892	617
36 month	2,221	1,290	931
48 month	2,523	1,456	1,067
60 month	1,516	900	616
Total	16,394	9,460	6,934

[a]There are gender data missing for 30 children.

Table C.2. Race/ethnicity comparison of ASQ:SE-2 normative sample (N = 14,137)[a] with 2010 U.S. Census Bureau estimates[b]

Race/ethnic category	Percentage: ASQ:SE-2 normative sample	Percentage: 2010 U.S. Census estimate[b]	Difference
White	72.9	72.4	+0.5
Black or African American	7.8	12.6	–4.8
Hispanic or Latino	7.3	N/A[c]	—
Asian	4.3	4.8	–0.5
Native American	0.8	0.9	–0.1
Native Hawaiian and other Pacific Islander	0.3	0.2	+0.1
Mixed race/ethnicity	6.6	N/A	—
Some other race	N/A	6.2	—
Two or more races	N/A	2.9	—

[a]There are race/ethnicity data missing for 2,287 cases.

[b]From U.S. Census Bureau (2010b).

[c]U.S. Census Bureau (2010b) reported Hispanic or Latino 16.3%, White Not Hispanic or Latino 83.7%; our demographic data were collected in different categories.

Note: The Pew Research Center report dated March 14, 2014, stated, "As many as 6.2% of census respondents selected only 'some other race' in the 2010 census, the vast majority of whom were Hispanic" (Krogstad & Cohn, 2014).

total scores across groups. We hypothesized that children with fewer risk factors would have lower scores on ASQ:SE-2, indicating social-emotional development in the typical range, and that as risk factors increased, ASQ:SE-2 scores would increase, indicating more potential social-emotional difficulties. The four groups are as follows: 1) No and Low Risk (i.e., children with no or one identified environmental/medical risk factor); 2) Risk (i.e., children with two or more environmental/medical risk factors); 3) Developmental Disability (i.e., children with established developmental disabilities who were receiving early intervention/early childhood special education services through IDEA); and 4) Social-Emotional Disability (i.e., children

Table C.3. Education level comparison of ASQ:SE-2 normative sample (N = 14,290)[a] with 2010 U.S. Census Bureau estimates

Highest level of education	Percentage: ASQ:SE-2 normative sample	Percentage: 2010 U.S. Census estimate[b]	Difference
Less than high school diploma	3.7	12.0	–8.3
High school diploma	22.2	48.0	–25.8
Associate degree	14.0	10.0	+4.0
4-year college degree or above	56.7	30.0	+26.7
Do not know	3.3	—[c]	—

[a]There are level of education data missing for 2,134 caregivers.

[b]Based on U.S. Census Bureau (2010a).

[c]The U.S. 2010 Census Bureau does not include a "Do not know" category.

Table C.4. Income level comparison of ASQ:SE-2 normative sample (N = 14,647)[a] with 2010 U.S. Census Bureau estimates

ASQ:SE-2		2010 U.S. Census Bureau estimates		
Income category	Percentage of ASQ:SE-2 normative sample	2010 U.S. Census income category[b]	Percentage of population	Difference
\$0–\$12,000	8.5	Less than \$9,999	7.8	+0.7
\$12,001–\$24,000	17.2	\$10,000–\$24,999	18.0	–0.8
\$24,001–\$40,000	14.2	\$25,000–\$39,999	15.9	–1.7
More than \$40,000	60.0	More than \$40,000	58.4	+1.6

[a]There are income level data missing for 1,777 children.
[b]Based on U.S. Census Bureau (2010a).

with identified social-emotional disabilities, according to IDEA Part B eligibility guidelines and *Diagnostic and Statistical Manual of Mental Disorders, Fourth Edition [DSM-IV]* diagnostic classifications). Variables used to determine level of risk for the Risk group included the following:

1. Family income less than \$12,000 per year
2. Mother younger than 18 years old when child was born
3. Mother's highest level of education less than high school diploma
4. Involvement of child protective services with family; or a child in foster care
5. Child's birth weight less than 3 pounds, 5 ounces
6. Child enrolled in Head Start or Early Head Start services

Children with developmental or social-emotional disabilities were classified in the Developmental Disability or Social-Emotional Disability group, regardless of the number of environmental risk factors. Table C.5 presents children in the normative sample by developmental status. (Developmental status information was missing for 6,039 children due to parents/primary caregivers choosing not to answer certain demographic questions; these were omitted from this analysis.)

PSYCHOMETRIC FINDINGS

This section describes how the cutoff scores for ASQ:SE-2 were developed. In addition, this section presents data collected from subgroups of the normative sample, which were used to examine the internal consistency, test–retest reliability, convergent validity, known groups validity (including comparisons related to ASD measures), and utility of ASQ:SE-2.

Establishing Reliability

This section explains how we established reliability, including internal consistency and test–retest reliability.

Table C.5. Number of questionnaires by developmental status for the ASQ:SE-2 normative sample (N = 10,385)[a]

		Developmental status							
		No risk[b]		At risk[c]		Developmental disability[d]		Social-emotional disability[e]	
ASQ:SE-2 age interval	N	n	Median	n	Median	n	Median	n	Median
2 month	160	125	20	34	10	1	50	—	—
6 month	1,121	1,010	20	103	10	8	60	—	—
12 month	1,279	1,148	30	103	35	25	65	3	155
18 month	1,309	1,133	36	110	35	55	95	11	115
24 month	1,127	953	35	108	35	51	60	15	135
30 month	937	766	50	88	45	69	80	14	132.5
36 month	1,514	1,043	60	311	40	104	90	56	157.5
48 month	1,876	1,079	55	627	35	98	77.5	72	145
60 month	1,062	659	50	307	35	43	95	53	165
Total/overall	10,385	7,916	40	1,791	35	454	80	224	150

[a]Developmental status data are missing for 6,039 children.
[b]No identified risk factors.
[c]One or more identified risk factors.
[d]Children receiving early intervention or early childhood special education services.
[e]Children with diagnosed social-emotional disabilities.

Internal Consistency

Internal consistency measures the extent to which the different items on the assessment tool measure the same underlying construct (Saliva, Ysseldyke, & Bolt, 2012). High internal consistency reflects items that assess the same characteristic or behavioral area. To measure internal consistency, coefficient alpha was calculated for each ASQ:SE-2 age interval using the variances of individual items and the variance of the total test scores (N = 11,489). Cronbach's coefficient alphas for the ASQ:SE-2 intervals are shown in Table C.6. Alphas ranged from .71 to .90, with an overall alpha of .84. An alpha of .70 is considered to be an adequate measure of internal consistency (Nunnally, 1978).

Test–Retest Reliability

Test–retest reliability measures the stability of child performance over time. Test–retest reliability for ASQ:SE-2 was determined by comparing the results of two of the same questionnaires completed by parents at 1- to 3-week intervals. A random sample of parents (N = 281) was asked to complete the same ASQ:SE-2 after returning the first completed questionnaire. The percent agreement between classifications of the child's performance on ASQ:SE at Time 1 (first questionnaire) and Time 2 (second questionnaire) was used to measure test–retest reliability.

Children were classified as Okay on ASQ:SE-2 if their scores were at or below the empirically derived cutoff point for that interval and no further evaluation of social-emotional competence was needed. Children were classified as At Risk on ASQ:SE-2 if their scores were above

Table C.6. Cronbach coefficient alpha by ASQ:SE-2 age interval (N = 11,489[a])

ASQ:SE-2 age interval	Number of questionnaires	Alpha
2 month	270	.71
6 month	1,857	.74
12 month	1,980	.79
18 month	1,956	.87
24 month	1,581	.87
30 month	719	.88
36 month	1,095	.90
48 month	1,236	.90
60 month	795	.90
Overall	11,489	.84

[a]There are data missing for 4,935 children.

the cutoff point and further evaluation of their social-emotional status was needed. Test–retest agreement between classifications was 89% between Time 1 and Time 2 questionnaires. Intraclass correlations also were calculated and were .91 across intervals.

Establishing Validity

The primary goal of a screening measure is to accurately discriminate between individuals who are typical or okay (i.e., do not have the problem or characteristic) on a targeted variable (e.g., social-emotional development) and individuals who appear atypical or not okay (i.e., potentially may have the problem or characteristic). Establishing the validity of a screening measure generally requires a two-step process. First, it is necessary to collect sufficient normative data to establish optimal cutoff scores for the screening test. Individuals whose scores are above the cutoff score are classified as At Risk and in need of follow-up, whereas individuals whose scores are below the cutoff score are classified as Okay and do not need follow-up.

There are no absolute scores that separate individuals who are typically developing from individuals who are not typically developing for any screening test. Rather, data must be collected and examined to determine the optimal cutoff scores that correctly classify children as needing or not needing follow-up evaluation. Finding optimal cutoff scores requires examining a range of alternatives to discover those scores that maximize the identification of individuals who should receive further testing (i.e., true positives) while minimizing the misidentification of individuals who do not require further testing (i.e., false positives) and minimizing the nonidentification of individuals who should receive further testing (i.e., false negatives).

After tentative cutoff scores are selected, the second step is to determine their accuracy and, thus, the validity of the screening measure. Determining the accuracy of the cutoff scores is done by comparing children's classification on the screening measure with their classification on a selected criterion or convergent measure(s). ASQ:SE-2 was examined by comparing children's classification (i.e., developmentally Okay, At Risk) on ASQ:SE-2 with their classification (i.e., developmentally Okay, At Risk/Disabled) on selected convergent measures that included the DECA-IT (Mackrain et al., 2007), ITSEA (Carter & Briggs-Gowan, 2006), CBCL (Achenbach & Rescola, 2000), and professional diagnosis of a social-emotional disability.

Receiver operating characteristic (ROC) curves were used to calculate optimal cutoff scores (i.e., those that yield high true positives, low false positives, and low false negatives for ASQ:SE-2). ROC analysis permits the systematic comparison of true positive probabilities against false positive probabilities for a range of possible cutoff scores (Swets & Picket, 1982). A sample of 2,862 children with completed ASQ:SE-2 questionnaires were given a concurrent

		Criterion measure classification	
		At Risk	Okay
Screening measure classification	At Risk	True positives A	False positives (overidentification) B
	Okay	False negatives (underidentification) C	True negatives D

Formulas for calculating:

Percent of children identified as needing further assessment:

$$\frac{A + B}{A + B + C + D}$$

Percent agreement: Proportion of agreement between the screening tool and standardized assessment:

$$\frac{A + D}{A + B + C + D} \times 100$$

Sensitivity: The proportion of children correctly identified by the questionnaires as needing further assessment:

$$\frac{A}{A + C}$$

Specificity: The proportion of children correctly identified by the questionnaires as developing typically:

$$\frac{D}{B + D}$$

Overidentification: The proportion of children (of the total number of children for whom a questionnaire was completed) incorrectly identified by the questionnaires as needing further assessment:

$$\frac{B}{A + B + C + D}$$

Underidentification: The proportion of children (of the total number of children for whom a questionnaire was completed) incorrectly excluded by the questionnaires:

$$\frac{C}{A + B + C + C}$$

Positive predictive value: The proportion of children identified by the questionnaires as needing further assessment who will, in fact, have intervention needs:

$$\frac{A}{A + B}$$

Figure C.1. Contingency table for comparing screening measure classification with criteria measure classification and formulas for deriving comparison data.

criterion measure—DECA-IT (Mackrain et al., 2007), ITSEA (Carter & Briggs-Gowan, 2006), CBCL (Achenbach & Rescola, 2000)—or had a professional diagnosis of a social-emotional disability to create these comparison data. Each child's classification (i.e., Okay, At Risk) on ASQ:SE-2 was then compared with the classification (i.e., Okay, At Risk/Disabled) of the child by one of the criterion measures. Figure C.1 shows a four-cell contingency table used to assess the agreement between the screening measure (i.e., ASQ:SE-2) and the criterion measure (i.e., DECA-IT, ITSEA, CBCL, diagnosis of social-emotional disability). In addition, this figure shows the formulas for calculating percentage of children identified as needing further assessment and the percent agreement, sensitivity, specificity, overidentification, underidentification, and positive predictive value of ASQ:SE-2.

Comparison of range of scored points, medians, interquartile ranges, and ROC cutoffs is shown in Table C.7. Note that ROC cutoff scores for most intervals were similar to scores derived from adding 1.5 semi-interquartile ranges to medians. The general trend of increasingly higher scores as children develop is reflected in median scores, except at 48 and 60 months.

Cutoff scores for screening tools frequently are set by using means and standard deviations. That is, the mean score plus one standard deviation is a likely choice for a cutoff score. Using means to calculate cutoff scores presumes a normal distribution of scores, however. Score distribution for ASQ:SE-2 questionnaires was positively skewed—that is, the majority of children obtained low scores (i.e., indicating no problem or Okay) and relatively few children obtained high scores (i.e., indicating a potential problem or risk). The majority of children had scores below 25. Figure C.2 shows the positively skewed distribution of scores for the 48 month ASQ:SE-2; other age intervals showed similar score distributions. Means and standard deviations were not used for determining cutoff points because of the positive skew of ASQ:SE-2 scores across intervals. Instead, ROC analyses were conducted to determine the best cutoff point for each interval.

Modifying Cutoff Scores

If programs want to modify cutoff scores, then semi-interquartile ranges [i.e., median + (Quartile 1 – Quartile 3)/2] should be used as the basis for modification. See www.agesandstages.com for additional discussion of guidelines for altering ASQ:SE-2 cutoff points.

Monitoring Zone

A monitoring zone has been designated to assist with ASQ:SE-2 score interpretation, as discussed in Chapter 6. The monitoring zone begins at the 65th percentile and ends at the referral cutoff. The monitoring zone identifies a group of children whose scores are close to the cutoff score. The range of points for each questionnaire's monitoring zone can be found in Table C.8.

Gender Differences

Scores for males and females were compared in order to examine gender differences. Mean and median scores by gender are presented in Table C.9. Box plots were then derived to examine the score distributions by gender. Box plots provide a visual picture of a distribution. Box plots for the 30 month and 36 month ASQ:SE-2 male and female score distributions are shown in Figure C.3. The bottom line of the box is the 25th percentile, or Quartile 1. The top line of the box is the 75th percentile, or Quartile 3. The middle line is the median, or Quartile 2; the

Table C.7. Range of points, medians, interquartile ranges, receiver operating characteristic (ROC) cutoffs, and percentages identified by ASQ:SE-2 interval (N = 16,424)[a]

ASQ:SE-2 age interval	N	Range of points	Median	Median + 1.5 semi-inter-quartile ranges	ROC cutoff score[a]	Percent identified
2 month	288	0–140	20	35.0	35	18.4
6 month	2,043	0–210	20	38.8	45	14.7
12 month	2,276	0–245	30	52.5	50	24.9
18 month	2,216	0–405	35	68.8	65	23.3
24 month	1,809	0–335	35	66.5	65	22.8
30 month	1,514	0–375	45	90.0	85	23.7
36 month	2,232	0–370	55	106.0	105	22.0
48 month	2,530	0–350	45	93.8	85	26.0
60 month	1,516	0–310	46	102.3	95	23.7

[a]ROC cutoff based on "best fit," maximizing true positives and true negatives.

mean is indicated by the "x." Whiskers (lines) extend to the highest and lowest observations but not further than 1.5 interquartile ranges. Outliers beyond 1.5 interquartile ranges are indicated by "o"; outliers beyond 3 interquartile ranges are indicated by "*."

As shown in Figure C.3, the majority of scores for males at the 30 month interval range between 25 and 75, with the 1.5 interquartile ranges extending to 180. Outliers extend upward to 370. For females, the range is between 20 and 61, with the 1.5 interquartile ranges extending to 150. Outliers extend upward to 325. A similar distribution for both males and females can be seen at the 36 month interval. Similar distribution patterns occurred at all test intervals and indicate, in general, that males tended to have greater dispersal of scores and more extreme scores.

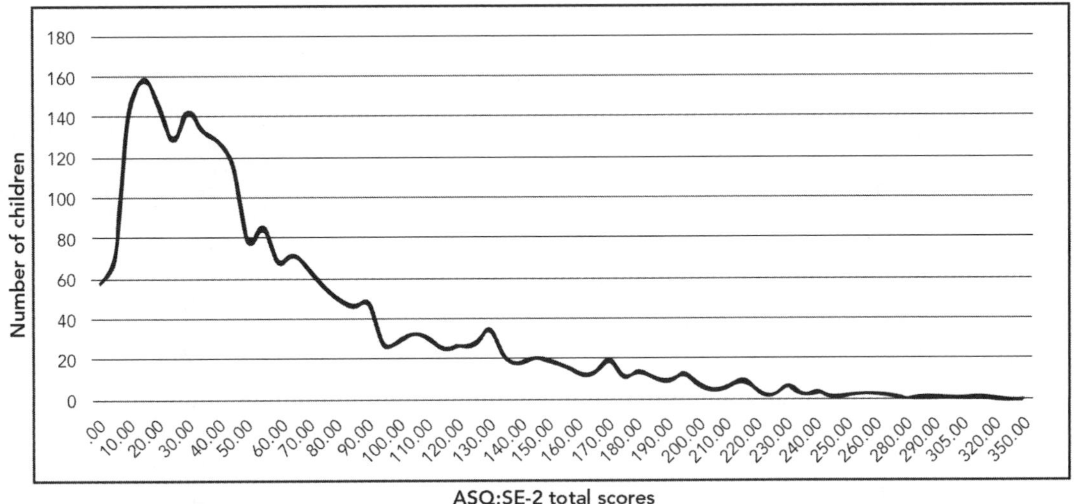

Figure C.2. ASQ:SE-2 total scores by number of children for the 48 month questionnaire (N = 2,530), showing a positively skewed distribution.

Table C.8. ASQ:SE-2 monitoring zone score ranges

ASQ:SE-2 interval	Monitoring zone
2 month	25–35
6 month	30–45
12 month	40–50
18 month	50–65
24 month	50–65
30 month	65–85
36 month	75–105
48 month	70–85
60 month	70–95

If gender group differences are compared using nonparametric tests (i.e., Kruskal-Wallis Test [Heiman, 1992]), significant differences are found at 12, 18, 24, 30, 36, 48, and 60 months, as shown in Table C.9. It is important to note that the validity sample did not have adequate numbers of girls identified with social-emotional problems to determine if separate cutoff scores for females are needed, especially at younger ages.

Gender differences also were compared using item response modeling (IRT), specifically differential item functioning (DIF). Differences between scores of boys and girls were analyzed across the nine ASQ:SE-2 age intervals using the Mantel (1963) approach (Dorans & Holland, 1993); 22 out of 295 items were identified with DIF or differential functioning for boys and girls. The majority of those 22 items were revised to include examples and/or modified wording.

Among all DIF items, one specific item across three age intervals was identified, potentially causing different responses based on the gender of the child being assessed. This item was "Does your child play with objects by pretending? For example by feeding a doll or talking on

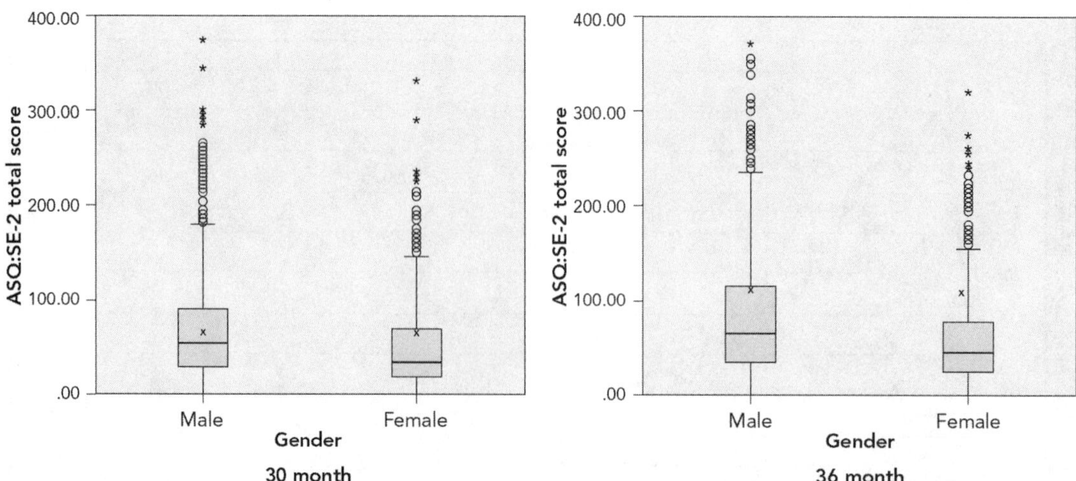

Figure C.3. Box plots for 30 month and 36 month ASQ:SE-2 by gender. Box plots illustrate the distribution of scores. The bottom line of the box is the 25th percentile, or Quartile 1. The top line of the box is the 75th percentile, or Quartile 3. The middle line is the median, or Quartile 2. Mean is indicted by an "x." Whiskers (lines) extend to the highest and lowest observations, but not further than 1.5 interquartile ranges. Outliers beyond 1.5 interquartile ranges are indicated by "O." Outliers beyond 3 interquartile ranges are indicated by "*." Box width varies by *n*. (*Note:* 30 month: male = 892, female = 617; 36 month: male = 1,290, female = 931).

Table C.9. ASQ:SE-2 means and medians for males and females by age interval (N = 16,394)[a]

ASQ:SE-2 age interval	Male			Female		
	N	Mean	Median	N	Mean	Median
2 month	148	26.0	20	139	22.8	20
6 month	1,066	28.1	21	976	26.6	20
12 month	1,278	42.8	35	996	34.6*	30
18 month	1,329	51.4	40	885	44.1*	30
24 month	1,101	53.4	40	707	41.8*	30
30 month	892	69.5	55	617	52.3*	35
36 month	1,290	81.3	65	931	59.2*	45
48 month	1,456	75.1	55	1,067	52.5*	35
60 month	900	70.7	51	616	58.7*	40
Total	9,460	—	—	6,934	—	—

[a]Gender data are missing for 30 children.
*Significant total at $p < .001$.

the phone?" Based on the analysis, we revised this item for subsequent versions to "Does your child play with objects by pretending? For example by talking on the phone, feeding a doll, or flying a toy airplane?" The order of items within the questionnaires was changed so that they followed the developmental order identified by the IRT analysis. Second, and perhaps most important, we included additional examples that might have more appeal to boys, with materials such as balls.

Furthermore, items with differential functioning indicated specific patterns in social-emotional competence areas across intervals by gender. For example, the scores of boys indicated a greater frequency of problem behaviors than girls on several items in social-communication and self-regulation areas; girls' scores indicated a greater frequency of problem behaviors than boys on items assessing sleeping and autonomy. The different patterns of scoring may have resulted from potential differences between genders or the parents' varying expectations for boys and girls.

As additional data are added to the validity sample, revised cutoffs, if necessary, will be shared via www.agesandstages.com. Based on our current normative sample, however, we recommend that programs carefully review with parents/caregivers ASQ:SE-2 results of girls with scores in the monitoring zone. Because girls in our normative sample in general had scores lower than boys, especially at 12 through 60 months of age, we believe that girls and their families may need to be considered for referral for further assessment and/or community services when their scores are near as well as above the screening cutoff points.

Examining Convergent Validity

A comparison with selected social-emotional measures was necessary to determine how accurately ASQ:SE-2 discriminates between children whose social-emotional development is proceeding without a problem from those children who have or are at risk for developing a social-emotional problem. DECA-IT (Mackrain et al., 2007), ITSEA (Carter & Briggs-Gowan, 2006), and CBCL (Achenbach & Rescola, 2000) were convergent measures chosen to examine the validity of ASQ:SE-2.

Parents or other primary caregivers of children in the validity sample (N = 2,862) completed the DECA-IT (Mackrain et al., 2007), ITSEA (Carter & Briggs-Gowan, 2006), and/or CBLC (Achenbach & Rescola, 2000) (depending on the age of their child) within 2–3 weeks of also completing ASQ:SE-2. Included in the validity sample was a group of 146 children ranging in age from 6 to 60 months who had been professionally diagnosed as having a social-emotional disability and were receiving intervention services. Each diagnosis was based on a multidisciplinary battery of diagnostic assessments. Table C.10 summarizes the numbers of children by convergent measure.

Children in the validity sample were classified as either Okay or At Risk based on their ASQ:SE-2 score using the established cutoffs and were independently classified as either Okay or At Risk/Disabled using their score on the DECA-IT (Mackrain et al., 2007), ITSEA (Carter & Briggs-Gowan, 2006), and/or CBLC (Achenbach & Rescola, 2000) or professional diagnosis. These two independent classifications were then compared for all children in the validity sample. One of four outcomes was possible: 1) ASQ:SE-2 and the criterion measure both classified the child as Okay (i.e., true negatives), 2) ASQ:SE-2 and the criterion measure both classified the child as At Risk/Disabled (i.e., true positives), 3) ASQ:SE-2 classified the child as Okay while the criterion measure classified the child as At Risk/Disabled (i.e., false negatives), and 4) ASQ:SE-2 classified the child as At Risk, whereas the criterion measure classified the child as Okay (i.e., false positives).

Contingency tables containing four cells (i.e., A = true positives, B = false positives, C = false negatives, and D = true negatives, as shown in Figure C.1) were developed for each ASQ:SE-2 age interval using the ROC cutoff scores (see Table C.7) to conduct these comparisons. Each contingency table contained in Figure C.4 shows the agreement for true positives, false positives, false negatives, and true negatives. Using the data contained in the contingency table, the sensitivity, specificity, false positive rate, false negative rate, percent agreement, underidentified rate, overidentified rate, and positive predictive value were calculated for each ASQ:SE-2 age interval. An overall comparison across all intervals is shown in Figure C.5.

Table C.10. Measures and *N* used for ASQ:SE-2 convergent validity analyses

ASQ:SE-2 interval	Autism diagnosis	CBCL	DECA-IT	ITSEA	Social-emotional diagnosis	Total
2 month	—	—	71	—	—	71
6 month	—	—	438	—	2	440
12 month	1	—	264	232	3	500
18 month	4	16	9	458	13	500
24 month	9	52	—	336	11	408
30 month	7	45	—	297	11	360
36 month	35	83	—	103	42	263
48 month	48	116	—	—	37	201
60 month	29	63	—	—	27	119
Total	133	375	782	1,426	146	2,862

Key: CBCL, Child Behavior Checklist (Achenbach & Rescola, 2000); DECA-IT, Devereux Early Childhood Assessment-Infant/Toddler (Mackrain, LeBuffe, & Powell, 2007); ITSEA, Infant Toddler Social Emotional Assessment (Carter & Briggs-Gowan, 2006).

Table C.11 presents a comparison of the sensitivity, specificity, percent agreement, false positive rate, false negative rate, underidentified rate, and overidentified rate across ASQ:SE-2 age intervals. Sensitivity ranged from a low of 77.8% at 2 months to a high of 84% at 24 months. Specificity ranged from 76.2% at 18 months to 98% at 60 months. Percent agreement ranged from 77% at 18 months to 89.1% at 60 months. The underidentified rate ranged from 1.8% at 6 months to 10.9% at 48 months, whereas the overidentified rate ranged from .8% at 60 months to 19.4% at 12 months. These findings suggest that ASQ:SE-2 is generally accurate in discriminating between children who are Okay and those who need follow-up. Because of the overidentification rate at 12 months (19.4%) and 18 months (19.0%), programs should consider rescreening in follow-up and referral actions.

2 month — **Criterion measure classification**[a]

ASQ:SE-2 classification		At risk	Okay	Total
	At risk	7	12	19
	Okay	2	50	52
	Total	9	62	71

Sensitivity	Specificity	False positive	False negative	Percent agreement	Under-identified	Over-identified	Positive predictive value
77.8%	80.6%	19.4%	22.2%	80.3%	2.8%	16.9%	36.8%

6 month — **Criterion measure classification**[b]

ASQ:SE-2 classification		At risk	Okay	Total
	At risk	29	47	76
	Okay	8	356	364
	Total	37	403	440

Sensitivity	Specificity	False positive	False negative	Percent agreement	Under-identified	Over-identified	Positive predictive value
78.4%	88.3%	11.7%	21.6%	87.5%	1.8%	10.7%	38.2%

Figure C.4. Contingency tables showing agreement between ASQ:SE-2 classification, criterion measure classification, and ASQ:SE-2 sensitivity, specificity, false positive rate, false negative rate, percent agreement, percent underidentified, percent overidentified, and positive predictive value by age interval (definitions and formulas are contained in Figure C.1). Criterion measure classification includes CBCL, DECA-IT, ITSEA, and professional diagnoses. (*Key:* [a]Includes DECA-IT; [b]Includes DECA-IT and professional diagnosis; [c]Includes DECA-IT, ITSEA, and professional diagnosis; [d]Includes DECA-IT, CBCL, ITSEA, and professional diagnosis; [e]Includes CBCL, ITSEA, and professional diagnosis; [f]Includes CBCL and professional diagnosis.)

(continued)

Figure C.4. *(continued)*

12 month — **Criterion measure classification**[c]

		At risk	Okay	Total
ASQ:SE-2 classification	At risk	40	97	137
	Okay	11	352	363
	Total	51	449	500

Sensitivity	Specificity	False positive	False negative	Percent agreement	Under-identified	Over-identified	Positive predictive value
78.4%	78.4%	21.6%	21.6%	78.4%	2.2%	19.4%	29.2%

18 month — **Criterion measure classification**[d]

		At risk	Okay	Total
ASQ:SE-2 classification	At risk	81	95	176
	Okay	20	304	324
	Total	101	399	500

Sensitivity	Specificity	False positive	False negative	Percent agreement	Under-identified	Over-identified	Positive predictive value
80.2%	76.2%	23.8%	19.8%	77.0%	4.0%	19.0%	46.0%

24 month — **Criterion measure classification**[e]

		At risk	Okay	Total
ASQ:SE-2 classification	At risk	63	39	102
	Okay	12	294	306
	Total	75	333	408

Sensitivity	Specificity	False positive	False negative	Percent agreement	Under-identified	Over-identified	Positive predictive value
84.0%	88.3%	11.7%	16.0%	87.5%	2.9%	9.6%	61.8%

30 month — **Criterion measure classification**[e]

		At risk	Okay	Total
ASQ:SE-2 classification	At risk	47	44	91
	Okay	12	257	269
	Total	59	301	360

Sensitivity	Specificity	False positive	False negative	Percent agreement	Under-identified	Over-identified	Positive predictive value
79.7%	85.4%	14.6%	20.3%	84.4%	3.3%	12.2%	51.6%

36 month		Criterion measure classification[e]		
		At risk	Okay	Total
ASQ:SE-2 classification	At risk	98	19	117
	Okay	27	119	146
	Total	125	138	263

Sensitivity	Specificity	False positive	False negative	Percent agreement	Under-identified	Over-identified	Positive predictive value
78.4%	86.2%	13.8%	21.6%	82.5%	10.3%	7.2%	83.8%

48 month		Criterion measure classification[f]		
		At risk	Okay	Total
ASQ:SE-2 classification	At risk	105	11	116
	Okay	22	63	85
	Total	127	74	201

Sensitivity	Specificity	False positive	False negative	Percent agreement	Under-identified	Over-identified	Positive predictive value
82.7%	85.1%	14.9%	17.3%	83.6%	10.9%	5.5%	90.5%

60 month		Criterion measure classification[f]		
		At risk	Okay	Total
ASQ:SE-2 classification	At risk	57	1	58
	Okay	12	49	61
	Total	69	50	119

Sensitivity	Specificity	False positive	False negative	Percent agreement	Under-identified	Over-identified	Positive predictive value
82.6%	98.0%	2.0%	17.4%	89.1%	10.1%	0.8%	98.3%

Known Groups Validity

This section describes the validity of known groups: risk and disability status, and ASD.

Risk and Disability Status

Examining the differences in scores across groups is another approach to assessing the validity of a screening measure suggested by Spector (1992). For this analysis, a subsample of children in the validity sample were divided into one of three groups based on developmental status—No Risk, Developmentally Disabled, and Socially-Emotionally Disabled. Children were assigned to the

Overall		**Criterion measure classification**[a]		
		Risk	Okay	
ASQ:SE-2 classification	Risk	527	365	892
	Okay	126	1,844	1,970
	Total	653	2,209	2,862

Sensitivity	Specificity	False positive	False negative	Percent agreement	Under-identified	Over-identified	Positive predictive value
80.7%	83.5%	16.5%	19.3%	82.8%	4.4%	12.8%	59.1%

[a]Includes CBCL, DECA-IT, ITSEA, and professional diagnosis.

Figure C.5. Contingency table showing overall agreement (combined across age intervals) between ASQ:SE-2 classification with criterion measure classification and ASQ:SE-2 sensitivity, specificity, false positive rate, false negative rate, percent agreement, percent underidentified, percent overidentified, and positive predictive value (definitions and formulas are contained in Figure C.1). Criterion measure classification includes CBCL, DECA-IT, ITSEA, and professional diagnosis.

No Risk group if caregivers reported no risk factors (*N* = 7,916); children were assigned to the Developmentally Disabled group if they were receiving general early intervention services (*N* = 454); and children were assigned to the Socially-Emotionally Disabled group if they had been diagnosed with a behavior or emotional problem and were receiving intervention services (*N* = 224). Risk factors included the following: 1) family income less than $12,000; 2) mother younger than 18 years old when child was born; 3) mother's level of education less than high school diploma; 4) involvement of child protective services with family or a child in foster care; 5) birth weight less than 3 pounds, 5 ounces; and 6) child enrolled in Early Head Start or Head Start services.

Figure C.6 presents the median scores for the four groups by interval. Score profiles by risk group indicate that ASQ:SE-2 can discriminate between children whose social-emotional development is typical and those who have disabilities. An example of box plots showing the

Table C.11. ASQ:SE-2 cutoff scores and classification statistics[a] by age interval based on receiver operating characteristic (ROC) cutoff score (*N* = 2,862)

ASQ:SE-2 age interval	N	Cutoff score	Sensitivity	Specificity	Percent agreement	False positive rate	False negative rate	Under-identified	Over-identified
2 month	71	35	77.8	80.6	80.3	19.4	22.2	2.8	16.9
6 month	440	45	78.4	88.3	87.5	11.7	21.6	1.8	10.7
12 month	500	50	78.4	78.4	78.4	21.6	21.6	2.2	19.4
18 month	500	65	80.2	76.2	77.0	23.8	19.8	4.0	19.0
24 month	408	65	84.0	88.3	87.5	11.7	16.0	2.9	9.6
30 month	360	85	79.7	85.4	84.4	14.6	20.3	3.3	12.2
36 month	263	105	78.4	86.2	82.5	13.8	21.6	10.3	7.2
48 month	201	85	82.7	85.1	83.6	14.9	17.3	10.9	5.5
60 month	119	95	82.6	98.0	89.1	2.0	17.4	10.1	0.8
Overall	2,862	—	80.7	83.5	82.8	16.5	19.3	4.4	12.8

[a]See Figure C.1 for formula used in calculating classification statistics.

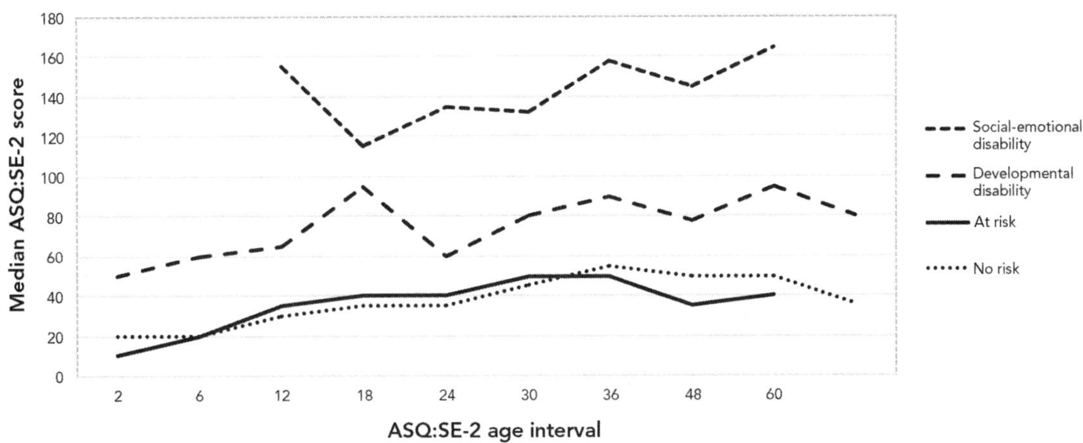

Figure C.6. Median ASQ:SE-2 scores by group risk status.

distribution of risk groups for the 48 month ASQ:SE-2 is presented in Figure C.7. The box plots show mean (marked with a "x") and median (middle horizontal line in each box) scores are elevated for children with developmental and social-emotional disabilities. In addition, there is almost no overlap in the distribution of scores between the No Risk and Social-Emotional Disability groups. Children with diagnosed social-emotional disabilities had the highest scores. There is an overlap in scores for the Risk and No Risk groups, possibly due to a selection factor involving a large number of parents with concerns for their child's social-emotional development who completed the ASQ:SE-2 online. The majority of these families experienced low or no risk. The No Risk and Low Risk groups could be collapsed for future analyses.

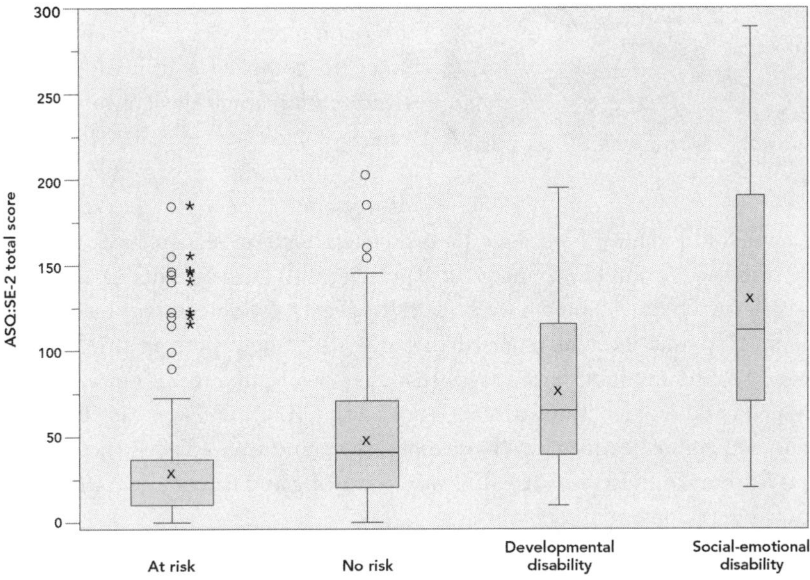

Figure C.7. Box plot distribution of total scores on the 48 month ASQ:SE-2 by developmental status. Box plots illustrate the spread of distribution. The bottom line of the box is the 25th percentile, or Quartile 1. The top line of the box is the 75th percentile, or Quartile 3. The middle line is the median, or Quartile 2. Mean is indicted by a "x." Whiskers (lines) extend to the highest and lowest observations but not further than 1.5 interquartile ranges. Outliers beyond 1.5 interquartile range are indicated by "O." Outliers beyond 3 interquartile ranges are indicated by "*." Box width varies with *n*.

Autism Spectrum Disorder

For comparisons related to ASD, the classification of children on ASQ:SE-2 was compared for 133 children between 18 and 60 months of age with a diagnosis of ASD. Overall, the ASQ:SE-2 classification (Okay, Risk) agreed 83.5% with the child's classification of ASD (Risk). These children had received a diagnosis of ASD through educational or medical diagnostic procedures, and their parents had completed an ASQ:SE-2 questionnaire.

These preliminary analyses suggest that ASQ:SE-2 will identify the majority of children with ASD. Ongoing research is being conducted in which in-depth ASD measures such as the Autism Diagnostic Observation Schedule, Second Edition (Lord, Rutter, DiLavore, & Risi, 2012) are used concurrently with ASQ:SE-2. These results may assist programs in making decisions regarding referral for ASD testing based on ASQ:SE-2 results. In addition, a summary of ASQ:SE-2 and ASQ-3 items related to behaviors associated with ASD appears in Table C.12. ASQ-3 items pertaining to autism are included to provide a better understanding of how to use the tools together.

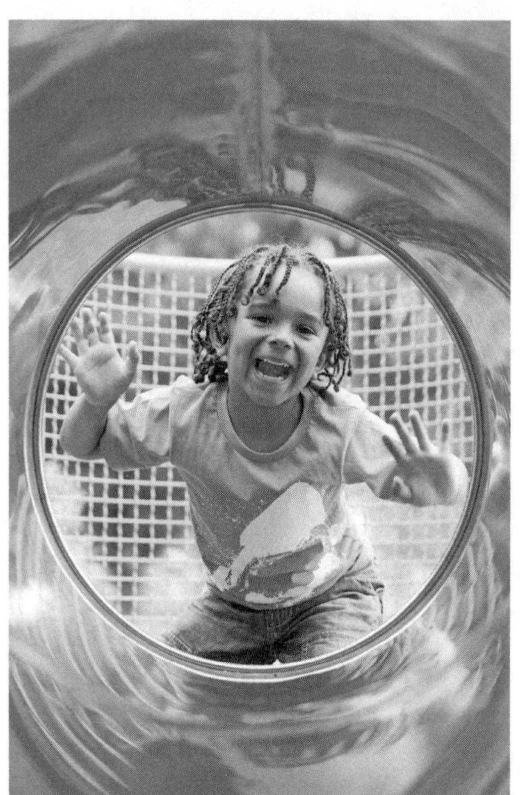

UTILITY SURVEY

Utility of a screening tool measures the usefulness or practicality of the test or procedure (Bricker & Squires, 1989). A random sample of parents ($N = 332$) who completed a paper version of ASQ:SE-2 was asked to complete a utility survey that requested their opinion about the length, appropriateness, and ease of completion of ASQ:SE-2. Summary results of the utility survey can be found in Table C.13. Thirty-one percent of the respondents indicated that it took less than 10 minutes to complete; thirty-nine percent indicated that it took 10–20 minutes to complete. Ninety-three percent of the respondents indicated that ASQ:SE-2 was easy to understand, and eighty percent felt that question content was appropriate for their child. Seventy-three percent reported that ASQ:SE-2 helped them think about their child's behavior, and ninety-four percent said that they would like to fill out another questionnaire when their child is older. Thus, parents reported that ASQ:SE-2 was easy to understand, it took little time to complete, questions were appropriate, and they enjoyed the process. In addition, parents felt that completing ASQ:SE-2 was interesting and helped them think about the social-emotional development of their children.

SUMMARY

Psychometric studies on ASQ:SE-2 are summarized in this technical report. Normative data are based on 16,424 completed questionnaires. Validity studies were conducted using 2,862

Table C.12. ASQ:SE-2 and ASQ-3 items related to autism spectrum disorder (ASD)

Item content (not exact wording)	ASD related skill/indicator	Intervals for 12–24 months	Intervals for 25–60 months
When you hold out your hand and ask for her toy, does your baby let go of it into your hand?**	Social reciprocity, social-communication, restricted/repetitive patterns	12	—
Does your baby like to play games such as Peekaboo?	Social reciprocity	12*	—
Does your baby look for you when a stranger approaches?	Social reciprocity	12, 18	—
When you talk to your baby, does he turn his head, look, or smile?	Social reciprocity	12, 18	—
Does your child respond to her name when you call her?	Social-communication	12, 18, 24	—
When you point at something, does your child look in the direction you are pointing?	Social reciprocity	12, 18, 24	30
Does your child try to show you things? (with point and check-in at later intervals)	Social reciprocity	12, 18, 24	30, 36
Does your child play with objects by pretending? (symbolic in later intervals)*	Social reciprocity	12**, 18, 24	30, 36
Does your baby roll or throw a ball back to you so you can return it to him?**	Social reciprocity	12, 14	—
Does your baby shake his head when he means "no" or "yes?"**	Social-communication	14	—
After you have shown your baby how, does he try to get a toy using a tool?**	Social reciprocity	14, 16, 18	—
Does your child come to you when she needs help?**	Social-communication	16, 18	—
Does your child look at you when you talk to him?	Social-communication	18, 24	30, 36, 48, 60
Does your child do things over and over and get upset when you try to stop her?	Restricted/repetitive patterns	18, 24	30, 36, 48, 60
Does your child let you know how she is feeling with gestures or words?	Social-communication	18, 24	30, 36, 48, 60
Does your child check to make sure you are near when exploring new places?	Social reciprocity	18, 24	30, 36
Does your child like to be around other children?	Social reciprocity	18, 24	—
Does your child copy specific gestures?**	Social reciprocity	20, 22	27, 30
Does your child copy or imitate you and line up blocks? (creating a bridge at later interval)**	Social reciprocity	20, 22, 24	27, 30, 33, 36, 42
Does he put a box on his head, pretending it is a hat?**	Social reciprocity	22, 24	27
Does your child correctly use at least two words such as *me* and *you*?**	Social-communication	22, 24	27

(continued)

Table C.12. *(continued)*

Item content (not exact wording)	ASD related skill/indicator	Intervals for 12–24 months	Intervals for 25–60 months
Does your child greet or say hello to familiar adults?	Social-communication	24	30
After your child watches you draw a line/circle, does your child copy your shape?**	Social reciprocity	—	27, 30, 33, 36, 42
When you point to the figure and ask your child, "What is this?" does your child say a word that means a person?**	Social reciprocity	—	27, 30, 33, 36, 42
Does your child do what you ask him to do?	Social reciprocity	—	30, 36, 48, 60
Does your child move from one activity to the next with little difficulty?	Restricted/repetitive patterns	—	30, 36, 48, 60
Does your child take turns and share when playing with an adult (other children at later intervals)?*	Social reciprocity	—	36**, 42**, 60
Can your child name a friend?*	Social reciprocity	—	36, 48, 54*
Do other children like to play with your child?	Social reciprocity	—	36, 48, 60
Does your child like to play with other children?	Social reciprocity	—	36, 48, 60
Does your child follow rules?	Restricted/repetitive patterns	—	48, 60
Does your child show concern for other people's feelings?	Social reciprocity	—	48, 60
Does your child have simple conversations with you?	Social reciprocity	—	48, 60
Can your child draw a picture of a person/girl/boy?**	Social reciprocity	—	54, 60

Note: No asterisk denotes ASQ:SE-2 item only. *Denotes ASQ-3 and ASQ:SE-2 item. **Denotes ASQ-3 only item. Wording may differ slightly between intervals and across measures. See questionnaires for exact wording.

children. Internal consistency measured by coefficient alpha was found to be high across intervals, ranging from .71 to .90, with an overall alpha of .84. Test–retest reliability, measured as the agreement between two ASQ:SE-2 questionnaires completed by parents at 1 day to 60 days apart was .89. Sensitivity ranged from .78 at 2 months to .84 at 24 months, with .81 overall sensitivity. Specificity of the questionnaires ranged from .76 at 18 months to .98 at 60 months, with .84 overall. Percent agreement between questionnaires and standardized assessments/disability status ranged from .77 at 18 months to .89 at 60 months with overall agreement at .83. The ability of ASQ:SE-2 to detect atypical social-emotional development (sensitivity) was generally less than specificity (i.e., the ability of ASQ:SE-2 to correctly identify typically developing children).

Research is continuing on ASQ:SE-2. Results of ASQ:SE-2 questionnaires completed by parents are being compared with in-depth ASD diagnostic evaluations to study the sensitivity and specificity of ASQ:SE-2 related to identifying young children with ASD. Additional research findings will be posted on the ASQ web site as they become available (www.agesandstages.com).

Table C.13. Parent responses to utility survey items (N = 332)

Question	Percent of parents reporting
1. How long to complete ASQ:SE-2?	
a. Less than 10 minutes	31.3
b. 10–20 minutes	39.5
c. 20–30 minutes	17.2
d. 30 minutes–1 hour	0.3
e. More than 1 hour	0.9
Missing	10.8
2. Was ASQ:SE-2 easy to understand?	
a. Yes	93.1
b. Sometimes	5.4
c. No	0.3
Missing	1.2
3. Were ASQ:SE-2 questions appropriate?	
a. Yes	80.4
b. Sometimes	8.7
c. No	1.2
Missing	9.7
4. The ASQ:SE-2 questionnaires was . . . (check all that apply)	
a. Fun to do	44.9
b. Interesting	62.0
c. Took too long	1.2
d. Helped me think about my child	73.2
e. Waste of time	1.2
f. Didn't tell me much	6.6
5. Would you fill out another ASQ:SE-2?	
a. Yes	94.3
b. No	1.5
Missing	4.2

REFERENCES

Achenbach, T., & Rescorla, L. (2000). *Manual for the ASEBA preschool forms and profiles.* Burlington: University of Vermont, Research Center for Children, Youth, and Families.

Beeber, L., Chazan Cohen, R., Squires, J., Jones Harden, B., Boris, N., Heller, S., & Malik, N. (2007). The early promotion and intervention research consortium (E-PIRC): Five approaches to improving infant/toddler mental health in Early Head Start. *Infant Mental Health Journal, 28*(2), 151–170.

Bricker, D., & Squires, J. (1989). The effectiveness of screening at-risk infants: Infant monitoring questionnaire. *Topics in Early Special Childhood Education, 3*(9), 67–85.

Bricker, D., Squires, J., Twombly, E., Yockelson, S., & Kim, Y. (1996). *Behavior–Ages and Stages Questionnaires.* Unpublished manuscript.

Carter, A., & Briggs-Gowan, M. (2006). *Manual for the Infant-Toddler Social & Emotional Assessment (ITSEA) and Brief-ITSEA (BITSEA).* San Antonio, TX: Psychological Corporation.

DelCarmen-Wiggins, R., & Carter, A. (Eds.). (2004). *Handbook of infant, toddler, and preschool mental health assessment.* New York, NY: Oxford University Press.

Dorans, N.J., & Holland, P.W. (1993). DIF detection and description: Mantel-Haenszel and standardization. In P.W. Holland & H. Wainer (Eds.), *Differential item functioning* (pp. 35–66). Hillsdale, NJ: Lawrence Erlbaum Associates.

Heiman, G. (1992). *Basic statistics for the behavioral sciences.* Boston, MA: Houghton Mifflin.

Krogstad, J., & Cohn, D. (2014). U.S. Census looking at big changes in how it asks about race and ethnicity. Retrieved from Pew Research Center web site: http://www.pewresearch.org/fact-tank/2014/03/14/u-s-census-looking-at-big-changes-in-how-it-asks-about-race-and-ethnicity/

Lord, C., Rutter, M., DiLavore, P., & Risi, S. (2012). *Autism Diagnostic Observation Schedule.* Los Angeles, CA: Western Psychological Services.

Mackrain, M., LeBuffe, P., & Powell, G. (2007) *Devereux Early Childhood Assessment for Infants and Toddlers (DECA-IT).* Lewisville, NC: Kaplan Early Learning.

Printz, P.H., Borg, A., & Demarree, M.A. (2003). *A look at social, emotional, and behavioral screening tools for Head Start and Early Head Start.* Newton, MA: Education Development Center, Center for Children & Families.

Saliva, J., Ysseldyke, J., & Bolt, S. (2012). Assessment. In *Special and inclusive education* (12th ed.). Belmont, CA: Wadsworth.

Spector, P.E. (1992). A consideration of the validity and meaning of self-report measures of job conditions (Paper 567). *Psychology Faculty Publications.* Retrieved from http://scholarcommons.usf.edu/psy_facpub/567

Swets, J.A., & Pickett, R.M. (1982). *Evaluation of diagnostic systems: Methods from signal detection theory.* San Diego, CA: Academic Press.

U.S. Census Bureau. (2010a). *Educational attainment in the United States: 2010—Detailed tables.* Retrieved from http://www.census.gov/hhes/socdemo/education/data/cps/2010/tables.html

U.S. Census Bureau. (2010b). *Overview of race and Hispanic origin: 2010.* Retrieved from http://www.census.gov/prod/cen2010/briefs/c2010br-02.pdf

Whitcomb, S., & Merrell, K. (2013). *Behavioral, social, and emotional assessment of children and adolescents* (4th ed.). New York, NY: Routledge.

D

Letters and Forms

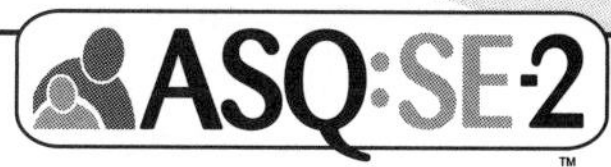

PARENT LETTERS/FORMS (IN ENGLISH)

What Is ASQ:SE-2? Parent Handout
ASQ:SE-2 Parent Welcome Letter
ASQ:SE-2 Consent Form
Demographic Information Sheet
ASQ:SE-2 Questionnaire Parent Cover Letter
ASQ:SE-2 Parent Feedback Letter: Typical
ASQ:SE-2 Parent Feedback Letter: Monitoring
Parent Feedback Survey

PARENT LETTERS/FORMS (IN SPANISH)

What Is ASQ:SE-2? Parent Handout
ASQ:SE-2 Parent Welcome Letter
ASQ:SE-2 Consent Form
Demographic Information Sheet
ASQ:SE-2 Questionnaire Parent Cover Letter
ASQ:SE-2 Parent Feedback Letter: Typical
ASQ:SE-2 Parent Feedback Letter: Monitoring
Parent Feedback Survey

PHYSICIAN/PROFESSIONAL LETTERS (IN ENGLISH)

ASQ:SE-2 Information for Health Care Providers
ASQ:SE-2 Physician Information Letter
ASQ:SE-2 Physician Results Letter

SCREENING/MONITORING PROGRAM FORMS

ASQ:SE-2 Master List (in English)
ASQ:SE-2 Implementation Progress Worksheet (in English)
ASQ:SE-2 Parent Conference Sheet (in English and Spanish)
ASQ:SE-2 Child Monitoring Sheet (in English and Spanish)

This appendix contains photocopiable versions of the sample forms and letters to parents and physicians of children participating in an ASQ:SE-2 screening/monitoring program that are described throughout the User's Guide. To assist program staff working with Spanish-speaking families, this appendix also provides Spanish versions of the sample forms and letters intended for use by parents. The forms and letters intended for use only by physicians and programs have not been translated into Spanish. ASQ:SE-2 purchasers are granted permission to photocopy the blank forms and letters (please see the Photocopying Release on p. xx).

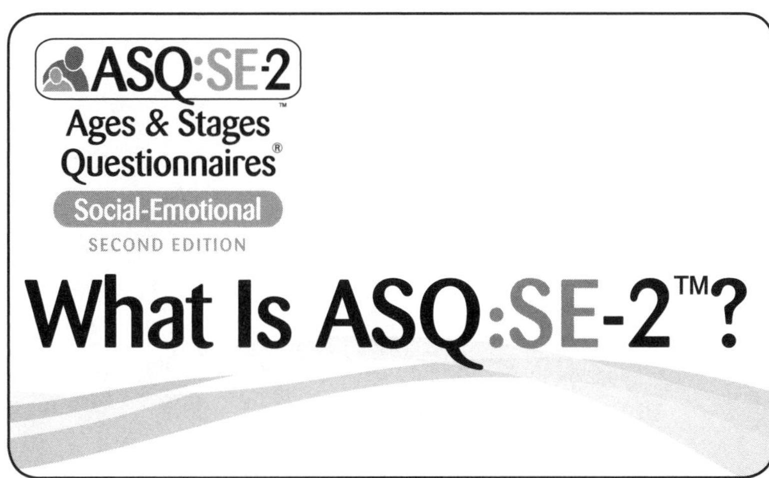

What Is ASQ:SE-2™?

The first 5 years of your child's life are very important. Your child's healthy social-emotional development forms a foundation for lifelong learning. ASQ:SE-2 is a set of questionnaires about behavior and social-emotional development in young children. There are nine questionnaires for different ages to screen children from 1 month to 6 years old.

ASQ:SE has been used by parents for more than 15 years. It makes sure that children's social-emotional development is on schedule. It helps you celebrate milestones while addressing any concerns as early as possible. ASQ:SE-2 can help identify your child's social-emotional strengths and areas where your child may need support.

As a parent or caregiver, you are the best source of information about your child. That's why ASQ:SE-2 is designed for *you* to complete. You will only need 10–15 minutes. It's that quick and easy. Here's how ASQ:SE-2 works:

- Answer each question by marking "often or always," "sometimes," or "rarely or never." Answer based on what you know about your child.
- Note if any behaviors concern you.
- Remember that your answers help show your child's strengths and areas where he or she may need support.
- After you finish, your child's provider will discuss the results with you.

If your child's social-emotional development is on target, then there is nothing more you need to do. If there are concerns, then the provider will help you with next steps. When children get support as early as possible for behavioral concerns, problem behaviors may be prevented from getting more difficult as children get older.

You play an important role in your child's learning and development. Completing ASQ:SE-2 questionnaires helps you make sure your child is off to a great start!

To find out more, please talk to your health care or education professional, or visit www.agesandstages.com.

Dear parent/caregiver:

Welcome to our social-emotional screening and monitoring program! The first 5 years of your child's life are very important. Social-emotional development within the first few years of life prepares your child to be confident, trusting, curious, and able to develop positive relationships with others. Your child's positive social-emotional development forms a foundation for learning throughout life.

As part of this service, we provide the Ages & Stages Questionnaires: Social-Emotional, Second Edition (ASQ:SE-2), to help you keep track of your child's social-emotional development. ASQ:SE-2 asks questions about your child's behaviors and social-emotional growth.

If the questionnaire shows that your child is developing without concerns, we will share some activities that you can do at home to encourage your child's social-emotional development. Then, we will give you a questionnaire every 6 months until your child is 3 years old, and then again at 4 and 5 years old.

If completing this questionnaire brings up any questions or concerns, we can talk about information and resources that can help. Information will be shared with other professionals or agencies only with your written consent.

We look forward to your participation in our program. Please call or e-mail me at any time if you have any questions or would like to discuss any concerns about your child's development.

Sincerely,

Program contact: ______________________________

Program name: ______________________________

Program telephone/e-mail: ______________________________

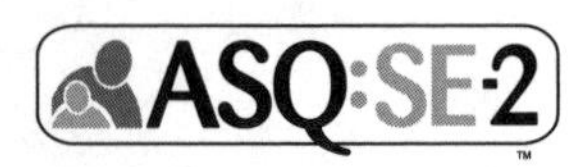

Consent Form

The first 5 years of life are very important. Social-emotional development within the first few years of life prepares your child to be confident, trusting, curious, and able to develop positive relationships with others. Your child's positive social-emotional development forms a foundation for learning throughout life.

Please read the text below and mark the desired space to indicate whether you will participate in the screening/monitoring program.

○ I have read the information provided about the Ages & Stages Questionnaires: Social-Emotional, Second Edition (ASQ:SE-2), and I wish to have my child participate in the screening/monitoring program. I will fill out questionnaires about my child's social-emotional development and will promptly return the completed questionnaires.

○ I do not wish to participate in the screening/monitoring program. I have read the provided information about the Ages & Stages Questionnaires: Social-Emotional, Second Edition (ASQ:SE-2), and understand the purpose of this program.

____

Parent's or guardian's signature

____

Date

Child's name: ______________________________

Child's date of birth: ____________________________

If child was born 3 or more weeks premature, # of weeks premature: ______________

Child's primary physician: ____________________________

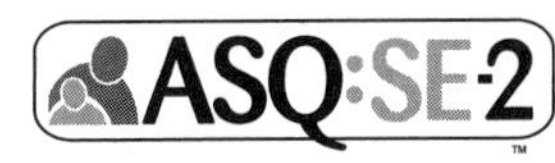

Demographic Information Sheet

Today's date: ______________________________

Child's name (first/middle/last): ______________________________

Child's date of birth (MM/DD/YYYY): ______ / ______ / ______

If child was born premature, # of weeks premature: ______________________________

Child's gender: ○ Male ○ Female

Child's race/ethnicity: ______________________________

Child's birth weight (pounds/ounces): ______________________________

Parent/primary caregiver's name (first/middle/last): ______________________________

Relationship to child: ______________________________

Street address: ______________________________

City: ______________________________

State/province: ____________________ ZIP/postal code: ____________________

Home telephone: ____________________ Work telephone: ____________________

Cell/other telephone: ______________________________

E-mail address: ______________________________

Child's primary language: ______________________________

Language(s) spoken in the home: ______________________________

Child's primary care physician: ______________________________

Clinic/location/practice name: ______________________________

Clinic/practice mailing address: ______________________________

City: ______________________________

State/province: ____________________ ZIP/postal code: ____________________

Telephone: ____________________ Fax: ____________________

E-mail address: ______________________________

Please list any medical conditions that your child has: ______________________________

____

Please list any other agencies that are involved with your child/family:

____

____

Program information

Child ID #: ______________________________

Date of admission to program: ______________________________

Child's adjusted age in months and days (if applicable): ______________________________

Program ID #: ______________________________

Program name: ______________________________

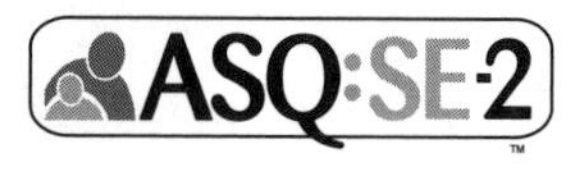

Dear parent/caregiver:

Thank you for participating in our child screening/monitoring program. Enclosed is a questionnaire from the Ages & Stages Questionnaires: Social-Emotional, Second Edition (ASQ:SE-2), which is a screening tool that will provide a quick check of your child's social-emotional development. This questionnaire asks questions about your child's behaviors and social-emotional growth. The information you supply will help reveal your child's strengths, uncover any areas of concern, and determine if there are community resources or services that may be useful for your child or your family. If completing this questionnaire brings up any questions or concerns, we can talk about information and resources that can help.

We'd like to ask you first to fill out the enclosed family information sheet, which helps us be sure we have the most up-to-date information possible. Please keep these tips and directions in mind while completing ASQ:SE-2.

Tips for completing ASQ:SE-2:

- ✓ Caregivers who know the child well and spend more than 15–20 hours per week with the child should complete ASQ:SE-2.
- ✓ Answer based on what you know about your child's behavior.
- ✓ Answer questions based on your child's *usual* behavior, not behavior when your child is sick, very tired, or hungry.

Directions for completing ASQ:SE-2:

1. Please read each question carefully and check the response that best describes your child's behavior:
    - **Often or always:** My child performs this behavior often or always.
    - **Sometimes:** My child sometimes performs this behavior (not consistently).
    - **Rarely or never:** My child rarely performs this behavior or has never performed the behavior.
2. **Concerns:** Check the circle to the right of a question if the behavior is a concern.
3. Some questions have blank spaces for you to provide examples of your child's behavior. Please be sure to explain your response(s).
4. The Overall section at the end of the questionnaire asks open-ended questions about your child's behaviors. Answer questions by marking ***yes*** or ***no*** and provide an explanation for your responses.

Please be sure to send back the questionnaire within 2 weeks. Please contact me if you have any questions or concerns.

Sincerely,

Program contact: ______________________________

Program name: ______________________________

Program telephone/e-mail: ______________________________

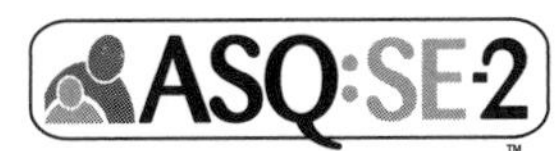

Dear parent/caregiver:

Thank you for completing the recent questionnaire from the Ages & Stages Questionnaires: Social-Emotional, Second Edition (ASQ:SE-2), for your child. Your responses on the questionnaire show that your child's social-emotional development is on schedule at this time.

Enclosed is some general information about social-emotional development specific to your child's age and activities that you can do together with your child to promote his or her social-emotional development.

You'll receive another questionnaire in ____ months. Please remember that it is very important to complete all items and return it as soon as you finish it.

Please call or e-mail us at any time if you have any questions or concerns about your child's behaviors or development. There is a lot of excellent information we can share with you, and resources are available in our community to support you on your parenting journey.

Sincerely,

Program contact: ____

Program name: ____

Program telephone/e-mail: ____________________________________

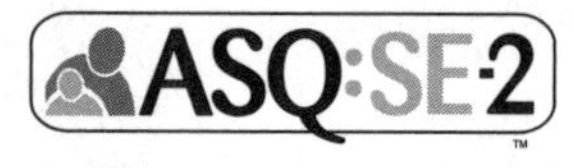

Dear parent/caregiver:

Thank you for completing the recent questionnaire from the Ages & Stages Questionnaires: Social-Emotional, Second Edition (ASQ:SE-2), for your child. Your responses on the questionnaire show that your child's social-emotional development should be monitored for a period of time.

Enclosed is some general information about the social-emotional development of children specific to your child's age and age-appropriate activities that you can do together with your child to promote his or her social-emotional development. Also included is specific information about some of the behaviors for which you have concerns.

We also suggest that you complete another ASQ:SE-2 questionnaire in ____ months. We will contact you with a reminder and send you an ASQ:SE-2 questionnaire at that time.

I will e-mail or call you in the next week to follow up about the concerns you mentioned in the questionnaire. There is a lot of excellent information we can share with you, and resources are available in our community to support you on your parenting journey.

I'm looking forward to talking to you soon.

Sincerely,

Program contact: ______________________________

Program name: ______________________________

Program telephone/e-mail: ______________________________

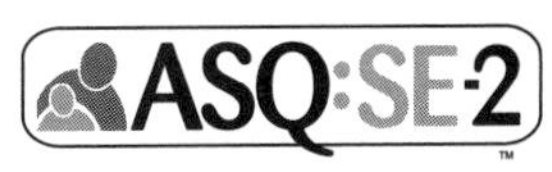

Dear parent/caregiver:

Would you please take a few minutes to evaluate our questionnaires? We appreciate your participation in our program and hope that our services have been helpful to you.

Please circle the number that best expresses your opinion.

1. Approximately how many minutes did it take you to fill out each questionnaire?
   ______ minutes.
   Did you consider this amount of time:

very little time			too much time
1	2	3	4

   Comments:

2. Did the questionnaires help you think about your child's behavior?

very little			very much
1	2	3	4

   Comments:

3. After filling out the questionnaires, did you learn any new things about your child?

very few			very many
1	2	3	4

   Comments:

4. Were any items unclear or difficult to understand?

very few			very many
1	2	3	4

   Comments:

5. Did you enjoy participating in this program?

very little			very much
1	2	3	4

   Comments:

If you have any further comments about the questionnaires, please write them on the back.

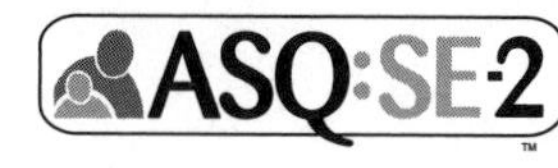

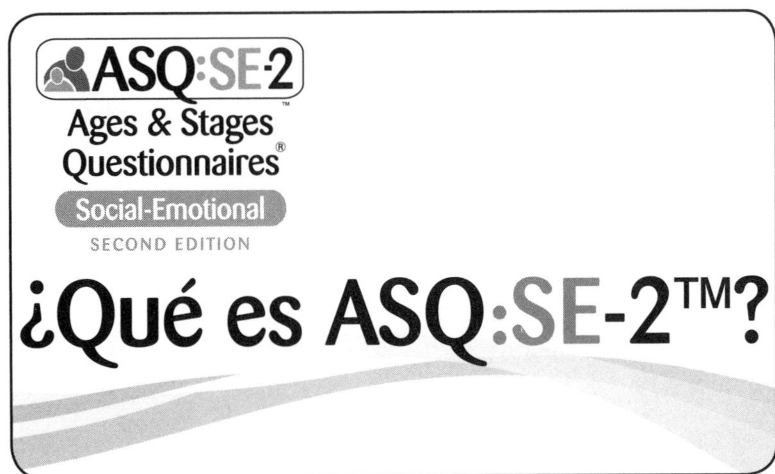

¿Qué es ASQ:SE-2™?

Los primeros 5 años de vida de su hijo/a son muy importantes. Un desarrollo socio-emocional sano en su hijo/a forma las bases del aprendizaje para toda la vida. El ASQ:SE-2 es una serie de cuestionarios para evaluar el comportamiento y el desarrollo socio-emocional de niños en su primera infancia. Hay nueve cuestionarios que cubren diferentes etapas para evaluar a los niños desde que tienen 1 mes de edad a los 6 años.

El ASQ:SE ha sido usado por padres y madres de familia por más de 15 años. Esta herramienta nos ayuda a asegurarnos de que el desarrollo socio-emocional de los niños se esté dando dentro de las expectativas. Le ayuda a usted a celebrar los logros que su hijo/a tiene en su desarrollo, así como a abordar cualquier preocupación que exista lo más pronto posible. El ASQ:SE-2 puede ayudarle a identificar cuáles son las fortalezas socio-emocionales de su hijo/a y cuáles son las áreas en las que podría necesitar más apoyo.

Como padre/madre o persona a cargo de un niño, usted es la mejor fuente de información sobre su hijo/a. Por esta razón, el ASQ:SE-2 ha sido diseñado para que usted lo conteste. Solamente necesitará 10–15 minutos para completarlo; es así de fácil. Esta es la manera en la que el ASQ:SE-2 funciona:

- Conteste cada pregunta marcando "a menudo o siempre", "a veces" o "rara vez o nunca". Conteste las preguntas basándose en lo que usted sabe sobre su hijo/a.
- Anote cualquier comportamiento que le preocupe.
- Recuerde que sus respuestas le ayudarán a saber cuáles son las fortalezas de su hijo/a y cuáles son las áreas en las que podría necesitar más apoyo.
- Una vez que termine, un profesional (ya sea el médico, maestro de su hijo/a u otra persona), hablará de los resultados con usted.

Si el desarrollo socio-emocional de su hijo/a está dentro de las expectativas, entonces usted no tiene que hacer nada más. Sin embargo, si existe alguna preocupación, un profesional le ayudará a saber qué pasos tomar para ayudar a su niño/a. Cuando los niños reciben apoyo lo más pronto posible en las áreas de desarrollo que nos preocupan, esta acción ayuda a que el comportamiento problemático no se agudice o se haga más difícil conforme va creciendo.

Usted cumple un rol muy importante en el desarrollo y aprendizaje de su hijo/a. ¡Al contestar los cuestionarios ASQ:SE-2, usted se asegura de que su hijo/a tenga el mejor comienzo posible!

Para más información, hable con un profesional de salud, con un especialista en educación, o visite el sitio Internet www.agesandstages.com.

Estimados padres de familia o guardián:

¡Bienvenidos a nuestro programa de evaluación y monitoreo socio-emocional! Los primeros 5 años de vida son muy importantes para su hijo/a. Un desarrollo socio-emocional sano en los primeros 5 años de vida preparará a su hijo/a a tener confianza en sí mismo/a y en otros, a tener curiosidad por conocer el mundo que lo/la rodea, así como a desarrollar relaciones positivas con otras personas. Un desarrollo socio-emocional positivo formará las bases del aprendizaje para el resto de su vida.

Como parte de este servicio, le ofrecemos los Ages & Stages Questionnaires: Social-Emotional, Second Edition (ASQ:SE-2), para ayudarle a llevar un registro del desarrollo socio-emocional de su niño/a. Los cuestionarios ASQ:SE-2 contienen preguntas sobre el comportamiento y crecimiento socio-emocional de su niño/a.

Si los resultados de un cuestionario muestran que su hijo/a se está desarrollando dentro de las expectativas, compartiremos con usted unas actividades que puede hacer en la casa para seguir fomentando un desarrollo socio-emocional sano en él/ella. Después le ofreceremos un cuestionario cada 6 meses hasta que su hijo/a cumpla 3 años, y nuevamente cuando cumpla 4 y 5 años.

Si surgen preguntas o preocupaciones al completar estos cuestionarios, podemos hablar con usted sobre los recursos disponibles y darle información que le podría ayudar. La información que usted nos proporciona solamente se compartirá con otros profesionales y agencias si usted nos da su consentimiento por escrito.

Nos da mucho gusto que usted haya elegido participar en nuestro programa. No dude en llamarme o mandarme un correo electrónico en cualquier momento si tiene preguntas o si le gustaría hablar conmigo sobre cualquier preocupación que tenga sobre el desarrollo de su hijo/a.

Cordialmente,

Nombre de la persona del programa que lo/la ayuda: ______________________________

Nombre del programa: ______________________________

Teléfono/correo electrónico del programa: ______________________________

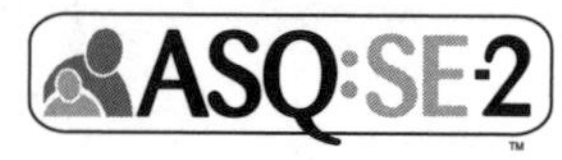

Hoja de autorización

Los primeros 5 años de vida son muy importantes para su hijo/a. Un desarrollo socio-emocional sano en los primeros 5 años de vida preparará a su niño/a a tener confianza en sí mismo/a y en otros, a tener curiosidad, así como a desarrollar relaciones positivas con otras personas. Un desarrollo socio-emocional positivo formará las bases del aprendizaje para el resto de su vida.

Favor de leer los siguientes párrafos y marcar el que corresponda para indicar si usted acepta participar en el programa de evaluación/monitoreo.

○ He leído la información provista sobre los Ages & Stages Questionnaires: Social-Emotional, Second Edition (ASQ:SE-2), y deseo que mi hijo/a participe en el programa de evaluación/monitoreo. Completaré los cuestionarios sobre el desarrollo socio-emocional de mi hijo/a y los devolveré al programa lo más pronto que pueda.

○ No deseo participar en el programa de evaluación/monitoreo. He leído la información provista sobre los Ages & Stages Questionnaires: Social-Emotional, Second Edition (ASQ:SE-2) y entiendo el propósito de este programa.

____

Firma del padre/madre o guardián

____

Fecha

Nombre del niño/a: ______________________________

Fecha de nacimiento del niño/a: ______________________________

Si nació 3 semanas o más antes de la fecha proyectada, # de semanas que se adelantó:

____

Médico familiar del niño/a: ______________________________

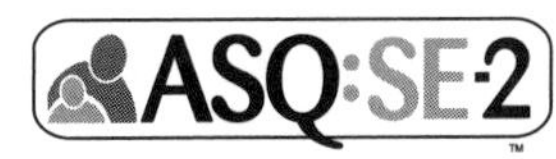

Hoja de información demográfica

Fecha de hoy: ______________________________

Nombre del niño/a (primero/segundo/apellidos): ______________________________

Fecha de nacimiento del niño/a (DD/MM/AAAA): ______ / ______ / ______

Si el niño/a nació prematuro, número de semanas que se adelantó: ______________________________

Sexo del niño/a: ○ Masculino ○ Femenino

Origen étnico o racial del niño/a: ______________________________

Peso del niño/a al nacer (libras/onzas): ______________________________

Nombre del padre/madre o adulto a cargo (primero/segundo/appellidos): ______________________________

Parentesco con el niño/a: ______________________________

Dirreción: ______________________________

Ciudad: ______________________________

Estado/provincia: ______________________________ ZIP/código postal: ______________________________

Teléfono de casa: ______________________________ Teléfono de trabajo: ______________________________

Teléfono celular/otro número: ______________________________

Dirección de correo electrónico: ______________________________

Idioma principal del niño: ______________________________

Idioma(s) que se habla(n) en casa: ______________________________

Nombre del médico familiar del niño/a: ______________________________

Nombre de la clínica o consultorio: ______________________________

Dirección de la clínica o consultorio: ______________________________

Ciudad: ______________________________

Estado/provincia: ______________________________ ZIP/código postal: ______________________________

Teléfono: ______________________________ Fax: ______________________________

Dirección de correo electrónico: ______________________________

Favor de anotar cualquier condición médica que tenga su hijo/a: ______________________________

____

Favor de escribir el nombre de cualquier otra agencia al servicio del niño/la familia:

____

____

Información del programa

de identificación del niño: ______________________________

Fecha de ingreso al programa: ______________________________

Edad ajustada del niño en meses y días (si corresponde): ______________________________

de identificación del programa: ______________________________

Nombre del programa: ______________________________

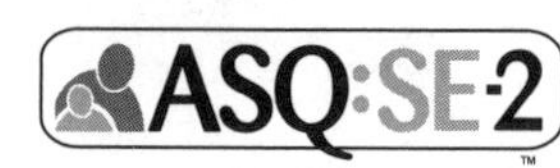

Estimados padres de familia o guardián:

Gracias por participar en nuestro programa de evaluación/monitoreo de desarrollo infantil. El cuestionario que usted encontrará adjunto es parte de la serie Ages & Stages Questionnaires: Social-Emotional, Second Edition (ASQ:SE-2), la cual es una herramienta de evaluación que le permitirá comprobar de manera rápida y fácil el desarrollo socio-emocional de su hijo/a. Este cuestionario contiene preguntas sobre el comportamiento y crecimiento socio-emocional de su hijo/a. La información que usted provea ayudará a detectar las áreas de fortaleza de su hijo/a, revelará si existen áreas que podrían ser motivo de preocupación y nos ayudará a determinar si existen recursos o servicios en su comunidad que podrían ser útiles para su hijo/a y su familia. Si surge alguna pregunta o preocupación al completar este cuestionario, podemos hablar con usted sobre los recursos disponibles y darle información que le podría ayudar.

Le pedimos que por favor complete primero la hoja de información sobre la familia, para asegurarnos de que los datos de nuestros archivos estén actualizados. Favor de ver las sugerencias que le damos a continuación antes de completar el cuestionario ASQ:SE-2.

Sugerencias para completar el ASQ:SE-2:

✓ Solamente las personas que cuidan al niño/a, que lo conocen bien y que pasan más de 15–20 horas por semana con él/ella deben completar un ASQ:SE-2.
✓ Para las preguntas que no sean específicas, favor de contestarlas basándose en lo que usted sabe sobre el comportamiento de su niño/a.
✓ Conteste las preguntas basándose en el comportamiento que su niño/a muestra comúnmente y no en el comportamiento que tiene cuando está enfermo/a, muy cansado/a o con hambre.

Instrucciones para completar el ASQ:SE-2:

1. Favor de leer cada pregunta con cuidado y marcar la respuesta que mejor describa el comportamiento de su niño/a:
    - **A menudo o siempre:** Mi niño/a muestra este comportamiento a menudo o siempre.
    - **A veces:** Mi niño/a muestra este comportamiento a veces (pero no con frecuencia).
    - **Rara vez o nunca:** Mi niño/a muestra este comportamiento en raras ocasiones o nunca lo ha mostrado.
2. **Preocupaciones:** Marque el círculo ubicado a la derecha de cada pregunta si el comportamiento es un motivo de preocupación para usted.
3. Algunas preguntas tendrán espacios en blanco para que usted nos dé ejemplos del comportamiento de su niño/a. Favor de explicar su(s) respuesta(s).
4. La sección de Observaciones generales al final del cuestionario contiene preguntas abiertas sobre el comportamiento de su niño/a. Conteste las preguntas marcando ***sí*** o ***no*** y dé una explicación para cada respuesta.

Favor de devolvernos este cuestionario a más tardar 2 semanas después de la fecha en que lo recibió. No dude en ponerse en contacto con nosotros para tratar cualquier pregunta o preocupación.

Cordialmente,

Nombre de la persona del programa que lo/la ayuda: ______________________

Nombre del programa: ______________________

Teléfono/correo electrónico del programa: ______________________

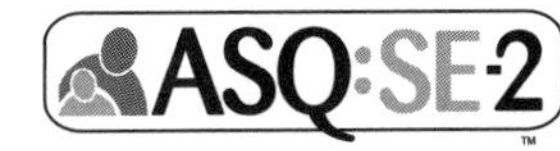

Estimados padres de familia o guardián:

Gracias por completar y devolver el cuestionario reciente de los Ages & Stages Questionnaires: Social-Emotional, Second Edition (ASQ:SE-2), sobre su hijo/a. Sus respuestas en el cuestionario indican que hasta ahora el desarrollo socio-emocional de su hijo/a se encuentra dentro de las expectativas.

Adjunto usted encontrará información general sobre el desarrollo socio-emocional de los niños de la edad de su hijo/a, así como actividades que pueden hacer juntos/as para seguir fomentando un desarrollo socio-emocional sano en él/ella.

Recibirá otro cuestionario en _____ meses. Recuerde que es muy importante contestar cada pregunta y devolver el cuestionario tan pronto como lo termine.

Por favor, no dude en llamarnos o mandarnos un correo electrónico si le surge cualquier pregunta o preocupación sobre el comportamiento de su hijo/a. Tenemos acceso a mucha información excelente que podemos compartir con usted, así como recursos en nuestra comunidad que le pueden ayudar a lo largo del proceso de criar a su hijo/a.

Cordialmente,

Nombre de la persona del programa que lo/la ayuda: ______________________________

Nombre del programa: ____

Teléfono/correo electrónico del programa: ___________________________________

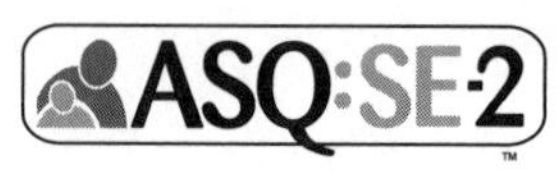

Estimados padres de familia o guardián:

Gracias por completar y devolver el cuestionario reciente de los Ages & Stages Questionnaires: Social-Emotional, Second Edition (ASQ:SE-2), sobre su hijo/a. Las respuestas que dio en el cuestionario indican que se debe monitorear el comportamiento socio-emocional de su hijo/a por un tiempo.

En este sobre, usted encontrará información general sobre el desarrollo socio-emocional de los niños de la edad de su hijo/a, así como actividades que pueden hacer juntos/as para promover un desarrollo socio-emocional sano en él/ella. También hemos incluido información específica sobre los comportamientos que usted marcó como motivo de preocupación.

Le sugerimos que complete otro cuestionario ASQ:SE-2 en ____ meses. Nos pondremos en contacto con usted para recordárselo y le mandaremos otro cuestionario ASQ:SE-2.

Dentro de esta semana le mandaré un correo electrónico o lo/la llamaré por teléfono para hablar sobre las preocupaciones que usted mencionó en el cuestionario. Tenemos acceso a mucha información excelente que podemos compartir con usted, así como recursos en nuestra comunidad que le pueden ayudar a lo largo del proceso de criar a su hijo/a.

Con gusto, quedo a la espera de hablar con usted.

Cordialmente,

Nombre de la persona del programa que lo/la ayuda: ______________________________

Nombre del programa: ____

Teléfono/correo electrónico del programa: ____

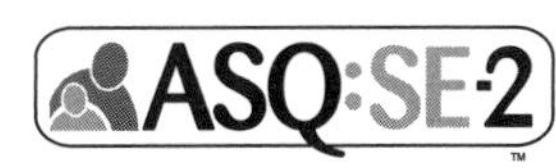

Estimados padres de familia o guardián:

¿Sería tan amable de tomar unos momentitos para evaluar nuestros cuestionarios? Le agradecemos su participación en el programa y esperamos que nuestros servicios le hayan sido de ayuda.

Favor de trazar un círculo alrededor del número que mejor expresa su opinión.

1. Aproximadamente, ¿cuántos minutos tardó en completar cada cuestionario?
   ______ minutos.
   ¿Le pareció que esto fue . . . ?

muy poco tiempo			demasiado tiempo
1	2	3	4

   Comentarios:

2. ¿El completar los cuestionarios le ayudó a pensar en el comportamiento de su hijo/a?

muy poco			mucho
1	2	3	4

   Comentarios:

3. Después de completar los cuestionarios, ¿se dio cuenta de algún comportamiento o cualidad de su hijo/a que no había notado anteriormente?

muy pocas cosas			muchas cosas
1	2	3	4

   Comentarios:

4. ¿Había preguntas que le parecieron difíciles de entender?

muy pocas			muchas
1	2	3	4

   Comentarios:

5. ¿Disfrutó de la experiencia de participar en el programa?

muy poco			mucho
1	2	3	4

   Comentarios:

Si usted tiene comentarios adicionales sobre los cuestionarios, favor de escribirlos al dorso.

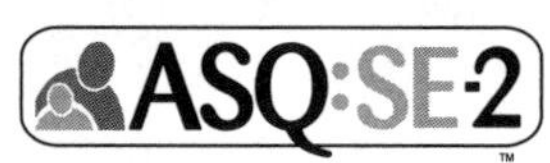

ASQ:SE-2 Information for Health Care Providers

The Ages & Stages Questionnaires: Social-Emotional, Second Edition (ASQ:SE-2), is a series of nine parent-completed questionnaires for screening children from 1 month to 6 years of age. ASQ:SE-2 assists with monitoring children's social-emotional development and identifying potential social or emotional issues. ASQ:SE-2 is a companion tool to the Ages & Stages Questionnaires, Third Edition (ASQ-3), which is designed to screen children's developmental skills.

ASQ:SE-2 CUTOFF GUIDANCE

There are three possible ASQ:SE-2 results based on the child's total score in relation to the cutoff. These are indicated as follows in the score interpretation section of the ASQ:SE-2 Information Summary:

- ***The child's total score is in the dark area. It is above the cutoff. Further assessment with a professional may be needed.*** A total score that is *above the cutoff* indicates a need for further evaluation and/or additional follow-up actions. This "refer" area on the scoring graphic is above the statistically derived cutoff score.
- ***The child's score is in the lightly shaded area. It is close to the cutoff. Review behaviors of concern and monitor.*** A total score in the lightly shaded area, called the *monitoring zone,* indicates a need for monitoring and may require follow-up actions for items of concern. The "monitor" area on the scoring graphic identifies children whose performance falls close to the cutoff score. *Note:* If the child being screened is a girl, consider a referral for further evaluation if her score is in the monitoring zone. Data collected in the renorming of ASQ:SE-2 indicated that girls' total scores overall were lower than boys.
- ***The child's total score is in the white area. It is below the cutoff. Social-emotional development appears to be on schedule.*** If there are no concerns about the child's behavior, a total score *below the cutoff* indicates that the child's social-emotional development is on schedule at this time. This is the "low or no risk" area on the scoring graphic.

ADDITIONAL RECOMMENDATIONS

Please carefully review the following important recommendations and considerations.

- This screening tool should be used in a preventive manner. For children whose ASQ:SE-2 scores are above cutoffs, respond immediately rather than waiting to see if children's social-emotional skills improve over time. Consider saying, "It's best not to wait. Let's play it safe and make a referral now."
- High scores on ASQ:SE-2 do not necessarily indicate a mental health diagnosis or eligibility for early intervention/early childhood special education (EI/ECSE) services. Carefully review with a child's parent or other primary caregiver a score above the cutoff, regardless of diagnoses or eligibility.
- Pay close attention to individual item scores of 10 points (indicated with an *X* beside the item response box) or 15 points (an *X* combined with a parent's checked concern for that item).
- When discussing concerns with caregivers, avoid using terms that may provoke anxiety, such as *abnormal* or *atypical*. Use phrases such as *above the cutoff* or *monitoring zone* when discussing results with concerns. The ASQ:SE-2 developers—and many health care providers—suggest a direct conversation with caregivers, ideally face to face, about any behavioral concerns.

(continued)

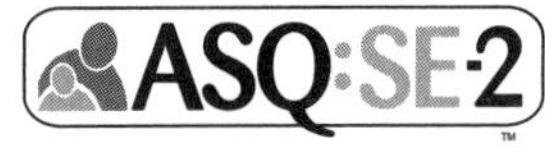

- Thoughtfully interpret ASQ:SE-2 results in combination with ongoing developmental-behavioral surveillance. It is important to
    - Elicit and address caregivers' concerns (e.g., "Can you tell me more about . . . ?")
    - Review the child's developmental milestones or ASQ-3 results over time
    - Consider pertinent biological factors (e.g., prematurity, low birth weight, in utero drug exposure), environmental risks (e.g., parental depression/anxiety, parental drug abuse, exposure to domestic violence), and protective/resiliency factors
    - Carefully observe parent–child interactions during the physical exam
    - Make observations while promoting healthy development and behavior (e.g., literacy promotion and other anticipatory guidance as recommended by the American Academy of Pediatrics)
- Be sure to interpret and make decisions about ASQ:SE-2 results with consideration to families' cultural contexts. Family expectations about behavior and child development may differ from those of professionals. In general, when parents complete ASQ:SE-2, the item responses should reflect the parents' beliefs, expectations, and concerns about their children. It is important to actively involve caregivers in any decision making to determine what next steps, if any, should be taken.
- The health care provider's ongoing surveillance decisions should *not* override the caregiver's concerns, or results above the cutoff, and thereby negate the need for parent-centered learning activities, a community-based referral, or other interventions.
- Recognize that there are many different actions that can be taken if ASQ:SE-2 scores are high or there are parent concerns. Examples include referrals to the following: the local EI/ECSE agency, an early childhood mental health provider or program, a multispecialty comprehensive evaluation, an evidence-based parenting program, family counseling, and in-office parent education/anticipatory guidance. When concerns arise, ongoing surveillance (or a care coordinator/patient navigator) should be used to work with the parent to determine the most effective next steps.
- Cross-sector collaboration and care coordination between health care providers and community-based agencies and other early childhood disciplines may be necessary to swiftly link children who are at risk and their families to a wide assortment of community resources.

BACKGROUND INFORMATION ON ASQ:SE-2

Normative data for ASQ:SE-2 were established based on a nationwide sample of more than 14,000 children. Research conducted on the validity of ASQ:SE-2 compared results with other parent-completed diagnostic measures, such as the Child Behavior Checklist, and/or a child's medical or behavior-related diagnoses (e.g., autism spectrum disorder, attention-deficit/hyperactivity disorder, anxiety disorder, oppositional defiant disorder).

The distribution of scores on this tool was positively skewed. For example, the 48 month questionnaire had a range of scores from 0 to 350—a median of 45. Cutoffs for questionnaires were determined using a statistical procedure (i.e., receiver operating characteristic curves) for nonnormal distributions.

Visit www.agesandstages.com for more information about ASQ:SE-2, including the technical report.

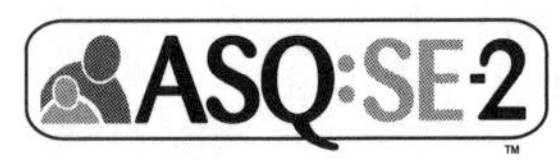

Dear physician or medical practitioner:

The parents or guardians of your patient, ________________________, have agreed to complete the Ages & Stages Questionnaires: Social-Emotional, Second Edition (ASQ:SE-2), as part of our screening/monitoring program. The purpose of this program is to monitor children's social-emotional development, refer as indicated by results, and provide support to caregivers when social-emotional/behavioral concerns are identified.

ASQ:SE-2—a series of nine parent-completed questionnaires for children from 1 month to 72 months (6 years) of age—screens children's social-emotional development and identifies potential social-emotional issues. ASQ:SE-2 is a companion tool to the Ages & Stages Questionnaires, Third Edition (ASQ-3), which is designed to screen children's developmental skills/milestones periodically over time.

Parents or guardians are asked at repeated intervals to respond to questions about their child's social-emotional behaviors. If the child obtains a score above an established cutoff point on a questionnaire, the parents/guardians and you will be notified so that further behavioral evaluation can be scheduled. More information on use of ASQ:SE-2 in a medical setting can be found at www.agesandstages.com.

Please contact me if you would like more information about this program.

Sincerely,

Program contact: ____

Program name: ____

Program telephone/e-mail: ______________________________________

Child's name: ____

Child's date of birth: ____

Parent/caregiver name(s): ______________________________________

ASQ:SE-2

Dear physician or medical practitioner:

Ages & Stages Questionnaires: Social-Emotional, Second Edition (ASQ:SE-2), is a series of nine parent-completed questionnaires developed for screening children from 1 month to 72 months (6 years). ASQ:SE-2 helps monitor children's social-emotional development and identify potential social-emotional/behavioral issues. ASQ:SE-2 is a companion tool to Ages & Stages Questionnaires, Third Edition (ASQ-3), which is designed to screen children's developmental skills/milestones. More information on use of ASQ:SE-2 in a medical setting can be found at www.agesandstages.com.

An ASQ:SE-2 questionnaire was recently completed for your patient as follows:

Child's name: ______________________________

Child's date of birth: ______________________________

Date completed: ______________________________

Questionnaire completed by: ______________________________

A copy of the ASQ:SE-2 Information Summary sheet is provided for your records.

The checked box below provides a brief summary of the results of that questionnaire:

☐ The child's ASQ:SE-2 score is **below the established cutoff,** indicating social-emotional development appears to be on schedule at this time.

☐ The child's ASQ:SE-2 score is **close to the established cutoff** (within the monitoring zone). We have provided information to the family and will monitor the child's development.

☐ The child's ASQ:SE-2 score is **above the established cutoff,** indicating a need for further social-emotional/behavioral evaluation. We have discussed referral options with the family.

The checked box below indicates the needed follow-up action:

☐ **No follow-up action needed.**

☐ **Follow-up action needed.** Attached is the completed ASQ:SE-2 with specific behavioral concerns highlighted. We hope you can discuss these concerns with the caregiver during the child's upcoming appointment to help the family determine the most effective next steps.

Please contact me if you have any questions.

Sincerely,

Program contact: ______________________________

Screening program name: ______________________________

Program telephone/e-mail: ______________________________

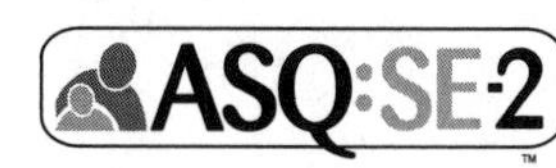

ASQ:SE-2 Master List

Program name/site: ____________________

Child's name	Child ID #	Parent consent on file	Demographic Information Sheet	Physician Information Letter	2 month ASQ:SE-2	6 month ASQ:SE-2	12 month ASQ:SE-2	18 month ASQ:SE-2	24 month ASQ:SE-2	30 month ASQ:SE-2	36 month ASQ:SE-2	48 month ASQ:SE-2	60 month ASQ:SE-2

Instructions: After filling in the program name and site, program staff should be diligent in keeping the ASQ:SE-2 Master List up-to-date. Every child who is participating in the program should be listed by name and ID number on this form or on one like it. In the spaces provided next to the child's name, record the date(s) any item in the top row was completed. For the questionnaires, program staff may also want to note an *S* after the date for a Spanish questionnaire or *IC* for a questionnaire that was returned incomplete and therefore could not be scored. Programs that use the ASQ Online management system (ASQ Pro, ASQ Enterprise) do not need to maintain an ASQ:SE-2 Master List on paper (the information is stored in the online system instead).

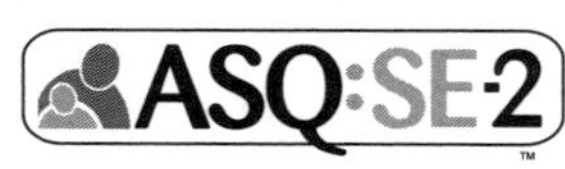

ASQ:SE-2 Implementation Progress Worksheet

Program name/site: ______________________________

Use the following scale for progress rating(s): 0 = not applicable; 1 = not begun; 2 = partially begun or implemented; 3 = fully completed or implemented.

Tasks	Actions								
	Personnel needs	Information needs	Supplies and equipment needs	Person/agency responsible	Projected completion date	Progress rating			
Phase I: Planning the screening/monitoring program									
1. Communicate with community partners.									
2. Include parent perspectives.									
3. Involve health and mental health providers.									
4. Determine target population.									
5. Finalize goals and objectives.									
6. Determine program resources.									
7. Determine administration methods and settings.									
8. Determine depth and breadth of program.									
9. Select referral criteria.									

(continued)

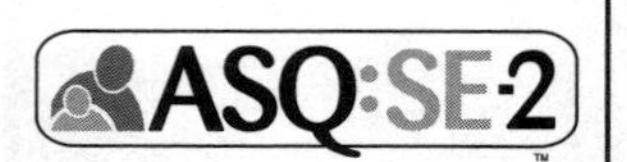

ASQ:SE-2 Implementation Progress Worksheet *(continued)*

Tasks	Actions								
	Personnel needs	Information needs	Supplies and equipment needs	Person/agency responsible	Projected completion date	Progress rating			
Phase II: Preparing, organizing, and managing the screening/monitoring program									
10. Create a management system.									
11. Prepare questionnaires.									
12. Develop forms, letters, and a referral guide.									
13. Articulate screening policies and procedures.									
14. Provide staff training and support.									
Phase III: Administering and scoring ASQ:SE-2 and following up									
15. Select the appropriate ASQ:SE-2 age interval.									
16. Support parent completion of ASQ:SE-2.									
17. Score ASQ:SE-2.									
18. Review written comments on scored and unscored sections of ASQ:SE-2.									
19. Interpret ASQ:SE-2 score.									
20. Communicate results with families.									
21. Determine appropriate follow-up.									
Phase IV: Evaluating the screening/monitoring program									
22. Assess progress in establishing and maintaining the screening/monitoring program.									
23. Evaluate the program's effectiveness.									

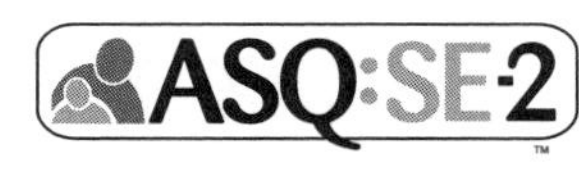

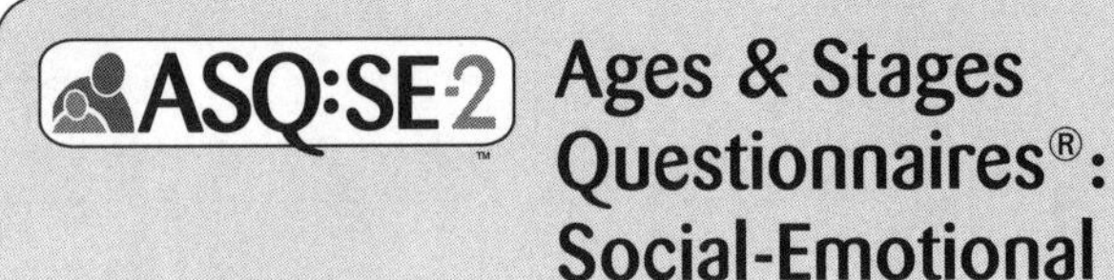

Parent Conference Sheet

Child's name: ______________________

Date of birth: ______________________

Date ASQ:SE-2 completed: ______________________

Child's age at screening (months/days): ______________________

ASQ:SE-2 questionnaire administered: ______________________

Date of conference: ______________________

Parent or caregiver attending: ______________________

Person conducting conference: ______________________

Others at conference: ______________________

____

CONFERENCE GOALS: The goal of this conference is to share results of ASQ:SE-2 with you and provide an opportunity to discuss your child's social-emotional development. Please let us know if you have additional goals for this meeting.

CHILD'S STRENGTHS: We will discuss your child's areas of strength identified through ASQ:SE-2 and shared by you and other team members.

BEHAVIORS OF CONCERN AND FOLLOW-UP CONSIDERATIONS: If there are behaviors of concern for you or other caregivers, then we will discuss factors that may affect your child's behavior. For example, we can talk about when, where, and with whom the behaviors are happening. We can also discuss your child's overall health and development.

FOLLOW-UP ACTION TAKEN: We will discuss the next steps (marked below) based on your child's ASQ:SE-2:

______ Try the activities provided and complete another ASQ:SE-2 in ________ months.
______ Share your child's ASQ:SE-2 results with his or her primary health care provider.
______ Refer your child to his or her primary health care provider for the following reason: ______________________
______ Contact the following community agency for information on parenting groups or other support.
List contact information here: ______________________
______ Have another caregiver complete ASQ:SE-2. Please bring results to next meeting.
List caregiver here (e.g., grandparent, teacher): ______________________
______ Complete a developmental screening for your child (e.g., ASQ-3).
______ Refer your child to early intervention/early childhood special education for further assessment.
List contact information here: ______________________
______ Refer your child for social-emotional, behavioral, or mental health evaluation.
List contact information here: ______________________
______ Other: ______________________

NOTES:

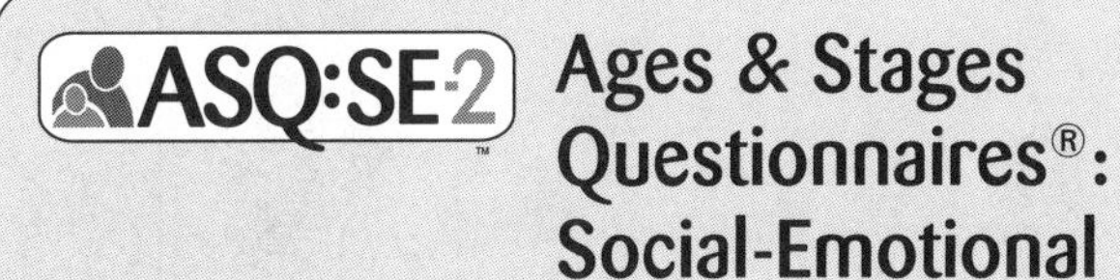

Hoja para la reunión con los padres

Nombre del niño/a: ______________________________

Fecha de nacimiento: ______________________________

Fecha en que se completó el ASQ:SE-2: ______________

Edad del niño/a cuando se completó el ASQ:SE-2 (meses y días): ______________________

Etapa del cuestionario ASQ:SE-2 que se usó: __________

Fecha de la reunión: ______________________________

El padre/madre o la persona que asiste a la reunión: ______________________________

La persona a cargo de la reunión: ______________

Otra(s) persona(s) en la reunión: ______________

____

____

OBJETIVOS DE LA REUNIÓN: El propósito de esta reunión es compartir con usted los resultados del ASQ:SE-2 y ofrecerle la oportunidad de hablar con nosotros acerca del desarrollo socio-emocional de su hijo/a. Le pedimos que nos avise si usted tiene objetivos adicionales para esta reunión.

FORTALEZAS DE SU HIJO/A: Hablaremos de las fortalezas de su hijo/a que fueron identificadas por medio de la evaluación ASQ:SE-2, tanto de las que usted identificó como de las que mencionaron otros miembros del equipo profesiona.

MOTIVOS DE PREOCUPACIÓN Y PROCESO DE SEGUIMIENTO: En el caso de que su hijo/a demuestre algún comportamiento que sea motivo de preocupación para usted o para las otras personas a cargo de él/ella, podremos hablar de los factores que puedan estar afectando su comportamiento. Por ejemplo, podremos hablar de cuándo, dónde y con quién(es) suelen ocurrir estos comportamientos, así como de la salud y del desarrollo de su hijo/a en términos generales.

SEGUIMIENTO: Hablaremos de los próximos pasos a seguir (señalados abajo) basándonos en los resultados del ASQ:SE-2 de su hijo/a:

______ Intentar las actividades infantiles provistas y completar otro cuestionario ASQ:SE-2 en ________ meses.

______ Compartir los resultados del ASQ:SE-2 con su proveedor/a de salud primario.

______ Referir a su hijo/a a su proveedor/a de salud primario por el siguiente motivo: ______________

______ Contactar a esta agencia de la comunidad para conseguir información sobre grupos de apoyo para padres u otras formas de asistencia. Anote la información de contacto aquí: ______________

______ Pedirle a otra de las personas a cargo de su hijo/a (por ej., abuelo, maestra) que complete el cuestionario ASQ:SE-2. Por favor traiga los resultados a nuestra próxima reunión. Anote el nombre de la persona aquí: ______________

______ Completar una evaluación de desarrollo infantil (por. ej., ASQ-3).

______ Referir a su hijo/a a un programa de intervención temprana/educación especial en la primera infancia para hacerle una evaluación adicional. Anote la información de contacto aquí: ______________

______ Referir a su hijo/a para que le hagan una evaluación socio-emocional, de comportamiento o de salud mental. Anote la información de contacto aquí: ______________

______ Otro: ______________

NOTAS:

Child Monitoring Sheet

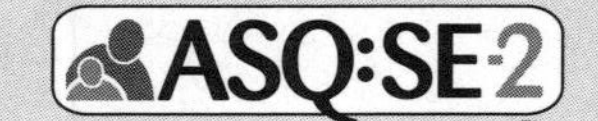

Child's name: ______________ Date of birth: ______________ Child ID #: ______________ Child gender: ○ Male ○ Female

Instructions: You may use this form to track a child's ASQ:SE-2 screening results over time. Write the date the ASQ:SE-2 was administered at the top of each column.

1. Mark the bubble that corresponds with the ASQ:SE-2 result (refer to the completed ASQ:SE-2 Information Summary). If a score is below the monitoring zone, mark the bubble for "Well Below." If a score is within the monitoring zone, mark "Monitor." If a score is above the cutoff, mark "Above."
2. Indicate the total number of scored items that the caregiver marked as a Concern.
3. Mark "Yes" or "No" to indicate whether there were items of Concern in the Overall section and whether there was a parent conference.
4. Record any follow-up action or notes.
5. **Optional:** Calculate an average item score* by dividing the ASQ:SE-2 total score by the number of answered scored items. (See page 117 of the *ASQ:SE-2 User's Guide* for more information.)

	ASQ:SE-2 **2 month** Date given ______	ASQ:SE-2 **6 month** Date given ______	ASQ:SE-2 **12 month** Date given ______	ASQ:SE-2 **18 month** Date given ______	ASQ:SE-2 **24 month** Date given ______	ASQ:SE-2 **30 month** Date given ______	ASQ:SE-2 **36 month** Date given ______	ASQ:SE-2 **48 month** Date given ______	ASQ:SE-2 **60 month** Date given ______
ASQ:SE-2 total score	○ Above ○ Monitor ○ Well Below	○ Above ○ Monitor ○ Well Below	○ Above ○ Monitor ○ Well Below	○ Above ○ Monitor ○ Well Below	○ Above ○ Monitor ○ Well Below	○ Above ○ Monitor ○ Well Below	○ Above ○ Monitor ○ Well Below	○ Above ○ Monitor ○ Well Below	○ Above ○ Monitor ○ Well Below
Number of scored items with Concern checked									
Overall concerns indicated	○ Yes ○ No	○ Yes ○ No	○ Yes ○ No	○ Yes ○ No	○ Yes ○ No	○ Yes ○ No	○ Yes ○ No	○ Yes ○ No	○ Yes ○ No
Parent conference	○ Yes ○ No	○ Yes ○ No	○ Yes ○ No	○ Yes ○ No	○ Yes ○ No	○ Yes ○ No	○ Yes ○ No	○ Yes ○ No	○ Yes ○ No
Follow-up action/ notes									
Optional: Average item score*									

Formulario para monitorear el desarrollo infantil

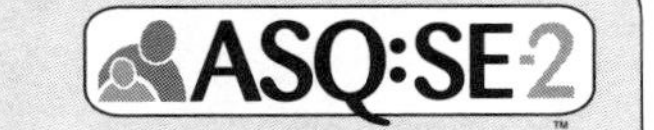

Nombre del niño/a: ______________ Fecha de nacimiento: ______________ # de identificación: ______________

Sexo del bebé: ○ Masculino ○ Femenino

Instrucciones: Usted puede usar esta ficha para llevar un registro de los resultados de todas las evaluaciones ASQ:SE-2 que se hayan hecho para su niño/a. Anote la fecha en la que se contestó el ASQ:SE-2 y la etapa (mes) del cuestionario en la parte superior de cada columna.

1. Marque el círculo que corresponda a los resultados del ASQ:SE-2 (tome este dato de la Compilación de datos del ASQ:SE-2). Si el puntaje se encuentra por debajo de la zona de monitoreo, entonces marque "Muy por debajo". Si el puntaje se encuentra dentro de la zona de monitoreo, entonces marque "Monitoreo". Si un puntaje está por encima del punto de corte, entonces marque "Por encima".
2. Indique la cantidad total de preguntas calificadas que se marcaron como motivo de preocupación.
3. Marque "Sí" o "No" para indicar si hubo respuestas que sean motivo de preocupación en la sección de Observaciones Generales.
4. **Opcional:** Calcule el puntaje promedio* dividiendo el puntaje total del ASQ:SE-2 entre la cantidad de preguntas calificadas. (Vea la página 117 del *ASQ:SE-2 User's Guide* para obtener más información.)

	ASQ:SE-2 **2 meses** Fecha en que se completó ______	ASQ:SE-2 **6 meses** Fecha en que se completó ______	ASQ:SE-2 **12 meses** Fecha en que se completó ______	ASQ:SE-2 **18 meses** Fecha en que se completó ______	ASQ:SE-2 **24 meses** Fecha en que se completó ______	ASQ:SE-2 **30 meses** Fecha en que se completó ______	ASQ:SE-2 **36 meses** Fecha en que se completó ______	ASQ:SE-2 **48 meses** Fecha en que se completó ______	ASQ:SE-2 **60 meses** Fecha en que se completó ______
Puntaje total del ASQ:SE-2	○ Por encima ○ Monitoreo ○ Muy por debajo	○ Por encima ○ Monitoreo ○ Muy por debajo	○ Por encima ○ Monitoreo ○ Muy por debajo	○ Por encima ○ Monitoreo ○ Muy por debajo	○ Por encima ○ Monitoreo ○ Muy por debajo	○ Por encima ○ Monitoreo ○ Muy por debajo	○ Por encima ○ Monitoreo ○ Muy por debajo	○ Por encima ○ Monitoreo ○ Muy por debajo	○ Por encima ○ Monitoreo ○ Muy por debajo
Cantidad de preguntas marcadas como motivo de preocupación									
Preocupaciones generales indicadas	○ Sí ○ No	○ Sí ○ No	○ Sí ○ No	○ Sí ○ No	○ Sí ○ No	○ Sí ○ No	○ Sí ○ No	○ Sí ○ No	○ Sí ○ No
Reunión con el padre/madre	○ Sí ○ No	○ Sí ○ No	○ Sí ○ No	○ Sí ○ No	○ Sí ○ No	○ Sí ○ No	○ Sí ○ No	○ Sí ○ No	○ Sí ○ No
Seguimiento: Pasos a seguir/ notas									
Opcional: Puntaje promedio*									

E

Social-Emotional Development Guides and Activities

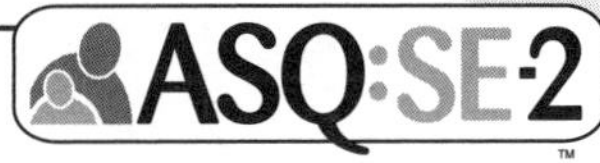

The following Social-Emotional Development Guides (on pp. 241–258) and Activities (on pp. 259–276) coordinate with the ASQ:SE-2 questionnaire intervals at 2, 6, 12, 18, 24, 30, 36, 48, and 60 months. After a child has been screened with ASQ:SE-2 and program staff have determined that there is no need to refer this child, staff may give the Development Guides and Activities to the family as additional resources. The Development Guides and Activities may also be shared with families who have been referred to provide some immediate information and ideas. The development guides provide parents with information about what types of behaviors they may expect from their growing child, whereas the activities provide ideas or ways to support their young child's social-emotional development. Please consider the following points when using these resources.

The ASQ:SE-2 Development Guides and Activities are not an intervention. Rather, these resources can be used in a preventive manner when children do not need further assessment. They are helpful for engaging parents in their child's development, with an overview of milestones to expect from the growing child as well as simple activities to try at home. The materials are not comprehensive, and they may include behaviors or suggestions that are inappropriate for certain cultures. The ASQ:SE-2 Development Guides and Activities may need to be modified to be appropriate for some families (e.g., adapted for cultural relevance, translated, shared verbally with families, illustrated).

In addition, parents may need other support and/or information about developmentally appropriate expectations and strategies to feel successful with their young child. Information about the following topics is not included in the development guides or activities and should be made available to families separately to help them support their child's social-emotional development.

- Positive feeding routines (including breast feeding)
- Typical sleeping patterns for different ages

- Toilet training
- Positive guidance
- Safety and childproofing home environments
- Health and nutrition

Please note that the handouts available separately in the *ASQ:SE-2™ Learning Activities* book help programs address these topics with families. This resource is available in English and Spanish and provides additional support and offers targeted guidance to parents.

Social-Emotional Development at 2 Months

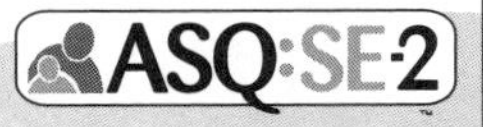

- Your baby is really smiling at you and others now.
- Your baby is not crying as much as she was as a newborn.
- Your baby uses different cries to tell you when he is hungry, uncomfortable, or sick.
- Your baby "talks" to you with noises and gurgles.
- Your baby looks at your face and may look in your eyes, but only for a few seconds at first.
- Your baby lets you know she is happy by cooing, smiling, laughing, and gurgling.
- Your baby likes to be with people and is becoming more interactive with you.
- Your baby is learning about eating and sleeping times, but it will take a few months for him to know the routine.
- Your baby likes to be picked up, hugged, and cuddled by people she knows.
- Sometimes your baby will be fussy only because he wants your attention.
- Your baby likes to play with her fingers, hands, feet, and toes.
- Your baby feels safe in your arms and enjoys your hugs.
- Your baby can recognize familiar people by their voices.

Social-Emotional Development at 6 Months

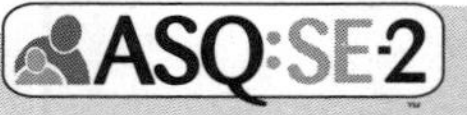

- Your baby responds to your smile and sometimes laughs when looking at you.
- Your baby responds to your soothing and comforting and loves to be touched or held close.
- Your baby responds to your affection and may begin to show you signs of affection.
- Your baby's vision is improving, and she is getting more curious about what she sees. She enjoys watching other babies and children.
- Your baby focuses on your voice and turns his head toward your voice. He may turn to you when you call his name.
- Your baby may be frightened by loud or unfamiliar noises.
- Your baby sometimes likes quiet and being soothed. Other times, she likes talking and playing.
- Your baby enjoys learning simple games such as Peekaboo.
- Your baby will sometimes stop crying when you talk to him rather than pick him up.
- Your baby sometimes sucks on her fingers or hands to calm herself down.
- Your baby plays with sounds and may babble by putting sounds together such as "ma-ma-ma," "ba-ba," and "da-da-da."
- A lot of the time, your baby wants you and no one else!

Social-Emotional Development at 12 Months

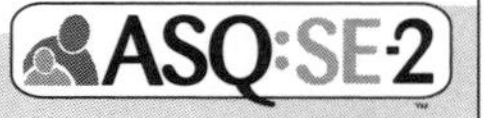

- Your baby responds to her name when you call her.
- Your baby is interested in other babies and children.
- Your baby shows many emotions, such as happiness, sadness, discomfort, and anger.
- Your baby may be shy around new people or seem jealous if you pay attention to someone else. He may need some time to watch and warm up to new people and new places.
- Your baby may have fears, such as fear of falling, darkness, large animals, loud sounds, or changes in routines.
- Your baby responds differently to strangers than she does to family members and friends she sees a lot.
- Your baby wants you in his sight all the time. He may get upset when you leave him with someone else.
- Your baby imitates other children and adults. She may imitate sounds, actions, and facial expressions.
- Your baby gives affection by hugging and kissing. He may hug or kiss you, familiar children and adults, pets, or stuffed animals.
- Your baby watches other people. She may respond to someone's pain by crying or showing distress.
- Your baby is beginning to show his likes and dislikes. He may push things away that he does not like. He may feel attached to a special toy or blanket.
- Your baby is becoming more independent. She may seem stubborn or frustrated when she cannot do something herself.

Social-Emotional Development at 18 Months

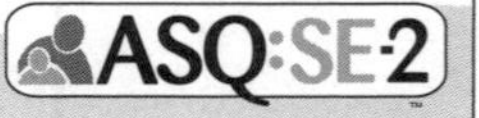

- Your toddler is generally happy and smiles at people, including other children.
- Your toddler likes to talk and is using more words every day.
- Your toddler likes to show affection and give hugs and kisses.
- Your toddler is showing different emotions such as fear, sympathy, modesty, guilt, or embarrassment.
- Your toddler likes to do things by himself. He may seem stubborn, but this is normal.
- Your toddler likes to help with simple household tasks.
- Your toddler turns to you for help when she is in trouble.
- Your toddler enjoys playing near other children but not with them yet.
- Your toddler may hand toys to other children, but he does not understand how to share and wants the toys right back.
- Your toddler can play by herself for short periods of time.
- Your toddler has specific likes and dislikes.
- Your toddler likes to say, "No!" He may have a quick temper and sometimes hits when frustrated.
- Your toddler loves to be held and read to and becomes upset when separated from you.
- Your toddler loves to imitate others.
- Your toddler likes to be the center of attention.
- Your toddler recognizes herself in pictures or mirrors.

Social-Emotional Development at 24 Months

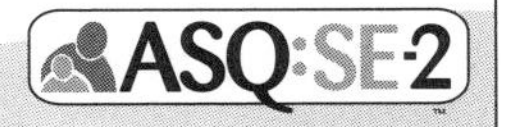

- Your toddler likes to imitate you, other adults, and her friends.
- Your toddler wants to do everything by himself, even though he can't!
- Some of your toddler's favorite words are *mine, no,* and *me do it.*
- Your toddler has many emotions, and her emotions can be very "big." She can get angry and have temper tantrums.
- Your toddler likes to imitate you doing household tasks. He can put some of his toys away with help from you.
- Your toddler loves to try new things and explore new places. But she wants to know you are nearby to keep her safe.
- Your toddler is very interested in other children. He is still learning how to play with them.
- Your toddler will play nearby other children but not really with them. She does not understand how to share her things yet.
- Your toddler has a hard time waiting and wants things right now.
- Your toddler loves attention from familiar adults and children but may act shy around strangers.
- Your toddler shows affection by returning a hug or kiss. He tries to comfort familiar people who are in distress.
- Your toddler knows her name and knows what she likes and dislikes. She may be very attached to certain things, such as a special book, toy, or blanket.
- Your toddler enjoys simple pretend play. He may like pretending to cook or talk on the telephone.
- Your toddler is learning about the routines in your home but often does not remember rules.

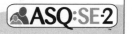

Social-Emotional Development at 30 Months

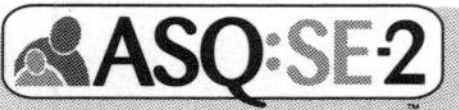

- Your child likes using her growing imagination. She likes to play with puppets, dress-up clothes, dolls, and play figures.
- Your child is beginning to understand others' feelings. He is learning to identify when another child is angry or happy.
- Your child is beginning to learn about sharing. She does not always share but can sometimes.
- Your child is getting louder and bossier at times. He may talk with a loud, urgent voice.
- Your child can follow simple routine directions such as "Bring me your cup" and "Please go in your room and get your socks."
- Your child enjoys hearing songs and stories—sometimes over and over again.
- Your child wants to be independent sometimes but also wants you nearby. She will now easily leave your side if she is in familiar surroundings.
- Your child can identify if he thinks he is a boy or a girl.
- Your child greets familiar adults and is happy to see friends.
- Your child sometimes screams and throws temper tantrums.
- Your child likes to be hugged and cuddled—but not in the middle of playtime.

Social-Emotional Development at 36 Months

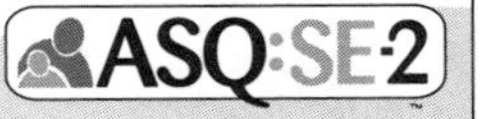

- Your child is more independent and can do many things for herself. Your child will tell you, "I can do it myself!"
- Your child is still learning to follow simple rules, although he sometimes needs gentle reminders.
- Your child now plays briefly *with* other children. She is still learning about sharing and taking turns.
- Your child likely has a special friend that he prefers playing with. Boys may prefer playing with boys, and girls with girls.
- Your child is becoming more independent. When you go on outings, she will not always hold your hand or stay by your side.
- Your child's emotions may shift suddenly, from happy to sad or from mad to silly. He's learning how to handle his emotions.
- Your child can sometimes use words to express her feelings.
- Your child is beginning to think about other people's feelings and is learning to identify their feelings, too.
- Your child uses imagination to create stories through pretend play with dolls, toy telephones, and action figures.
- Your child sometimes bosses people around and makes demands. This shows that he is independent and values himself. He might do something that he is asked to do, but he is more willing if he thinks it is his idea.
- Your child may be fearful and sometimes has nightmares. Scary images and sounds, even cartoons, can give her nightmares.
- Your child's attention span is increasing. She often stays with an activity for at least 5 minutes.

Social-Emotional Development at 48 Months

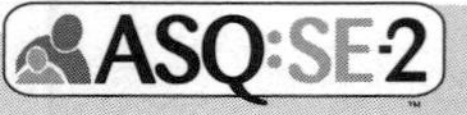

- Your child likes to play with other children and has favorite games and playmates.
- Your child is beginning to share. He takes turns but is possessive of favorite toys.
- Your child expresses extreme emotions at times—happiness, sadness, anger, silliness. She may be able to label her own feelings.
- When your child plays, he often uses real-life situations, such as going to the store, school, and gas station.
- Your child may have imaginary friends when playing games, sleeping at night, and going to preschool.
- Your child now understands short and simple rules at home.
- Your child is starting to understand danger. She knows when to stay away from dangerous things.
- Your child loves silly jokes and has a sense of humor.
- Your child is beginning to control his feelings of frustration.
- Your child may use her imagination a lot, and she can be very creative.
- Your child is becoming more independent and adventurous. He may like to try new things.
- With her new independence, your child can be boastful and bossy at times.
- Your child shows concern and sympathy for younger siblings and playmates when they are hurt or upset. His ability to empathize—to put himself in someone else's shoes—is increasing.
- Your child's attention span is increasing. She often stays with an activity for at least 10 minutes.

Social-Emotional Development at 60 Months

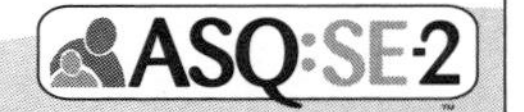

- Your child likes to play best with one or two other children at a time.
- Your child likes to choose his own friends and may have a best friend.
- Your child now plays simple games such as Candy Land and Go Fish.
- Your child may play with small groups of children at the park or at school.
- Your child understands and can follow simple rules at home and at school.
- Your child shows a variety of emotions. She may be jealous of other children at times, especially of a younger brother or sister who is getting attention.
- Your child is now very independent and likes to make his own choices about clothes to wear, foods to eat, and activities in which to be involved.
- Your child is sensitive to other children's feelings. She can identify other people's feelings: "She's sad."
- Your child likes to talk with familiar adults and children.
- Your child understands how to take turns and share at home and at school, but he may not want to all of the time.
- Your child is beginning to understand the meaning of right and wrong. She does not always do what is right, though.
- Adult approval is very important to your child. Your child looks to adults for attention and praise.
- Your child is showing some self-control in group situations and can wait for his turn or stand in a line.
- Your child is usually able to respond to requests such as "Use your quiet voice" or "Inside is for walking."
- Your child's attention span is increasing. She is able to focus her attention for a necessary length of time, such as listening to directions or a story.

Desarrollo socio-emocional a los 2 meses

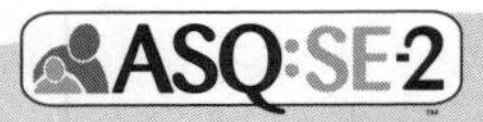

- Su bebé ya le sonríe a usted y a otras personas.
- Su bebé ya no llora tanto como cuando era recién nacida.
- Su bebé llora de maneras diferentes para avisarle que tiene hambre, que está incómodo o enfermo.
- Su bebé le "habla" haciendo ruidos y balbuceos.
- Su bebé lo/la ve a la cara y quizá lo/la vea a los ojos, pero solamente por unos cuantos segundos al principio.
- Su bebé le dice que está feliz por medio de una sonrisa, la risa, sonidos suaves y balbuceos.
- A su bebé le gusta estar con personas y cada vez interactúa más con usted.
- Su bebé está aprendiendo cuáles son las horas de dormir y de comer, pero tardará algunos meses en saber la rutina.
- A su bebé le gusta que la tomen en brazos, y que la acurruquen las personas que ella conoce.
- Su bebé se muestra inquieto o irritable a veces solamente para llamar su atención.
- A su bebé le gusta jugar con sus manos, dedos de la mano, pies y dedos del pie.
- Su bebé se siente segura en sus brazos y disfruta que usted la abrace.
- Su bebé puede reconocer a la gente que conoce por la voz.

Desarrollo socio-emocional a los 6 meses

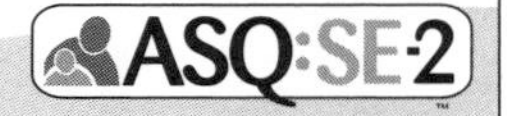

- Su bebé responde a la sonrisa de usted y algunas veces se ríe cuando lo/la ve.
- Su bebé responde cuando usted la calma o la conforta y le encanta que usted la toque o la abrace.
- Su bebé responde al cariño que usted le da y podría empezar a mostrar señales de cariño.
- La vista de su bebé va mejorando y cada vez muestra más curiosidad hacia las cosas que ve. Le gusta ver a otros bebés y niños.
- Su bebé le pone atención a la voz de usted y voltea la cabeza cada vez que escucha su voz. Es posible que voltee su cabecita hacia usted cuando lo llama por su nombre.
- Su bebé se asusta cuando oye ruidos fuertes o sonidos que no le son familiares.
- A su bebé le gustan los momentos tranquilos y ser confortada a veces y otras veces le gusta hablar y jugar.
- A su bebé le gustan los juegos sencillos como "¿Dónde está el nene?".
- Su bebé para de llorar a veces cuando usted le habla en lugar de abrazarlo.
- Su bebé se chupa los dedos o las manos a veces para calmarse a sí misma.
- Su bebé juega con sonidos que produce y es posible que balbucee juntando algunos sonidos como "ma-ma-ma", "ba-ba", y "da-da-da".
- ¡Su bebé quiere estar con usted y con nadie más una gran parte del tiempo!

Desarrollo socio-emocional a los 12 meses

ASQ:SE-2

- Su bebé responde a su nombre cuando usted la llama.
- Su bebé muestra interés en otros bebés y niños.
- Su bebé muestra muchas emociones tales como felicidad, tristeza, incomodidad y enojo.
- Su bebé puede ser tímido cuando está con gente que no conoce o mostrarse celoso si usted le pone atención a otra persona. Es posible que su bebé necesite tiempo para observar y sentirse cómodo con personas o lugares nuevos.
- Su bebé puede tener muchos miedos, tales como el miedo de caerse, miedo a la oscuridad, a animales grandes, a sonidos fuertes o a cambios en su rutina.
- Su bebé responde de manera diferente a gente desconocida que a miembros de la familia o amigos que ve muy frecuentemente.
- Su bebé quiere que usted esté cerca todo el tiempo. Es posible que se moleste si usted la deja con otra persona.
- Su bebé imita a otros niños y adultos. Es posible que imite sonidos, acciones y expresiones faciales de otras personas.
- Su bebé muestra cariño a través de abrazos y besos. Podría abrazarlo/la o besarlo/la a usted o a niños que conoce o a sus animales de peluche.
- Su bebé observa a otras personas. Es posible que llore o que se muestre angustiado cuando observa dolor en otra persona.
- Su bebé empieza a mostrar lo que le gusta y lo que no le gusta. Es posible que aviente las cosas que no le gustan o que tenga un apego a una cobija o a un juguete en particular.
- Su bebé se hace cada vez más independiente. Es posible que muestre terquedad o frustración cuando no puede hacer las cosas por sí misma.

Desarrollo socio-emocional a los 18 meses

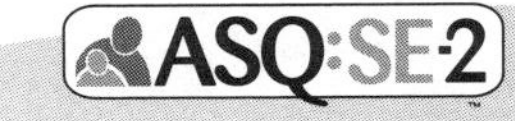

- Su niño se muestra feliz por lo general y le sonríe a otras personas, incluyendo niños.
- A su niña le gusta hablar y cada vez usa más palabras.
- A su niño le gusta mostrar cariño y dar abrazos y besos.
- Su niña muestra diversas emociones tales como miedo, empatía, modestia, culpa o vergüenza.
- A su niño le gusta hacer las cosas sin ayuda; podría parecer terco, pero este es un comportamiento normal.
- A su niña le gusta ayudar con los quehaceres de la casa.
- Su niño le pide ayuda cuando tiene un problema.
- A su niña le gusta jugar cerca de otros niños, pero todavía no juega con ellos.
- Es probable que su niño le dé juguetes a otros niños, pero todavía no entiende cómo compartir y quiere que le regresen los juguetes inmediatamente.
- Su niña puede jugar solita por períodos de tiempo cortos.
- A su niño le gustan o no le gustan cosas específicas.
- A su niña le gusta decir "¡No!". Es posible que tenga mal genio y que pegue cuando se siente frustrada.
- A su niño le encanta que lo abracen y que le lean un cuento, y a veces se molesta o se enoja cuando es separado de usted.
- A su niña le encanta imitar a otros.
- A su niño le gusta ser el centro de atención.
- Su niña se reconoce a sí misma en fotos o en el reflejo del espejo.

Desarrollo socio-emocional a los 24 meses

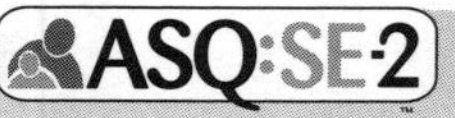

- A su niño le gusta imitarlo/la a usted, a otros adultos y a sus amigos.
- Su niña quiere hacer todo solita, aunque no pueda.
- Algunas de las palabras favoritas de su niño son: *Mío, no* y *yo solito* o *yo puedo.*
- Su niña muestra muchas emociones y pueden ser muy fuertes. Puede mostrarse muy enojada y hacer berrinches.
- A su niño le gusta imitar los quehaceres de la casa que usted realiza. Puede recoger algunos de sus juguetes si usted lo ayuda.
- A su niña le encanta hacer cosas nuevas y explorar nuevos lugares, pero siempre quiere saber que usted está cerca y sentirse segura porque usted está ahí.
- Su niño se muestra muy interesado en otros niños, pero todavía está aprendiendo cómo jugar con ellos.
- Su niña juega cerca de otros niños, pero no con ellos. Todavía no entiende cómo compartir sus cosas.
- A su niño se le dificulta esperar y quiere que le den las cosas en el momento en que las pide.
- A su niña le encanta la atención que le dan los adultos y niños que conoce, pero es posible que se muestre tímida con personas que no conoce.
- Su niño muestra cariño al reciprocar un abrazo o un beso. Trata de reconfortar a las personas que muestran angustia o dolor, siempre y cuando las conozca.
- Su niña sabe su nombre y sabe lo que le gusta o lo que no le gusta. Es posible que tenga mucho apego hacia ciertas cosas que son especiales para ella, tales como un libro, juguete o cobija.
- A su niño le gustan los juegos sencillos que usan la imaginación. Es posible que haga como que está hablando por teléfono o que se imagine que es un cocinero.
- Su niña está aprendiendo cuáles son las rutinas de la casa, pero a menudo no recuerda las reglas.

Desarrollo socio-emocional a los 30 meses

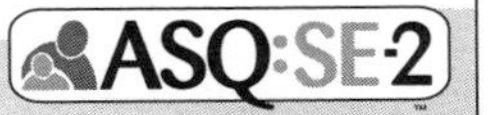

- A su niño le gusta usar su imaginación, que se va expandiendo conforme crece. Le gusta jugar con títeres, muñecas y otros juguetes, así como disfrazarse.
- Su niña está empezando a entender los sentimientos de los demás. Está aprendiendo a saber cuándo otro niño está enojado o feliz.
- Su niño está empezando a saber cómo compartir. No comparte siempre, pero lo hace a veces.
- Su niña cada vez expresa más su opinión y se muestra exigente a veces. Es posible que hable en voz muy alta y expresando mucha urgencia.
- Su niño puede seguir instrucciones simples con respecto a una rutina tales como "Tráeme tu taza" o "Ve a tu cuarto y tráeme tus calcetines, por favor".
- A su niña le gusta escuchar canciones y cuentos; a veces le gusta escucharlos una y otra vez.
- Su niño quiere ser independiente a veces, pero también quiere que usted esté cerca de él. Ahora puede separarse de usted fácilmente siempre y cuando esté en situaciones o lugares que le son familiares.
- Su niña puede decir si ella es una niña o un niño.
- Su niño saluda a adultos que le son familiares y se muestra feliz cuando ve a sus amigos.
- Su niña grita y hace berrinches a veces.
- A su niño le gusta que lo abracen y lo acurruquen, pero no cuando está jugando.

Desarrollo socio-emocional a los 36 meses

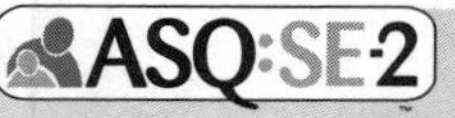

- Su niño es más independiente y puede hacer muchas cosas solito. Su niño le dice "¡Puedo hacerlo solito!".
- Su niña todavía está aprendiendo a seguir reglas sencillas, y necesita que usted se las recuerde a veces.
- Su niño ahora juega brevemente *con* otros niños. Todavía está aprendiendo a compartir y a tomar turnos.
- Es muy probable que su niña tenga un/a amigo/a especial con el/la que prefiere jugar. Es probable que los niños prefieran jugar con otros niños y que las niñas prefieran jugar con otras niñas.
- Su niño se hace cada vez más independiente. Cuando ustedes salen a la calle, es probable que no siempre lo/la tome de la mano o que se quede a su lado.
- Las emociones de su niña podrían cambiar muy rápidamente de feliz a triste o de enojada a eufórica. Ella todavía está aprendiendo a manejar sus emociones.
- Es posible que su niño use palabras para expresar sus sentimientos a veces.
- Su niña empieza a considerar los sentimientos de otras personas y también está aprendiendo a identificar sus propios sentimientos.
- Su niño usa su imaginación para crear historias usando muñecas, teléfonos de juguete o figuras de acción.
- Su niña se muestra exigente con otras personas y pide cosas de manera autoritaria a veces. Esto muestra que es independiente y que se valora a sí misma. Es posible que haga algo que usted le pida, pero prefiere hacerlo si siente que es idea de ella.
- Es probable que su niño tenga miedos y pesadillas a veces. Los programas de televisión y los videos (incluyendo caricaturas) que le den miedo, podrían causarle pesadillas.
- La capacidad de concentración va creciendo en su niña y frecuentemente se queda haciendo la misma actividad por al menos 5 minutos.

Desarrollo socio-emocional a los 48 meses

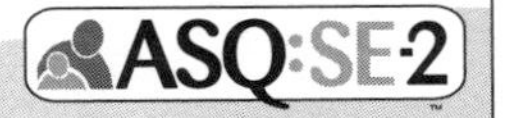

- A su niño le gusta jugar con otros niños y tiene juegos y compañeros de juego favoritos.
- Su niña está empezando a compartir y puede tomar turnos aunque se muestra posesiva de algunos de sus juguetes favoritos.
- Su niño muestra emociones fuertes—felicidad, tristeza, enojo, euforia—a veces. Es posible que pueda identificar algunas de sus emociones por su nombre.
- Cuando su niña juega, lo hace frecuentemente imitando situaciones de la vida diaria, tales como ir a la tienda, a la escuela o a la gasolinera.
- Es posible que su niño invente amigos imaginarios cuando juega, cuando duerme o cuando va a la escuela.
- Su niña ahora entiende reglas de la casa que sean simples y cortas.
- Su niño empieza a entender lo que es el peligro y sabe cuándo apartarse de situaciones o cosas que son peligrosas.
- A su niña le encantan los chistes y tiene sentido del humor.
- Su niño está empezando a controlar sus sentimientos de frustración.
- Es posible que su niña use mucho su imaginación y puede ser muy creativa.
- Su niño se hace cada vez más independiente y aventurero, y es posible que le guste probar cosas nuevas.
- La independencia que siente ahora su niña podría hacerla comportarse de manera presuntuosa y autoritaria a veces.
- Su niño muestra preocupación y empatía hacia sus hermanos menores o compañeros de juego cuando se lastiman o están enojados. Su capacidad de tener empatía—de ponerse en el lugar de otros—va incrementando cada día.
- La capacidad de concentración de su niña va incrementando cada día y con frecuencia puede quedarse haciendo una actividad por al menos 10 minutos.

Desarrollo socio-emocional a los 60 meses

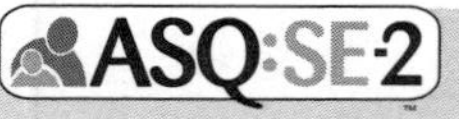

- A su niño le gusta más jugar con uno o dos niños a la vez.
- A su niña le gusta elegir con quién juega y es probable que tenga un/a mejor amigo/a.
- Su niño ahora puede participar en juegos sencillos como lotería y "A pescar".
- Es posible que su niña juegue en grupos pequeños de niños en el parque o en la escuela.
- Su niño entiende y puede seguir reglas simples en la casa y en la escuela.
- Su niña muestra una variedad de emociones. Es posible que se sienta celosa de otros niños a veces, sobre todo si se trata de un hermano o hermana menor que esté recibiendo atención.
- Su niño es ahora muy independiente y le gusta tomar sus propias decisiones sobre la ropa que va a usar, la comida que va a comer o las actividades en las que va a participar.
- Su niña es sensible a los sentimientos de otros niños; puede identificar esos sentimientos y decir: "Ella está triste".
- A su niño le gusta hablar con los adultos y niños que conoce.
- Su niña entiende cómo tomar turnos y compartir en la escuela y en la casa, pero es posible que no lo quiera hacer siempre.
- Su niño está empezando a entender el significado de lo que está bien o mal, aunque no siempre hace lo que es correcto.
- La aprobación de un adulto es muy importante para su niña. Su niña busca la atención y el elogio de los adultos.
- Su niño muestra algo de autocontrol en situaciones de grupo y puede esperar su turno o quedarse en una fila.
- Generalmente su niña responde a peticiones como "Baja la voz" o "Cuando estamos adentro de un edificio, hay que caminar".
- La capacidad de concentración de su niño va incrementando y puede poner atención, por el tiempo que sea necesario, para escuchar una historia o instrucciones.

Social-Emotional Activities for Babies 2 Months Old

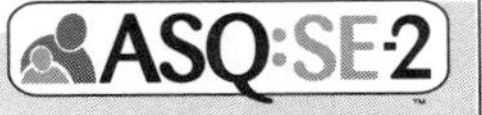

Sing songs you remember from childhood to your baby. Hold your baby close in your arms or in a baby carrier. Gently dance with your baby.	With your baby on her back, take a tissue and wave it above your baby for her to see. Tissues also can fly, float, and tickle parts of your baby's body. See how your baby responds. If she fusses, then stop playing.	Let your baby hear new, gentle sounds. Quiet musical toys or soft bells will be interesting to him. Ask, *"Did you hear those bells? Do you like how they sound?"*	Your face, smile, voice, and touch are the most important things for your baby right now. You do not need fancy toys. She wants to play and get to know you!
If your baby cries, find out what he needs. He is letting you know something with his cry. When you respond, he learns to trust you are there for him. You cannot spoil your baby at this age.	Hold your baby and put your face close to hers. Make silly faces. Smile at your baby. Stick out your tongue. Yawn. Wait a few seconds and see if she tries to repeat your actions back to you.	Step back from your baby so he cannot see you. Gently call his name. Watch what he does. Does he stop moving for a moment? Does he try to move his head toward your voice? Pick him up. Say, *"Here I am."*	Let your baby lie on a blanket on the floor and get down on the floor with her. See the world from her point of view. Talk to her about what she is seeing. Say, *"There is the light."*
Make life interesting for your baby. Go for a walk. Introduce new sounds and places to him from the safety of your arms.	Talk to your baby about what she is doing, seeing, hearing, and feeling. Say, *"I am changing your diaper. You will like being nice and dry. I love you!"*	You can begin to play simple games with your baby such as Peekaboo. Put a cloth over *your* head and peek out. Say, *"There you are!"*	Introduce new, safe* objects for your baby to explore. Simple objects such as plastic cups and big wooden spoons are all new to him.
Place interesting things close to her bed for her to look at. Hang objects or toys out of reach. Tape simple pictures from magazines on the wall.	It is never too early to start reading books with your baby. Choose simple board books at first and talk about the pictures she sees. Cuddle up close.	Learn your baby's special language. He will "talk" to you with sounds and gestures and let you know when he is happy, uncomfortable, hungry, or lonely.	Give your baby a little massage after a bath or diaper change. Rub her tummy very gently. Talk to her. Say, *"Rub-a-dub, I'm rubbing your tummy. Do you like how that feels?"*

*Be sure to review safety guidelines with your health care provider.

Social-Emotional Activities for Babies 6 Months Old

ASQ:SE-2

Learn your baby's special rhythms, and try to settle into a regular routine for eating, sleeping, and diapering. Talk to your baby about his routines. This will help your baby feel secure and content.	Your baby likes to hear new sounds. Bells, whistles, and barking dogs are all new and interesting. Talk to your baby about what she is hearing.	Get down on the floor with your baby and play with him on his level. Look at toys, books, or objects together. Have fun, laugh, and enjoy your time together.	When your baby cries, respond to her. Whisper in her ear to quiet her. Hold her close and make soft sounds. This will help her know that you are always there and that you love her.
Play Peekaboo and Pat-a-cake with your baby. Be playful, have fun, and laugh with your baby. He will respond with smiles and laughs.	Read to your baby. Snuggle up close, point to pictures, and talk about what you are seeing. Your baby will begin to choose favorite books as she gets a bit older.	Bring your baby to new places to see new things. Go on a walk to a park or in the mall, or just bring him shopping. He will love to see new things while you keep him safe.	Place your baby in new areas or in new positions when you are at home. The world looks very different from a new spot!
Let your baby begin to feed herself bits of food and use a spoon and a cup. She will begin to enjoy doing things herself.	Use your baby's name when you dress, feed, and diaper him. Say, *"Here is Dusty's finger. Here is Dusty's foot."*	Provide new, safe objects for your baby to explore.* Everything is interesting to her. Large wooden spoons and a soft baby brush are new things to learn about.	"Talk" with your baby. When your baby makes a sound, imitate the sound back to him. Go back and forth as long as possible.
Sing songs to your baby and tell her nursery rhymes. Make up songs about your baby using her name. This will make her feel special and loved.	Bath time* is a wonderful time to have fun and be close with your baby. Sponges, plastic cups, and washcloths make simple, inexpensive tub toys.	Enjoy music with your baby. Pick him up, bounce him gently, and twirl with him in your arms. Dance to new and different types of music.	Visit a friend who has a baby or young child. Stay close to your baby and let her know that these new people are okay. It takes a little time to warm up.

*Be sure to review safety guidelines with your health care provider.

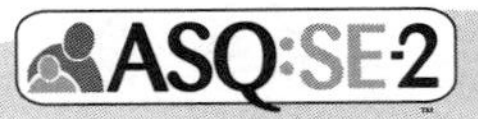

Social-Emotional Activities for Babies 12 Months Old

Keep a home routine for eating, sleeping, diapering, and playtime. Talk to your baby about routines and what will be next. This will help her feel secure.	Let your baby know every day how much you love him and how special he is—when he wakes up in the morning and when he goes to sleep at night.	Play on the floor with your baby every day. Crawl around with her, or just get down and play on her level. She will really enjoy having you to herself.	Play simple games with your baby, such as Pat-a-cake, Peekaboo, and Hide and Seek, or chase each other. Laugh and have fun together!
Your baby can "help" you while you are making dinner. Have a drawer or cupboard that is full of safe kitchen items, such as measuring cups and big spoons, that he can empty.	Play gentle tickle games with your baby, but make sure to stop when she lets you know she has had enough. Watch her carefully and you will know.	Dance to music with your baby. Hold his hands while he bends up and down. Clap and praise him when he "dances" by himself.	Play name games with your baby, such as "Where is Rita?"
Go on a walk to a park or a place where children play. Let your baby watch them and visit a little if he is ready.	Play with child-safe mirrors* with your baby. Make silly expressions and talk to your baby about what she is seeing in the reflection.	Twirl your baby around. He will enjoy a little rough-and-tumble play, but make sure you stop when he has had enough.	Read together with your baby. Before naptime and bedtime are great times to read together. Let your baby choose the book and snuggle up!
Let your baby have as many choices as possible about foods, clothing, toys, and events. She will enjoy making choices.	Invite a friend over who has a baby or young child. Make sure you have enough toys for both children. It is a little early for them to know about sharing.	Sit on the floor with your baby and roll a ball back and forth. Clap your hands when your baby pushes the ball or "catches" the ball with his hands.	When you are dressing or diapering your baby, talk about her body parts and show her your body parts. Say, *"Here is Daddy's nose. Here is Destiny's nose."*

*Be sure to review safety guidelines with your health care provider.

Social-Emotional Activities for Toddlers 18 Months Old

ASQ:SE-2

Your toddler likes to have a regular daily routine. Talk to him about what you are doing now and what will be happening next. Give him time to be active and time to be quiet.	Your toddler loves to have a lot of hugs and kisses. Give big hugs, little hugs, loud kisses, and soft kisses. Tell her you love her so much!	Your toddler will enjoy gentle tickling games. Make sure he can let you know when he has had enough. He will like quiet snuggle times, too.	Have a pretend party with stuffed animals or dolls. You can cut out little "presents" from a magazine, make a pretend cake, and sing the birthday song.
Your toddler needs a lot of time to move around and exercise. Go for a walk, visit a playground, or take a trip to a shopping mall.	Your toddler will love to help with daily tasks. Give her simple "jobs" to do and let her know what a big girl she is. She can wipe off a table, put her toys away, or help sweep up.	Play simple games such as Hide and Seek and Chase with your toddler. Have fun and laugh together.	Dance with your toddler. Make a simple instrument out of a large plastic food tub (for a drum) or a small plastic container filled with beans or rice (for a shaker).
Help your child learn about emotions. Make happy faces, sad faces, mad faces, and silly faces in front of a mirror. This is fun!	Let your toddler help during mealtimes by bringing some things to the table or setting a place.	Your child might enjoy having a little place to hide. Use a blanket or sheet to make a tent or secret spot for him to play in.	Your child can help clean up after play-times. Make it simple by putting things in a big tub or box and help her clean. Clap and praise her for her help.
Make playhouse furniture for your child out of boxes. For a stove, turn a box upside down and draw "burners." Use simple containers for pots, and use wooden spoons or sticks to stir the "soup."	Set up playtimes with other children. Your child doesn't understand how to share yet, so make sure there are plenty of toys. Stay close by and help him learn how to play with other chil-dren.	Your toddler is getting big and wants to do things by herself! Let her practice eating with a spoon and drinking with a sippy cup during mealtimes. Be ready for some spilling!	Storytimes, especially before naptime and bedtime, are a great way to settle down before sleep. Let your child choose books to read and help turn pages. Help him name what he sees.

Social-Emotional Activities for Toddlers 24 Months Old

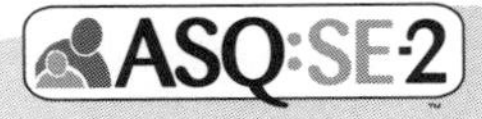

Try to have set routines during the day, and let your child know what will be happening next. Say, *"Remember, after we brush your hair, we get dressed."*	Your child is learning about rules but will need a lot of reminders. Keep rules short and simple, and be consistent.	Have a special reading time every day with your toddler. Snuggle up and get close. Before bedtime or naptime is a great time to read together.	Let your toddler know how special she is! She will love to be praised for new things she learns how to do. Say, *"You are so helpful. Wow, you did it yourself!"*
Stay nearby to help your child learn about taking turns during play with friends. It is early to know how to share. Talking about turns will help him learn.	Give your toddler choices, but keep them simple. Let her choose a red or a blue shirt while dressing. Let her choose milk or juice at lunch.	Provide a lot of time to play with other children. Your child may be very active but needs rest times, too. Try to learn your child's rhythms and go with his flow.	Let your child do more things for herself.* Put a stool near the sink so she can wash her hands and brush her teeth. Let her pick out clothes and help dress herself.
Get down on the floor and play with your child. Try to follow your child's lead by playing with toys he chooses and trying his ideas.	Encourage your child to pretend play. Put a few small chairs in a row to make a "bus." Cut up some paper "money" to pay the driver. Ask, *"Where will we go today?"*	Everything is new to your toddler. She can observe some weeds growing on a path or a bird pecking for seeds. Take some time to see the little things with her.	Your toddler is learning all about emotions. Help him label his feelings when he is mad, sad, happy, or silly. Say, *"You are really happy"* or *"You seem really mad."*
Play Parade or Follow the Leader with your toddler. Your child will love to copy you—*and* be the leader!	If your child has a temper tantrum, then stay calm and talk in a quiet tone. If possible, let her calm down by herself.	Don't forget to tell your child how much you love him! Give him hugs and kisses and soft touches to let him know.	Teach your child simple songs and finger plays, such as "The Itsy-Bitsy Spider."

*Be sure to review safety guidelines with your health care provider.

Social-Emotional Activities for Young Children 30 Months Old

ASQ:SE-2

Make a "Me Book" with your child. Take some pieces of paper and glue in pictures of your child, family members, pets, or other special things. Tape or staple the pages together.	Tell your child funny stories about things he did when he was a baby. Begin a favorite story and see if he can tell what happens next.	Show your child family photos. Talk about the people in the pictures and who they are. Say, *"That is your Uncle Ling."* Can your child tell you who the people are?	Tell your child a favorite nursery rhyme, and ask her how the characters in the story felt.
Give your child directions that have two steps. Say, *"Put all of the LEGOs in the box, and then put the box in the closet."* Let him know what a big help he is!	Let your child help when you are cooking and cleaning.* She can do things such as helping to stir, putting flour in a cup, or putting away spoons and forks in the drawer.	Your child loves to imitate you. Try new words, animal sounds, and noises, and see if your child can imitate what you say or how you sound.	Encourage creative play, such as drawing with crayons, painting, and playing with playdough. Playing with chalk on the sidewalk is fun.
Let your child do more things for himself. He can put on his shoes and coat when you go out. Make sure you give him plenty of time to work on these new skills. Say, *"What a big boy!"*	Draw and cut out faces that show different feelings, such as angry, frustrated, and happy. Encourage your child to use the faces to tell you how she is feeling.	Tell your child every day how much you love him. Give him little kisses on his nose, ears, and fingers. Say, *"I love your nose! I love your ear! I love your finger. I love you!"*	Have a special reading time every day. Snuggle up and get close. Look in the library for books about children with big feelings. Ask, *"What do you do when you get mad?"*
Play with your child and help her learn how to share. Show her how to share and praise her when he shares with you. This is a new thing for her, so do not expect too much at this age.	Encourage your child to tell you his name and age. Sometimes making up a rhyme or song about his name will help him remember. See if he can tell you the names of friends and teachers.	Sing songs and dance with your child. Play different types of music from the radio. Make simple instruments from boxes, oatmeal canisters, or yogurt tubs.	Invite a friend with a child over for a playdate. Keep it short, such as 1 or 2 hours. Have some playtime with enough toys for two, snack time, and some outdoor play. Say, *"That was fun! See you next time."*

*Be sure to review safety guidelines with your health care provider.

Social-Emotional Activities for Young Children 36 Months Old

ASQ:SE-2

Tell your child a simple story about something she did that was funny or interesting. See if your child can tell a different story about herself.	Encourage your child to identify and label his emotions and those of other children or adults.	Provide opportunities for your child to play with other children in your neighborhood or at a park.	Many children this age have imaginary friends. Let your child talk and play with these pretend playmates.
At dinner time, let family members talk about their day. Help your child tell about her day. Say, *"Latoya and I went to the park today. Latoya, tell your sister what you did at the park."*	Give your child directions that have at least two steps when you and he are cooking, dressing, or cleaning. Say, *"Put that pan in the sink, and then pick up the red spoon."*	Write a letter together to grandparents, a pen pal, or a friend. See if your child can tell you what to write about herself to include in the letter.	Play games with your child that involve taking turns, such as Follow the Leader and Hopscotch.
Create a pretend argument between stuffed animals or dolls. Talk with your child about what happened, feelings, and how best to work out problems when they come up.	Have a special reading time each day. Snuggle up and get close. Slowly increase the length of the stories so your child can sit and listen a little longer.	Let your child know every day that you love him and how great he is. Give him a "high five," a big smile, a pat on the back, or a hug. Tell him he is super, cool, sweet, and fun.	Tell your child a favorite story, such as the *Three Little Pigs* or *Goldilocks and the Three Bears.* See if your child can tell you how the animals felt in the story.
Draw simple pictures of faces that show happy, sad, excited, or silly expressions. Cut them out and glue them on a Popsicle stick or pencil. Let your child act out the different feelings with the puppets.	Get down on the floor and play with your child. Try to follow your child's lead by playing with toys she wants to play with and trying her ideas.	Play games that involve following simple rules, such as Mother May I and Red Light, Green Light.	Tell silly jokes with your child. Simple "What am I?" riddles are also fun. Have a good time and laugh with your child.

Social-Emotional Activities for Young Children 48 Months Old

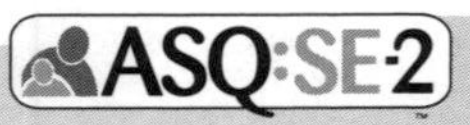

Introduce a new feeling each day, such as *bored*. Use pictures, gestures, and words. Encourage your child to use a variety of words to describe how he feels.	Encourage activities that involve sharing, such as building with blocks, coloring with crayons, and playing dress up. Teach your child how to ask a friend for a turn. Give your child a lot of time to play with other children.	Provide opportunities for your child to be creative. Empty containers, glue, newspapers, rubber bands, and magazines can be used to make new inventions.	Take your child to the store, a restaurant, or the library. Explore new places. Talk with her about how people are alike and how they are different.
When doing housework or yard work, allow your child to do a small part on his own. Let him empty the wastebasket or clean crumbs off the table.	Talk with your child about possible dangers in your home, such as electrical outlets and stovetops. Talk about outdoor dangers, too, such as crossing the street or talking with strangers.*	Encourage your child's independence. Let her fix something to eat, such as a peanut butter and jelly sandwich. At bedtime, let her choose her clothes to wear the next day.	Use stuffed animals to act out an argument. Talk first about how the different animals are feeling. Then, talk about different ways to come to an agreement.
Tell a favorite nursery rhyme or story. Talk about what is make-believe and what is real.	Make puppets out of Popsicle sticks by gluing on paper faces, adding yarn for hair, and so forth. Put on a show about two children who meet and become friends.	Find a children's book at your library about anger. Talk to your child about how his body feels when he gets angry. Then, discuss what your child can do when he is angry.	Take your child to the library for story hour. She can learn about sitting in a group and listening to stories.
Your child is learning more about rules but will still need reminders. Talk about your family rules. Keep rules short and simple, and be consistent.	Have simple props such as old clothes, boxes, and folding chairs for playing store, fire station, or school.	Remember at least once a day to hug and cuddle and to praise your child for new skills. Praise independence, creativity, expressing emotions, and sharing toys.	Try to have clear routines during the day. Let your child know what will happen next. Have a reading time and quiet time each day.

*Be sure to review safety guidelines with your health care provider.

Social-Emotional Activities for Young Children 60 Months Old

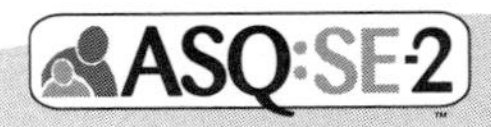

Tell simple jokes and riddles. Your child will love it when you laugh at her jokes—the sillier, the better.	Gather old shirts, hats, and other clothes from friends or a thrift store. Encourage dramatic play—acting out stories, songs, and scenes from the neighborhood.	Encourage your child to make choices as often as possible. Ask, *"Do you want to go to the park or play at home?"* He will like having some control over what he does.	Most of the time, your child will feel good about doing small jobs around the house. Give her a lot of praise when she does a good job, and tell her what a big help she is.
Your child may need some help when he argues or disagrees with a friend or sibling. Remind him to express his feelings with words and that he can come to you for help.	Make sure your child has plenty of rest and quiet and alone time when she needs it.	When your child has friends over, encourage them to play games that require working together. Try building a tent out of old blankets, playing catch, or acting out stories.	Tell your child a favorite nursery rhyme that involves the idea of "right" and "wrong." Discuss what kinds of choices the characters made in the story.
Let your child know how special he is. Give him a lot of love, praise, and hugs every day.	Show your child pictures in magazines of people from different cultures. Talk about things that are the same or different between your family and other families.	Ask your child her birthday, telephone number, and first and last name. Practice what she would do if she was separated from you at the store.	Play games with your child such as Go Fish, Checkers, or Candy Land. Board games or card games that have three or more rules are great.
Have a special time for reading each day. Talk about what happens in the story. Ask your child questions. Listen to his answers. He has a lot to share.	Talk about real dangers (fire, guns, cars) and make-believe dangers (monsters under the bed) using hand-drawn pictures or pictures cut out from a magazine.	Build a store, house, puppet stage, or fire truck out of old boxes. Your child can invite a friend over to play store or house, have a puppet show, or be firefighters.	Encourage your child to talk about the different rules at home and at school. Talk about why there are rules.

Actividades para el desarrollo socio-emocional en bebés de 2 meses de edad

ASQ:SE-2

Cántele a su bebé las canciones de cuna que usted recuerda de su niñez. Tómelo en sus brazos y sosténgalo cerca de su cuerpo (puede usar un rebozo o cangurera). Baile suavemente con él.	Acueste a su bebé sobre su espalda. Tome un paño suave y muévalo de un lado a otro por encima de ella para que lo mire. Haga que el paño vuele, o que le haga cosquillas en diferentes partes de su cuerpo. Observe cómo responde su bebé. Si empieza a llorar, pare el juego.	Deje que su bebé descubra nuevos sonidos suaves. Los juguetes musicales o campanitas le llamarán la atención. Pregúntele: *"¿Oíste las campanitas? ¿Te gusta como suenan?"*	La cara, sonrisa, voz y tacto de usted son las cosas más importantes para su bebé a esta edad. No es necesario tener juguetes sofisticados. Lo que su bebé quiere es jugar con usted y conocerla/lo.
Si su bebé está llorando, trate de averiguar qué es lo que necesita. Con su llanto le está comunicando algo. Cuando usted lo atiende, él empieza a confiar en que usted lo cuidará. La atención que usted le dé a esta edad no lo hará un niño mimado.	Sostenga a su bebé de manera que pueda verle la cara de cerca. Hágale caras divertidas, sonríale, saque la lengua y bostece. Espere unos segundos y observe si su bebé intenta imitarlo/la.	Póngase de manera que su bebé no lo/la vea. Con un tono dulce, llame su nombre y observe lo que hace. ¿Deja de moverse por un momentito? ¿Intenta girar la cabeza hacia donde oye su voz? Tómelo en sus brazos y dígale: *"Aquí estoy"*.	Ponga a su bebé sobre una cobija en el suelo y acuéstese a su lado. Vea el mundo desde su punto de vista. Hable con ella sobre lo que está viendo. Dígale: *"Ahí está la luz"*.
Procure que la vida sea interesante para su bebé. Sáquelo de la casa a pasear. Dele la oportunidad de conocer nuevos sitios y sonidos desde sus brazos reconfortantes.	Hable con su bebé sobre lo que ella hace, ve, escucha y siente. Dígale: *"Estoy cambiándote el pañal. Te encantará sentirte seca. ¡Te amo!"*	Puede comenzar a jugar juegos sencillos con su bebé, como "¿Dónde está el nene?". Tápese la cabeza con una toallita, asómese por un lado y dígale: *"¡Ahí estás!"*	Dele nuevos objetos que sean seguros* a su bebé para que los explore. Los objetos sencillos tales como vasos de plástico o cucharones de madera son todos nuevos para ella.
Coloque objetos interesantes cerca de la cuna de su bebé de modo que los pueda mirar, pero asegúrese de colocarlos fuera de su alcance. Pegue ilustraciones sencillas de revistas en la pared.	Nunca es demasiado temprano para empezar a leerle cuentos a su bebé. Al principio, elija libros sencillos de cartón grueso laminado y háblele de las ilustraciones. Acurruque a su bebé mientras leen.	Aprenda a reconocer el lenguaje especial de su bebé. Él le "hablará" usando sonidos y gestos, y le avisará cuando esté contento o incómodo, cuando tenga hambre o se sienta solito.	Dele un masaje a su bebé después de bañarla o de cambiarle el pañal. Frótele el vientre suavemente. Hable con ella: *"Mmmm. Te estoy dando un masaje en la barriguita. ¿Te gusta cómo se siente?"*

*Asegúrese de revisar las medidas de seguridad con su proveedor/a de servicios de salud.

Actividades para el desarrollo socio-emocional en bebés de 6 meses de edad

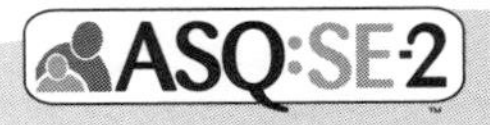

Aprenda a reconocer el ritmo de actividad que tiene su bebé, e intente establecer una rutina para comer, dormir y cambiarle los pañales. Hable con él sobre su rutina. De esta manera, se sentirá seguro y contento.	A su bebé le encantará escuchar nuevos sonidos. Las campanas, los silbidos y el ladrido de los perros le llamarán la atención. Hable con ella sobre los sonidos que oye.	Póngase en el suelo a un lado de su bebé y juegue con él a su altura. Miren juntos los juguetes, libros u otros objetos. Diviértanse, ríanse y disfruten de su tiempo juntos.	Cuando su bebé esté llorando, atiéndala. Susúrrele palabras agradables al oído para calmarla. Abrácela y hágale sonidos suaves. De esta manera sabrá que usted la ama y que siempre la cuidará.
Juegue a las palmaditas y a "¿Dónde está el nene?" con su bebé. Muéstrese juguetón/a, ría con su bebé y diviértase. Él le responderá con sonrisas y risitas.	Lea con su bebé. Acurrúquense los/las dos, señale las ilustraciones y háblele de lo que están mirando. Conforme vaya creciendo su bebé, empezará a escoger sus libros favoritos.	Lleve a su bebé a conocer nuevos lugares y a ver cosas nuevas. Paséense en el parque o en un centro comercial, o simplemente llévelo con usted cuando vaya de compras. Le encantará ver cosas nuevas mientras se sienta seguro con usted.	Coloque a su bebé en posturas y en áreas diferentes de la casa. ¡El mundo se ve muy distinto desde un nuevo sitio!
Deje que su bebé empiece a comer trocitos de comida sola. Dele una taza para niños y una cuchara. Le encantará empezar a hacer las cosas por sí misma.	Llame a su bebé por su nombre al darle de comer, vestirlo o cambiarle el pañal. Dígale: *"Éste es el dedo de Beto. Éste es el piecito de Beto"*.	Procure darle nuevos objetos que sean seguros* a su bebé. Todo lo nuevo le fascinará. Un cucharón de madera o un cepillo blando para bebés son buenos objetos para que explore y aprenda.	"Hable" con su bebé. Cuando su bebé haga un sonido, responda imitándoselo. Mantenga esta "conversación" el más tiempo que pueda.
Cántele canciones y rimas infantiles a su bebé. Invente canciones sobre su bebé usando su nombre. Esto la hará sentirse especial y querida.	La hora del baño* es un buen momento para jugar y estar cerca de su bebé. Las esponjas, tazas de plástico y toallitas son juguetes sencillos y económicos con los que puede jugar cuando lo bañe.	Disfrute de la música con su bebé. Tómela en sus brazos y salte o dé vueltas con ella. Ponga diferentes estilos de música.	Visite a un amigo/a que tenga un bebé o niño pequeño. Quédese cerca de su bebé y hágale saber que estas nuevas personas son amigos. Puede que necesite un tiempito para acostumbrarse a ellos.

*Asegúrese de revisar las medidas de seguridad con su proveedor/a de servicios de salud.

Actividades para el desarrollo socio-emocional en bebés de 12 meses de edad

ASQ:SE-2

Establezca una rutina en casa para comer, dormir, cambiar los pañales y jugar. Hable con su bebé sobre la rutina y dígale qué actividad harán a continuación. Esto le ayudará a sentirse segura.	Dígale a su bebé todos los días lo tanto que lo ama y lo precioso que es —cuando se despierta en la mañana y cuando se acuesta por la noche.	Póngase en el suelo a jugar con su bebé todos los días. Gatee con ella, o simplemente siéntese cerca de ella en el suelo para que esté a su altura. Le encantará pasar estos momentos a solas con usted.	Juegue juegos sencillos con su bebé, tales como las tortillitas, "¿Dónde está el nene?", o un juego de perseguirse el uno al otro. ¡Ríanse y diviértanse juntos!
Deje que su bebé "ayude" a preparar la cena. Procure tener un cajón o una alacena especial en la cocina con objetos seguros para niños, tales como cucharones o tazas medidoras que pueda llenar y vaciar.	Hágale cosquillas a su bebé, pero asegúrese de hacerlo suavemente y de dejar el juego si su bebé se muestra molesta. Obsérvela cuidadosamente para saber si está disfrutando el juego.	Ponga música y baile con su bebé. Tome sus manos y deje que él se mueva hacia arriba y hacia abajo. Aplauda y festéjelo cuando él "baile" solito.	Juegue a los juegos de nombres con su bebé, tales como "¿Dónde está Rita?".
Lleve a su bebé a dar un paseo al parque o a un sitio donde haya otros niños jugando. Deje que su bebé los observe y que se les acerque si quiere.	Use un espejo para bebés* para hacer un juego. Ponga caras divertidas y hable con su bebé sobre lo que está viendo en el espejo.	Tome a su bebé de las manos y hágala girar. Le encantará un poco de juego brusco, pero asegúrese de parar si nota que su bebé se cansa del juego.	Léale cuentos a su bebé antes de la siesta o antes de acostarlo a dormir por la noche. ¡Deje que su bebé escoja el libro y acurrúquense!
Deje que su bebé seleccione sus propios alimentos, ropa, juguetes y actividades la mayor parte del tiempo. Le encantará poder escoger por sí misma.	Invite a una amiga que tenga un bebé o niño pequeño a su casa. Procure tener suficientes juguetes para ambos niños ya que a esta edad todavía no saben compartir.	Siéntese en el suelo frente a su bebé y ruede una pelota hacia él. Aplauda cuando su bebé empuje la pelota o la "agarre" con sus manos.	Cuando usted vista a su bebé o le cambie el pañal, hable con ella sobre las partes de su cuerpo. Nombre las partes de su propio cuerpo y dígale: *"Ésta es la nariz de papá. Ésta es la nariz de María"*.

*Asegúrese de revisar las medidas de seguridad con su proveedor/a de servicios de salud.

Actividades para el desarrollo socio-emocional en niños de 18 meses de edad

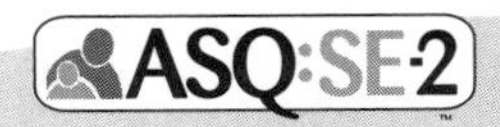

A su niño le gustará tener una rutina diaria predecible. Hable con él acerca de lo que están haciendo en ese momento y de lo que vendrá después. Dele tiempo de estar activo y también de tener momentos tranquilos.	A su niña le encantará que usted le demuestre su cariño. Dele abrazotes de oso, abrazos más suaves, besotes ruidosos y besitos suaves. ¡Dígale lo mucho que la quiere!	Su niño disfrutará que usted le haga cosquillas y también un poco de juego brusco. Asegúrese de parar cuando vea que se ha cansado del juego. A su niño también le gustará tener momentos tranquilos y acurrucarse con usted.	Organicen una "fiesta" para las muñecas o animales de peluche. Puede recortar fotos de cajas de regalo de una revista, preparar un "pastel" de mentira y cantar la canción de Feliz Cumpleaños o Las Mañanitas.
Su niño querrá tener mucho tiempo y libertad para moverse y estar activo. Llévelo a dar un paseo, al parque o al centro comercial.	A su niña le encantará ayudar con los quehaceres domésticos. Dele tareas sencillas y dígale que parece una niña muy grande. Puede limpiar la mesa, guardar sus juguetes o ayudar a barrer.	Jueguen al escondite o a atraparse el uno al otro en casa. Diviértanse y ríanse juntos.	Baile con su niña. Haga un tambor sencillo con un recipiente grande de plástico o haga unas maracas con un envase pequeño lleno de frijoles o arroz.
Ayude a su niño a reconocer las emociones. Frente a un espejo haga caras alegres o tristes, caras enojadas o caras tontas. ¡Es muy divertido!	Deje que su niña lleve cosas a la mesa o que coloque los cubiertos en la mesa a la hora de comer.	A su niño le encantará tener un escondite secreto donde pueda jugar. Use una manta o sábana para hacer una tienda de campaña o lugar en donde pueda esconderse.	Su niña puede ayudar a recoger los juguetes después de jugar. Ponga una caja o cesto grande para facilitar la tarea y ayúdele a guardar las cosas. Aplauda y elógiela por haber ayudado.
Haga muebles de cocina con cajas de cartón para su hija. Para hacer la estufa, dibuje unas "hornillas" en un lado de una caja. Use recipientes de plástico para las ollas y cucharas de madera para revolver la sopa.	Reúnase con otras familias para que los niños puedan jugar juntos. Su hijo todavía no sabrá compartir, por lo tanto debe asegurarse de tener suficientes juguetes disponibles. Quédese cerca de él y ayúdelo a aprender a jugar con otros niños.	¡Su niña está creciendo ahora y querrá hacer cosas por sí misma! Deje que coma sola con una cucharita y que beba de su taza para bebé sin ayudarla a la hora de la comida. ¡Tenga una esponja o trapo a la mano para limpiar lo que derrame!	Leer con su niño, especialmente antes de la siesta o de la hora de dormir, es una excelente actividad para calmarlo y prepararlo para que se duerma. Deje que él escoja el libro. Ayúdelo a darle vuelta a las páginas y a nombrar lo que ve en las ilustraciones.

Actividades para el desarrollo socio-emocional en niños de 24 meses de edad

ASQ:SE-2

Intente tener rutinas predecibles durante el día, y dígale a su niño la actividad que viene enseguida. Dígale: *"Recuerda que después de cepillarte el pelo, debes ponerte la ropa y yo te voy a ayudar"*.	Su hija está aprendiendo a seguir las reglas, pero usted tendrá que recordárselas muchas veces todavía. Procure que las reglas sean breves, sencillas y constantes.	Establezca la costumbre de leer con su niño todos los días. Acurrúquense. Los mejores momentos para leer son antes de acostarse o antes de la siesta.	¡Dígale a su niña lo preciosa que es! Le encantará ser alabada por las nuevas habilidades que aprende. Dígale: *"Eres una ayudante magnífica. ¡Qué bien lo hiciste tú solita!"*
Quédese cerca de su niño cuando esté jugando con sus amigos y enséñele cómo tomar turnos. Todavía está muy chiquito para saber compartir, pero si usted le habla sobre cómo tomar turnos, esto le ayudará a aprender.	Dele opciones a su niña, pero asegúrese de que sean sencillas. Por ejemplo, deje que escoja entre ponerse una camisa roja o una azul, o que decida entre tomar leche o jugo con el almuerzo.	Dele a su niño muchas oportunidades para jugar con otros pequeños. Probablemente, su niño jugará hasta agotarse y por lo tanto necesitará tener momentos tranquilos también. Ponga atención a los ritmos de actividad que tiene su niño y deje que los siga.	Deje que su niña haga más cosas solita.* Coloque un taburete frente al lavabo para que pueda lavarse las manos y cepillarse los dientes sin ayuda. Ella sola podrá escoger su ropa y ayudar a vestirse.
Siéntese en el suelo a jugar con su niño. Deje que él escoja los juguetes y que dirija el juego. Tome en cuenta las ideas de su niño para jugar.	Motive a su niña a jugar juegos que usen su imaginación. Coloque unas sillas en fila para hacer un "autobús". Recorte trozos de papel de colores para hacer "dinero" para pagarle al chofer. Dígale: *"¿A dónde vamos hoy?"*	El mundo es nuevo para su niño. Le parecerá fascinante ver la maleza que crece por un sendero o una paloma comiendo semillas. Tome tiempo para detenerse y disfrutar de los detalles con él.	Su niña está aprendiendo a reconocer sus emociones. Ayúdele a decir lo que siente cuando está enojada, triste, contenta o graciosa. Dígale: *"Te ves muy contenta."* o *"Parece que estás muy enojada"*.
Juegue al "desfile" o a "Sigan al líder" con su niño. A su niño le encantará imitarla/lo—¡*y también* le gustará ser el líder cuando sea su turno!	Si su niña hace berrinches, mantenga la calma y hable con ella en un tono tranquilo. Si se puede, deje que se calme por sí misma.	¡No olvide decirle a su niño lo mucho que lo ama! Demuéstrele su cariño dándole muchos besos y abrazos, y haciéndole caricias.	Enséñele a su niña canciones sencillas como "Witsi, witsi araña". Enséñele los movimientos que se hacen con las manos al cantar estas canciones.

*Asegúrese de revisar las medidas de seguridad con su proveedor/a de servicios de salud.

Actividades para el desarrollo socio-emocional en niños de 30 meses de edad

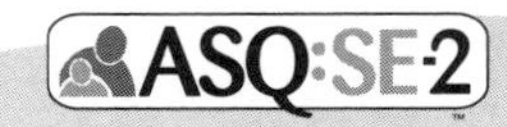

Construya un "libro personal" con su hijo. Tome unas hojas de papel y pegue fotos de él, de miembros de la familia, de mascotas o de otras cosas que le gusten. Una las páginas con grapas o cinta adhesiva.	Háblele a su hija de las cosas divertidas que hacía cuando era bebé. Cuéntele el comienzo de una historia y vea si ella la puede continuar.	Muéstrele a su hijo fotos de la familia. Hable sobre las personas de las fotos y dígale quiénes son: *"Él es tu tío José"*. ¿Su hijo puede decirle quiénes son las personas de las fotos?	Cántele a su niña una de sus rimas infantiles favoritas y pregúntele sobre las emociones de los personajes.
Dele a su niño instrucciones que tengan dos pasos, por ejemplo: *"Pon todos los legos en la caja y luego guarda la caja en el clóset"*. Dígale que es muy buen ayudante.	Cuando esté cocinando o limpiando la casa, deje que su niña le ayude.* Puede hacer cosas como ayudar a revolver la comida, poner harina en una taza, o guardar las cucharas y tenedores en el cajón.	A su niño le encantará imitarlo/la. Dígale nuevas palabras o haga sonidos de animales o ruidos diferentes para ver si su niño puede repetir lo que usted dice o imitar los sonidos.	Motive a su niña a jugar de manera creativa, ya sea dibujando con crayolas, pintando o jugando con plastilina. Dibujar sobre la acera con gises de muchos colores es muy divertido.
Deje que su niño haga más cosas por sí mismo conforme vaya creciendo. Deje que se ponga los zapatos y el abrigo sin ayuda cuando salgan a la calle. Procure darle suficiente tiempo de practicar estas nuevas habilidades. Dígale: *"¡Qué niño más grande!"*	Haga dibujos de caras que expresen una gama de emociones como enojo, frustración y alegría, y después recórtelas. Su hija puede usar las caras para comunicarle cómo se siente.	Dígale a su hijo lo mucho que lo ama todos los días. Dele besitos en la nariz, las orejas y los dedos. Dígale: *"¡Amo tu nariz! ¡Amo tu orejita! ¡Amo tu dedo! ¡Te amo!"*	Dedique unos momentos cada día para leer con su niña. Acurrúquense mucho. Vayan a la biblioteca a buscar libros sobre niños que expresan sus emociones fuertemente. Dígale: *"¿Qué haces tú cuando te enojas?"*
Juegue con su niño y ayúdelo a aprender a compartir. Comparta las cosas con él y elógielo cuando él comparta las cosas con usted. Esta es una nueva habilidad para su niño, por lo tanto, no debe esperar mucho de él a esta edad.	Pregúntele a su niño su nombre y su edad. Para ayudarlo a recordar su nombre y su edad, usted podría inventar una rima o canción que lleve su nombre. Pídale también que le diga los nombres de sus amigos y sus maestros.	Cante canciones y baile con su niña. Ponga la radio para escuchar diferentes estilos de música. Elaboren instrumentos musicales sencillos usando cajas de avena o cereal, o recipientes de yogur.	Invite a un amigo de su niño a la casa para que jueguen. La visita puede ser corta—1 o 2 horas bastarán. Asegúrese de tener suficientes juguetes para los dos y deles tiempo de jugar. Después deles algo para comer y un tiempito para jugar afuera en el jardín. Dígales: *"¡Qué bien lo pasamos! ¡Nos vemos la próxima vez!"*

*Asegúrese de revisar las medidas de seguridad con su proveedor/a de servicios de salud.

Actividades para el desarrollo socio-emocional en niños de 36 meses de edad

ASQ:SE-2

Cuéntele a su hija una historia sencilla sobre algo chistoso o interesante que ella haya hecho. Pídale que cuente otra historia sobre sí misma.	Motive a su niño a identificar y nombrar sus sentimientos y también los de otros niños o adultos.	Ofrézcale a su hija oportunidades para jugar con otros niños en su vecindario o en un parque.*	Muchos niños de esta edad tienen amigos imaginarios. Deje que su niño hable y juegue con sus amiguitos de fantasía.
Escuche a otros miembros de la familia hablar sobre su jornada a la hora de la comida. Ayúdele a su hija a hablar de lo que ella hizo ese día. Por ejemplo: *"Carolina y yo fuimos al parque hoy. Carolina, dile a tu hermana lo que hicimos en el parque"*.	Dele a su niño instrucciones que tengan por lo menos dos pasos cuando ustedes estén preparando la comida, limpiando la casa o vistiéndose. Por ejemplo: *"Pon la sartén en el fregadero y luego agarra la cuchara roja"*.	Escríbanle una carta a los abuelos o a un amigo. Pregúntele a su hija qué le gustaría escribir acerca de sí misma e inclúyalo en la carta.	Haga juegos con su niño en los que se debe tomar turnos, tales como "Sigan al líder" o "Rayuela".
Utilice muñecos o animales de peluche para que actúen situaciones conflictivas. Hable con su niño de lo que ocurrió, pregúntele qué sintieron los personajes y cómo se pueden solucionar problemas cuando surgen.	Dedique un tiempo especial para la lectura todos los días. Acurrúquese con su niña. Vaya aumentando la duración de los cuentos cada día para que ella aprenda a permanecer sentada y a escuchar un poco más de tiempo.	Dígale a su hijo lo mucho que lo ama y lo fabuloso que es todos los días. Dígale, "¡chócala!", sonría mucho, frote su espalda o dele un abrazo. Dígale que es lo máximo, que es precioso y divertido.	Cuéntele a su hija una de sus historias favoritas, como *"Los tres cochinitos, Ricitos de oro* o *Los tres osos"*. Pídale a su niña que describa los sentimientos de los personajes del cuento.
Haga dibujos de caras que expresen diferentes sentimientos. Luego recórtelas y péguelas en palitos de madera. Deje que su niño use las figuras para actuar las diferentes emociones.	Póngase en el suelo para jugar con su niña. Deje que ella escoja los juguetes y que ella determine las reglas y dirija el juego.	Jueguen a juegos que tengan reglas sencillas, como "Simón dice" o "Luz roja, luz verde".	Cuéntele chistes sencillos a su hija. También es divertido jugar a las adivinanzas, tales como "Adivina quién soy". Diviértase y ría con su niña.

Actividades para el desarrollo socio-emocional en niños de 48 meses de edad

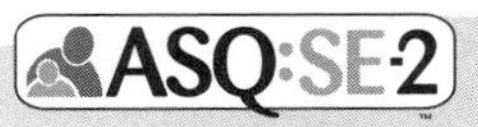

Enséñele a su hijo una nueva emoción (por ej.: aburrimiento) cada día a través de fotos, gestos o palabras. Dele a escoger de una variedad de palabras para describir cómo se siente.	Ofrézcale a su hija muchas actividades que le enseñarán a saber compartir con otros niños. Por ejemplo: colorear con crayolas, hacer torres con bloques, modelar con plastilina o jugar a disfrazarse. Dele a su niña mucho tiempo para jugar con otros niños.	Procure que su hijo tenga muchas oportunidades para desarrollar su creatividad. Podría usar recipientes vacíos, pegamento, periódicos viejos, ligas y revistas para hacer muchas creaciones.	Explore nuevos lugares con su hija. Llévela a la tienda, a un restaurante o a la biblioteca. Hable con ella sobre las semejanzas y diferencias que hay entre las personas que vean.
Cuando usted esté limpiando la casa o trabajando en el jardín, deje que su niño haga un quehacer solito. Por ejemplo: vaciar el cesto de la basura o limpiar las migajas de la mesa.	Hable con su niña sobre los posibles peligros que hay adentro de la casa, tales como los enchufes de la electricidad o las hornillas de la estufa. También hable de los peligros que hay en el exterior, por ejemplo: hablar con personas desconocidas o cruzar la calle.*	Fomente la independencia en su hijo. Deje que se prepare un sándwich solo. Antes de dormir, deje que escoja la ropa que se pondrá al día siguiente.	Hagan una representación de un conflicto o problema usando animales de peluche. Hable primero de cómo se sienten los animales. Después hablen sobre las diversas soluciones que podría haber para resolver su problema.
Cuéntele una historia o una rima infantil a su niña. Hable con ella acerca de lo que es real y de lo que es fantasía.	Hagan muñequitos con palos de paleta. Pueden usar cartoncillo para hacer las caras y estambre para el cabello, etc. Después hagan una representación en la que dos niños se conocen y se hacen amigos usando los muñequitos.	Cuéntele a su niña una historia o rima infantil sobre "el enojo". Hable con ella sobre las maneras positivas en las que actuaron los personajes para manejar su enojo o resolver su problema.	Lleve a su niño a la "hora de cuentos" de la biblioteca. Ahí aprenderá a formar parte de un grupo y a escuchar la lectura.
Su niña está aprendiendo más acerca de las reglas de la casa, pero usted tendrá que recordárselas todavía. Hable sobre las reglas de la familia; éstas deben ser sencillas, breves y predecibles.	Tenga a mano accesorios sencillos como ropa vieja, cajas y sillas para jugar a la tienda, a la estación de bomberos o a ir al colegio.	Procure abrazar, acurrucar y alabar a su niño al menos una vez por día para elogiar habilidades que sean nuevas. Elógielo por su independencia y creatividad, por expresar sus emociones y por compartir juguetes.	Intente establecer una rutina diaria para su niña. Cada que cambien de actividad, dígale cuál es la que sigue. Reserve unos momentos tranquilos para leer y descansar con ella todos los días.

*Asegúrese de revisar las medidas de seguridad con su proveedor/a de servicios de salud.

Actividades para el desarrollo socio-emocional en niños de 60 meses de edad

ASQ:SE-2

Cuéntele chistes y adivinanzas sencillas a su niña. Le encantará ver que usted se ríe de sus bromas—cuanto más tontas sean, mejor.	Reúna camisas viejas, sombreros y otras prendas de ropa (de una tienda de segunda mano o de sus amigos). Anime a su niño a hacer representaciones de cuentos, canciones y escenas tomadas de lo que pasa en su vecindario.	Deje que su niña tenga oportunidades para elegir sus actividades lo más que se pueda. Pregúntele: *"¿Quieres ir al parque o jugar en casa?"* A ella le gustará tener algo de control sobre sus actividades.	A su niño le gustará ayudarla/lo en casa la mayor parte del tiempo.* Elógielo mucho cuando lo hace bien y dígale que es un ayudante magnífico.
Puede que su hijo necesite ayuda para resolver conflictos, sobre todo con sus amigos. Recuérdele cómo expresar sus emociones con palabras y que siempre puede acudir a usted si necesita ayuda.	Procure que su hija tenga suficientes momentos de tranquilidad para descansar o estar a solas cuando lo necesite.	Cuando su hijo esté jugando con sus amigos, sugiérales juegos que requieran cooperación entre ellos. Podrían montar una tienda de campaña con mantas viejas, jugar a la pelota o actuar cuentos.	Cuéntele a su hija una historia infantil que incluya ideas sobre lo "correcto" o lo "incorrecto". Hable con ella sobre las decisiones que tomaron los personajes del cuento.
Hágale saber a su hija lo preciosa que es. Dele mucho cariño y amor, y hágale elogios todos los días.	Muéstrele a su niño fotos de gente de diferentes culturas recortadas de revistas. Hable con él sobre las semejanzas y diferencias entre su familia y otras familias.	Enséñele a su hija a decir su nombre y apellido, el día de su cumpleaños y su número de teléfono. Practique lo que debe hacer en caso de que se separe de usted en la tienda.	Juegue juegos de mesa con su hijo, tales como "A pescar", damas o lotería. Los juegos de mesa o de naipes que tengan tres reglas o más son ideales.
Procure reservar unos momentos para leer con su hija todos los días. Hable con ella sobre lo que pasa en el cuento. Hágale preguntas y escuche sus respuestas. Ella tiene mucho que compartir.	Hable con su hijo sobre los peligros reales (como el fuego, las armas o los autos) y los peligros imaginarios (los monstruos debajo de la cama). Use dibujos o recorte ilustraciones de una revista para hablar de estos temas.	Con unas cajas viejas, monte un escenario para títeres, haga un camión de bomberos, una tienda o una casa. Su hija puede invitar a sus amiguitas a casa para jugar a la tienda, a la casa, a ser bomberos o a tener una función de títeres.	Pregúntele a su hijo sobre las diferentes reglas que hay en casa y en el colegio. Explíquele por qué existen las reglas.

*Asegúrese de revisar las medidas de seguridad con su proveedor/a de servicios de salud.

F

Resources

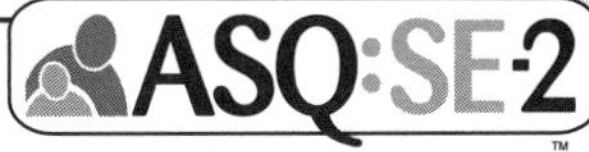

DEVELOPMENTAL SCREENING TOOLS

Ages & Stages Questionnaires®, Third Edition (ASQ-3™): A Parent-Completed Child Monitoring System

Jane Squires and Diane Bricker, with assistance from Elizabeth Twombly, Robert Nickel, Jantina Clifford, Kimberly Murphy, Robert Hoselton, Lawanda Potter, and Jane Farrell (2009); Paul H. Brookes Publishing Co.; http://www.brookespublishing.com; http://agesandstages.com

ASQ-3 is an accurate, family-friendly way to screen children for developmental delays from 1 month to 5½ years. The tool can be filled out by, or with, caregivers to report on their children's development related to communication, gross motor, fine motor, problem-solving, and personal-social skills.

Brigance Early Childhood Screens III

Albert H. Brigance and Brian F. French (2013); Curriculum Associates; http://www.curriculumassociates.com

These screening tools—which cover the age ranges of birth through 35 months, 3 through 5 years, and kindergarten and first grade—provide quick and accurate measures of children's physical, language, academic/cognitive, self-help, and social-emotional skills. Teachers can use results to identify children's developmental needs, determine children's school readiness, and guide instructional planning.

Early Screening Inventory–Revised (ESI-R)

Samuel J. Meisels, Dorothea B. Marsden, Martha S. Wiske, and Laura W. Henderson (2008); Pearson Education; http://www.pearsonclinical.com

ESI-R is a brief developmental screening tool designed to be individually administered to preschool and kindergarten children. It identifies children who may need special education services in order to perform successfully in school. ESI-R addresses developmental, sensory, and behavioral concerns in the following areas: visual motor/adaptive, language and cognition, and gross motor skills.

Parents' Evaluation of Developmental Status (PEDS)

Frances Page Glascoe (2010); http://www.PEDStest.com

PEDS is a screening tool that elicits and addresses parents' concerns about their children's language, motor, self-help, early academic skills, behavior, and social-emotional/mental health. It helps determine when parents' concerns suggest problems requiring referral.

PARENT–CHILD AND TEACHER–CHILD INTERACTION SCALES

Classroom Assessment Scoring System (CLASS)

Robert C. Pianta, Karen M. La Paro, and Bridget K. Hamre (2008); Paul H. Brookes Publishing Co.; http://www.brookespublishing.com

CLASS is an observational assessment tool used to measure the quality of teacher–child interactions. It addresses factors such as positive and negative classroom climate, teacher sensitivity, language modeling, and behavior management. There are infant, toddler, pre-K, and K–3 versions. Training is required for reliable use of CLASS.

Keys to Interactive Parenting Scale (KIPS)

Marilee Comfort and Philip R. Gordon (2006); Comfort Consults; http://www.comfortconsults.com

KIPS is an assessment scale used to measure 12 key parenting behaviors through observation of parent–child interactions. Results can be used to help create individualized support for families and track parent progress. Training is required.

Parent–Child Interaction (PCI) Feeding and Teaching Scales

Nursing Child Assessment Satellite Training (NCAST; 1995); University of Washington; http://www.washington.edu

These scales assess parent–child interactions in feeding and teaching situations. Public health nurses, researchers, social workers, psychologists, early intervention workers, and other professionals can use the results to identify strengths of and ways to further promote parent–child relationships, offering specific ways to guide intervention. A companion video series, *Keys to Caregiving,* offers information for professionals working with families with newborns. Training is required.

Parenting Interactions with Children: Checklist of Observations Linked to Outcomes (PICCOLO™)

Lori A. Roggman, Gina A. Cook, Mark S. Innocenti, Vonda Jump Norman, and Katie Christiansen (2013); Paul H. Brookes Publishing Co.; http://www.brookespublishing.com

PICCOLO is a quick, reliable observational tool designed to help family support professionals assess and monitor the quality of parent–child interactions. Developed for use with parents of children ages 10–47 months, it measures 29 developmentally supportive parenting behaviors in 4 domains—affection, responsiveness, encouragement, and teaching. It helps professionals assess which parenting behaviors are working, develop individualized interventions, and track the positive outcomes of parent support programs. The training DVD is recommended for scoring reliability.

ENVIRONMENTAL/PROGRAM ASSESSMENT TOOLS

Environment Rating Scales

Teachers College Press; http://www.teacherscollegepress.com

These assessment tools are designed to evaluate the quality of settings for young children in early childhood, family child care, and infant-toddler environments. Training is required.

- *Early Childhood Environment Rating Scale–Third Edition (ECERS-3):* Thelma Harms, Richard M. Clifford, and Debby Cryer (2014)
- *The Family Child Care Environment Rating Scale–Revised (FCCERS-R):* Thelma Harms, Debby Cryer, and Richard M. Clifford (2007)
- *Infant/Toddler Environment Rating Scale–Revised (ITERS-R):* Thelma Harms, Debby Cryer, and Richard M. Clifford (2015)

Preschool-Wide Evaluation Tool™, Research Edition (PreSET™)

Elizabeth A. Steed, Tina M. Pomerleau, and Robert H. Horner (2012); Paul H. Brookes Publishing Co.; http://www.brookespublishing.com

The PreSET helps assess the use of programwide positive behavior interventions and support (PBIS) in early childhood settings. Conducted twice a year by an outside observer—such as a behavior consultant, inclusion coordinator, or school psychologist—PreSET takes an accurate snapshot of a program's PBIS through a review of program documents, classroom observations, and interviews with the administrator, teachers, and a few children from each classroom.

Teaching Pyramid Observation Tool (TPOT™) for Preschool Classrooms, Research Edition

Lise K. Fox, Mary Louise Hemmeter, and Patricia Snyder (2014); Paul H. Brookes Publishing Co.; http://www.brookespublishing.com

Early childhood care and education programs use the TPOT to measure how well teachers are implementing the three-tiered Pyramid Model of practices that support children's social competence and prevent challenging behaviors. TPOT results can be used to reinforce interactions that promote social-emotional competence in young children, implement strategies to prevent and address challenging behavior, and compare implementation across early childhood classrooms, teachers, and programs.

FUNCTIONAL BEHAVIOR ASSESSMENT

Prevent-Teach-Reinforce for Young Children:
The Early Childhood Model of Individualized Positive Behavior Support

Glen Dunlap, Kelly Wilson, Philip S. Strain, and Janice K. Lee (2013); Paul H. Brookes Publishing Co.; http://www.brookespublishing.com

This book provides in-depth information on how to individualize positive behavior support for young children. It includes forms and guidance for conducting functional behavioral assessments.

SOCIAL-EMOTIONAL TRAINING AND CURRICULUM

See Diane Powell and Glen Dunlap's (2009) *Evidence-Based Social-Emotional Curricula and Intervention Packages for Children 0–5 Years and Their Families* (available at http://challengingbehavior.fmhi.usf.edu/do/resources/documents/roadmap_2.pdf) for a list of social-emotional curricula.

The Incredible Years (Parent, Teacher, and Child Training Series)

Carolyn Webster-Stratton; The Incredible Years; http://www.incredibleyears.com

The Incredible Years, a series of three different curricula for parents, teachers, and children, is focused on preventing and addressing problem behaviors in young children. These curricula can be used separately or in combination and have additional components, such as a troubleshooting guide for parents. The Incredible Years BASIC Parent Training Program targets parents of children who are at high risk or are displaying behavior problems. The Incredible Years ADVANCE Parent Training Program addresses interpersonal skills, such as how to handle stress, anger, and depression and how to communicate effectively with your children and other adults. The Incredible Years Child Training Program is composed of the Dina Dinosaur Social Skills and Problem-Solving Curriculum. It is designed to promote social competence and reduce challenging behaviors.

PATHS (Promoting Alternative THinking Strategies) Program, Preschool/Kindergarten Edition

C. Domitrovich, M. Greenberg, R. Cortes, & C. Kusche (2011); Channing Bete Company; http://www.channing-bete.com

PATHS is a preschool and kindergarten classroom curriculum focused on social-emotional learning. It concentrates on helping young children learn to resolve conflicts, handle their emotions, empathize with others, and make responsible decisions.

ADDITIONAL SOCIAL-EMOTIONAL RESOURCES

Bowman, B., & Moore, E.K. 2006. *School readiness and social-emotional development: Perspectives on cultural diversity.* Washington, DC: National Black Child Development Institute.

Brazelton, T.B. (2006). *Touchpoints: Birth to 3: Your child's emotional and behavioral development* (2nd ed.). Cambridge, MA: Da Capo Lifelong Books.

Brazelton, T.B., & Sparrow, J. (2001). *Touchpoints: 3 to 6: Your child's emotional and behavioral development.* Cambridge, MA: Perseus.

Bricker, D., Macy, M., Squires, J., & Marks, K. (2013). *Developmental screening in your community: An integrated approach for connecting children with services.* Baltimore, MD: Paul H. Brookes Publishing Co.

Dombro, A.L., Jablon, J., & Stetson, C. (2011). *Powerful interactions: How to connect with children to extend their learning.* Washington, DC: National Association for the Education of Young Children.

Durand, V.M. (2011). *Optimistic parenting: Hope and help for you and your challenging child.* Baltimore, MD: Paul H. Brookes Publishing Co.

Epstein, A.S. (2009). *Me, you, us: Social-emotional learning in preschool.* Washington, DC: National Association for the Education of Young Children.

Honig, A.S. (2010). *Little kids, big worries: Stress-busting tips for early childhood classrooms.* Baltimore, MD: Paul H. Brookes Publishing Co.

Hyson, M. (2004). *The emotional development of young children: Building an emotion-centered curriculum.* New York, NY: Teachers College Press.

Landy, S. (2009). *Pathways to competence: Encouraging healthy social and emotional development in young children* (2nd ed.). Baltimore, MD: Paul H. Brookes Publishing Co.

Landy, S., & Thompson, E. (2006). *Pathways to competence for young children: A parenting program.* Baltimore, MD: Paul H. Brookes Publishing Co.

Marion, M. (2014). *Guidance of young children* (9th ed.). New York, NY: Pearson.

Merrell, K.W., Parisi, D.M., & Whitcomb, S.A. (2007). *Strong Start-K-2: A social and emotional learning curriculum.* Baltimore, MD: Paul H. Brookes Publishing Co.

Merrell, K.W., Whitcomb, S.A., & Parisi, D.M. (2009). *Strong Start-Pre-K: A social and emotional learning curriculum.* Baltimore, MD: Paul H. Brookes Publishing Co.

Perry, D.F., Kaufmann, R.K., & Knitzer, J. (Volume eds.). (2007). *Social and emotional health in early childhood: Building bridges between services and systems.* Baltimore, MD: Paul H. Brookes Publishing Co.

Raikes, H.H., Edwards, C.P., & Gandini, L. (2009). *Extending the dance in infant and toddler caregiving: Enhancing attachment and relationships.* Baltimore, MD: Paul H. Brookes Publishing Co.

Serna, L.A., Nielsen, M.E., & Forness, S.R. (2007). *Social skills in pictures, stories, and songs: A multisensory program for preschool and early elementary students: Teacher's guide.* Champaign, IL: Research Press.

Squires, J., & Bricker, D. (2007). *An activity-based approach to developing young children's social emotional competence.* Baltimore, MD: Paul H. Brookes Publishing Co.

Squires, J., Bricker, D., Waddell, M., Funk, K., Clifford, J., & Hoselton, R. (2014). *Social-Emotional Assessment/Evaluation Measure (SEAM™), research edition.* Baltimore, MD: Paul H. Brookes Publishing Co.

ORGANIZATIONS

American Academy of Pediatrics (AAP)

http://www.aap.org—AAP offers a variety of materials, including a Healthy Children site (http://www.healthychildren.org) that includes information on breastfeeding, crying and colic, sleep, social-emotional development, and many other topics.

Center for Early Childhood Mental Health Consultation

http://www.ecmhc.org—This organization focuses on helping Head Start programs build a strong mental health foundation for children, families, and staff. The site offers free resources for families, educators, and administrators, including resources to help reduce stress, self-assessment and teaching tools, best practice tutorials, and implementation toolkits.

Collaborative for Academic, Social, and Emotional Learning (CASEL)

http://www.casel.org—CASEL works to advance students' development of academic and social-emotional competence through research, policy, and practice. It help makes evidence-based social-emotional learning an integral part of education from preschool—including child care and Head Start programs—through high school.

Devereux Center for Resilient Children

http://www.centerforresilientchildren.org—Devereux Center for Resilient Children works to establish partnerships among early childhood educators, mental health professionals, and families to promote young children's social-emotional development, resilience, and school readiness. Devereux offers training for practitioners and families and an assessment program for infants and toddlers, preschoolers, and school-age children.

Division for Early Childhood (DEC) of the Council for Exceptional Children

http://www.dec-sped.org—DEC is an international membership organization that promotes policies and evidence-based practices that support families and enhance the development of young children, birth to 8 years, who have or are at risk for developmental delays and disabilities.

Early Childhood Technical Assistance Center (ECTA)

http://www.ectacenter.org—ECTA is a national center funded by the Office of Special Education Programs (OSEP) within the U.S. Department of Education to support early intervention and preschool special education programs and practitioners. It helps states build effective systems and provide services, and promotes research-based interventions for infants, toddlers, and preschoolers with disabilities and their families.

National Association for the Education of Young Children (NAEYC)

http://www.naeyc.org—NAEYC is a nonprofit organization that promotes high-quality early learning for all children, birth through age 8, by connecting practice, policy, and research. Its web site includes position statements on best early childhood education practices, a blog, the NAEYC For Families site, and a members only site with early care and education resources, including electronic issues of *Young Children*—NAEYC's peer-reviewed, professional journal.

National Head Start Association (NHSA)

http://www.nhsa.org—NHSA is a nonprofit organization committed to the belief that every child, regardless of life circumstances, has the ability to succeed. NHSA is the voice for more than 1 million children, 200,000 staff, and 1,600 Head Start grantees in the United States. Its web site includes a Head Start program locator tool, links to resources for children and families, and research about the positive impact of Head Start.

The Pyramid Model Consortium

http://www.pyramidmodel.org—The Pyramid Model Consortium promotes the high-fidelity use of a positive behavior intervention and support framework that early educators can use to promote young children's social-emotional development and prevent and address challenging behavior—the Pyramid Model for Supporting Social Emotional Competence in Infants and Young Children. This nonprofit organization continues the work of the Technical Assistance Center on Social Emotional Intervention for Young Children (TACSEI) and the Center on the Social and Emotional Foundations for Early Learning (CSEFEL).

ZERO TO THREE

http://www.zerotothree.org—ZERO TO THREE is a national nonprofit organization that provides parents, professionals, and policy makers with information about nurturing young children's early development. Its web site provides resources on promoting social-emotional development, mental health screening and assessment, early childhood mental health, and more.

G

Translation and Adaptation Guidelines for ASQ:SE-2

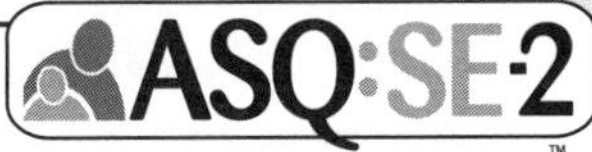

As ASQ has become accepted and established in the early childhood field, there has been an increasing demand in the United States and abroad for translated versions. A Spanish translation of ASQ:SE-2 is available through Brookes Publishing, and translations of ASQ:SE-2 are in development in a number of languages. Brookes Publishing considers requests to translate questionnaires as needed for successful implementation within a community. Please visit www.agesandstages.com for further information.

Translating, or *adapting,* ASQ:SE-2 into other languages brings up several issues and considerations, both linguistic and cultural. Linguistic issues include proper translation of items so that the words impart the same meaning while still being accessible to caregivers who may have minimal levels of education. A translation process, which ensures that the intent of items is maintained, is outlined at the end of this appendix. It is important to use simple words and phrases to ensure that parents understand each item, and it may be helpful to consider adding or modifying examples to improve caregiver understanding.

The cultural appropriateness of items is another important issue. Specific skills that ASQ:SE-2 covers may develop at different developmental stages or ages across various cultures. People from different cultures may have varied expectations about what behaviors are developmentally on track at a given age. Some behaviors may not be encouraged in young children. For example, the item "Does your child look at you when you talk to him?" asks for the demonstration of a behavior that is not encouraged in young children across all cultural groups. This item may need adaptation to reflect cultural norms and expectations so that false concerns are not raised for children for whom this is not the cultural norm or expectation. Items may be omitted and scoring adjusted if an appropriate adaptation cannot be developed that reflects the intent of the item.

Research conducted by Lyman, Njoroge, and Willis (2007) on the use of ASQ:SE with culturally diverse families indicated that there may be cultural variation in items related to parent-guided activities such as sleeping, feeding, and toilet training, as well as attachment and self-regulation. For example, the item that asks whether a parent and child enjoy mealtimes together may not be relevant to cultures where feeding is the ultimate goal of mealtimes, not the quality of time together. Cultural bias may be present in items that involve judgment of what constitutes an ordinary or long period of time, such as "Does your baby cry, scream, or have tantrums for long periods of time?" Parents who do not leave their very young children with other caregivers may be confused by the item "When you leave, does your child remain upset and cry for more than an hour?" Whenever possible, potential cultural discrepancies must be taken into consideration so that adaptations to or omissions of items can be made when administering ASQ:SE-2 with families.

Strategies for working effectively with culturally diverse families include administering ASQ:SE-2 through an interview as well as involving professionals with experience with or from the same cultural background as the families. Using an interview approach rather than having parents fill out paper questionnaires on their own is highly recommended when working with culturally diverse families (Lyman et al., 2007). Employing staff who are familiar with or members of a specific culture often leads to better results as well. Providers can reframe questions for parents and discuss culturally imbued perspectives on development, thereby minimizing opportunities for cross-cultural confusion.

Another issue arises when using a translated or adapted version of ASQ:SE-2, as the norms and cutoffs were developed using the English or Spanish versions of the questionnaire on a population reflective of U.S. Census data. In general, a child's total score should be considered with the family's cultural context in mind before making any follow-up decisions. Behaviors of concern that are raised by parents during the screening process should be addressed, such as if the parent indicates that getting the child to sleep is very difficult. Parents should lead the process of determining what type of follow-up, if any, is appropriate for the child and family. A culturally sensitive process to screening with ASQ:SE-2 is possible by following the parent's lead in administering, interpreting, and following up on the screening.

Based on research and recommendations for adapting educational and psychological assessments into other languages (Beaton, Bombardier, Guillemin, & Ferraz, 2000; Hambleton, Merenda, & Spielberger, 2005), we have established guidelines for programs that are interested in adapting ASQ:SE-2 or ASQ-3 for use with speakers of non-English languages. Translating an assessment tool requires a series of translation and validation steps. Before beginning the translation process, however, we encourage programs to contact the publisher to find out what, if any, work has been done toward adapting ASQ:SE-2 into the target language. As previously mentioned, there is much demand for translations of ASQ:SE-2, both within and outside of the United States. Although not available commercially, unpublished adaptations of ASQ:SE questionnaires exist in many languages. Programs interested in learning more about translations can visit www.agesandstages.com and may find the *Guidelines for Cultural and Linguistic Adaptation of ASQ-3 and ASQ:SE-2* posted there to be useful.

RECOMMENDED TRANSLATION PROCESS

Step 1: Translate forward. Identify a native speaker who has an excellent grasp of American English and who is familiar with the early childhood field and child development. This native speaker translates ASQ:SE-2 from English into the target language.

Step 2: Translate back. Use a different translator who is proficient in both languages and unfamiliar with ASQ:SE-2 to translate back into English, without reference or exposure to the original English version of ASQ:SE-2.

Step 3: Compare the back translation with the original ASQ:SE-2. A native English speaker who has a strong familiarity with ASQ:SE-2 (in some cases, this may be one of the ASQ:SE-2 developers) compares the back translation from Step 2 with the original ASQ:SE-2 to identify items in which discrepancies occur. Notes are made regarding discrepant items.

Step 4: Modify the forward translation. Based on discrepancies identified in Step 3, items in the initial translation should be modified according to notes from the ASQ:SE-2 expert. This step ideally is done with the translator from Step 1 or at least with a native speaker who is familiar with child development.

Step 5: Pilot the translated version. Using the latest version of the adapted ASQ:SE-2 developed in Step 4, the ASQ:SE-2 translation can be pilot tested with caregivers who are native speakers of the target language. Caregivers should be asked to provide feedback on any items that were difficult to understand or observe because they were uncertain of item wording, and feedback on items they thought were culturally inappropriate.

Step 6: Modify the pilot version. After considering the feedback from caregivers in Step 5, make modifications as needed to the pilot version. This final version of the ASQ:SE-2 translation is now ready for general use and can be used to establish local norms and develop cutoff scores for the intended population.

REFERENCES

Beaton, D.E., Bombardier, C., Guillemin, F., & Ferraz, M.B. (2000). Guidelines for the process of cross-cultural adaptation of self-report measures. *Spine, 25*(24), 3186–3191.

Lyman, D., Njoroge, W., & Willis, D. (2007). Early childhood psychosocial screening in culturally diverse populations: A survey of clinical experience with the Ages & Stages Questionnaires: Social-Emotional. *Zero to Three, 27*(5), 46–54.

Hambleton, R.K., Merenda, P.F., & Spielberger, C.D. (2005). *Adapting educational and psychological tests for cross-cultural assessment.* Boston, MA: Lawrence Erlbaum Associates.

Index

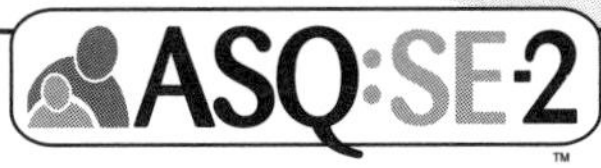

Tables and figures are indicated by *t* and *f*, respectively.

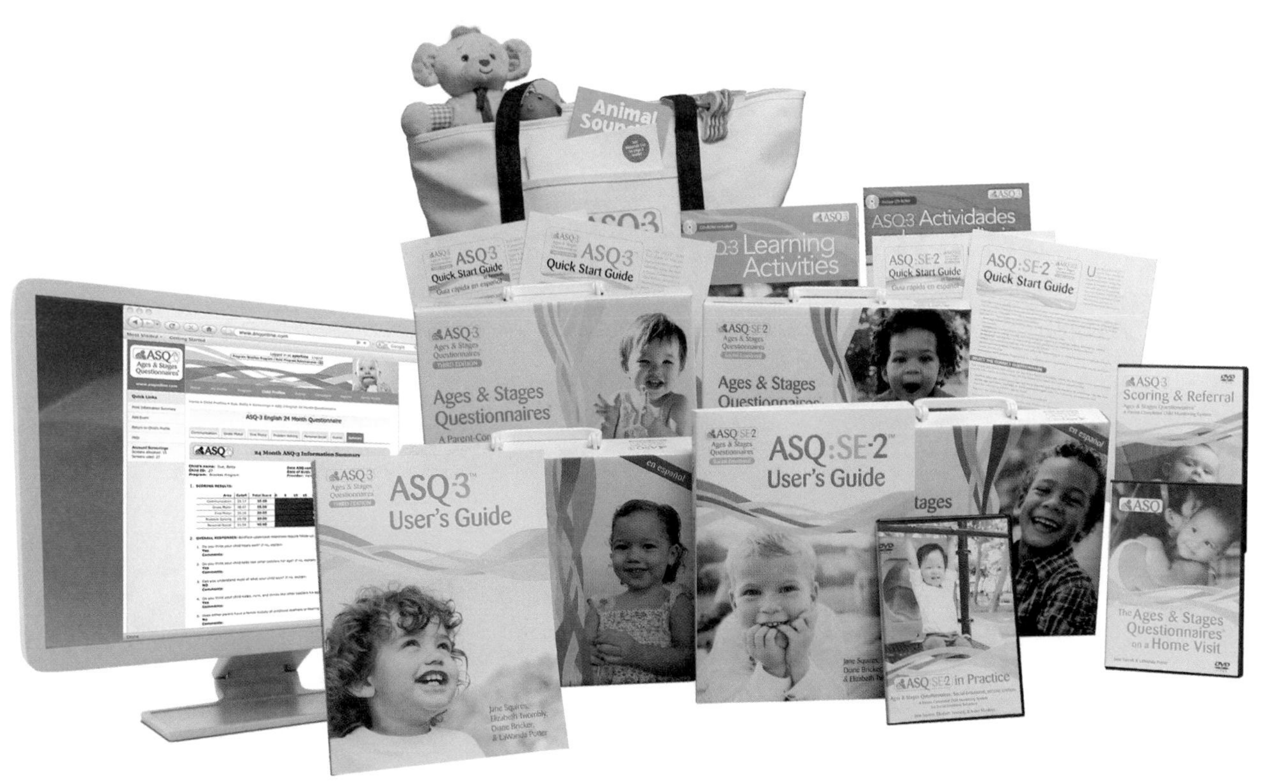

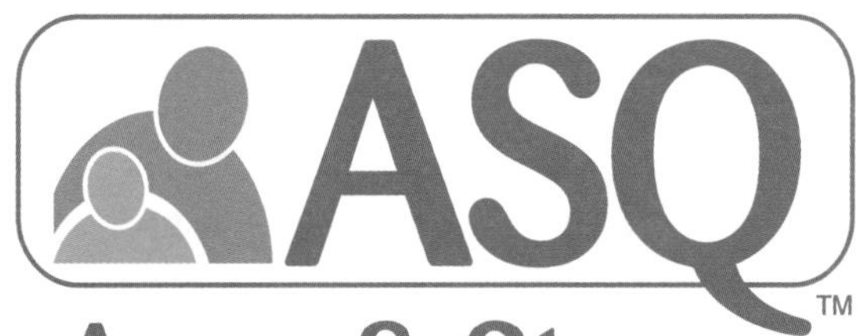

Ages & Stages Questionnaires®

Ordering Guide

ORDER FORM

Name ______________________ Savings code __________

Address ______________________
❍ residential ❍ commercial

City______________ State _____ ZIP__________ Country__________

Phone ______________________

Email ______________________

❍ **Yes!** I want to receive email about new titles & special offers. (Your email address will not be shared.)

Specialty
❍ Birth to Five ❍ K–12 ❍ Clinical/Medical Personnel
❍ 4-year College/Grad. ❍ Comm. College/Vocational
❍ Association/Foundation ❍ Comm. Services

Stock #	Title	Qty	Price
BA-_ _ _ _ _			
BA-_ _ _ _ _			
BA-_ _ _ _ _			
BA-_ _ _ _ _			

Product subtotal (in U.S. dollars) ________

Shipping (see chart) ________

Order subtotal ________

PA, WA, TX, IN, MD state sales tax or GST (for CAN residents)** ________

Grand total ________

PAYMENT METHOD

❍ Check enclosed (payable to Brookes Publishing Co.)

❍ Purchase Order (bill my institution—P.O. MUST be attached)*

❍ Credit card

Credit card account number _ _ _ _ _ _ _ _ _ _ _ _ _ _ _ _

Security code (3 or 4 digit code on back of card) _ _ _ _

Expiration date _ _ /_ _ **Signature** ______________________

** We reserve the right to add an additional 2% order processing fee on all orders that require special processing.*

***PA, WA, TX, IN, and MD residents: Please add state sales tax. Canadian residents: please add your GST. Sales tax should be calculated based on the total order (including shipping) in U.S. dollars. If sales tax is calculated incorrectly, Customer Service will correct it prior to processing your order and the adjusted total will appear on your invoice.*

STANDARD GROUND SHIPPING & HANDLING

(For other shipping options and rates, call 1-800-638-3775, in the U.S.A. and Canada, and 410-337-9580, worldwide.)

USA

For subtotal of	Add*
$50.00 and under	$6.50
$50.01 and over	13%**

*Calculate percentage on product subtotal.
**AK, HI, PR: Please add a $12.00 surcharge for any order over $55.01

Canada

For subtotal of	Add*
$70.00 and under	$10.50
$70.01 and over	15%

Orders for Canada are consolidated for shipping twice each month. Orders must be submitted by 5 PM ET on the 9th or 24th of any given month to be included in our bi-monthly shipments.

MAIL form to Brookes Publishing Co.
P.O. Box 10624; Baltimore, MD 21285-0624

PHONE 1-800-638-3775

FAX 410-337-8539

WEBSITE www.brookespublishing.com

ASQ Discounts

Buy 6 or more copies of the same ASQ family product and SAVE:

6-10 copies: 5%
11-20 copies: 10%
21-50 copies: 15%
51-100 copies: 20%
101-200 copies: 25%
200+ copies: Call for pricing.

(Please note: ASQ Pro, ASQ Enterprise, and ASQ Family Access are not discounted.)

Your Listcode is BA

Prices subject to change.
6/16

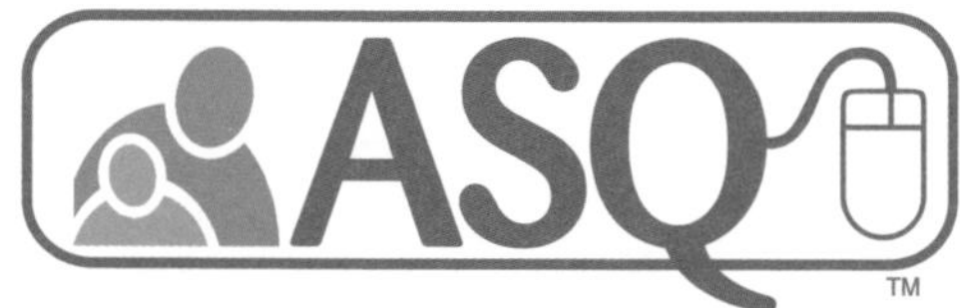

Online data management & questionnaire completion

Join our growing family of ASQ Online users, and you'll be able to score automatically, eliminate data entry errors, run child and program reports in seconds, and allow parents to easily fill out questionnaires online.

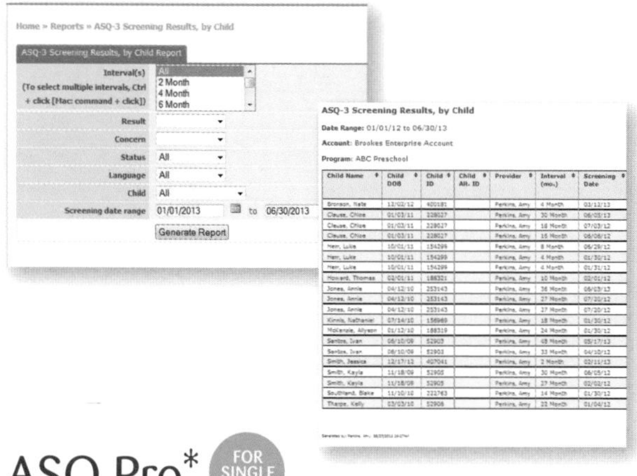

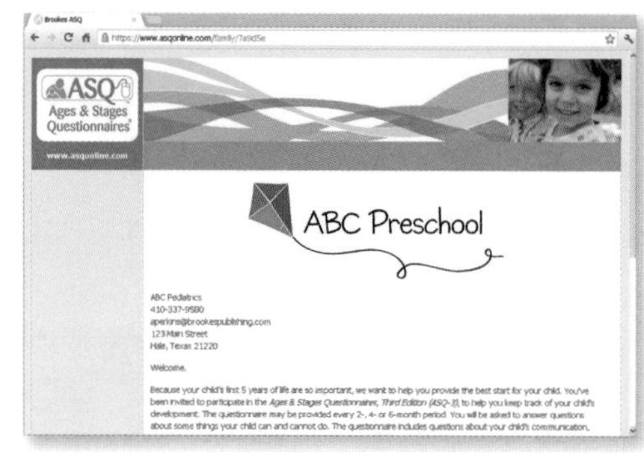

ASQ Pro* FOR SINGLE SITES

Online Data Management

Ideal for single-site programs, this online management option is your key to managing your ASQ-3™ and ASQ:SE-2™ data and ensuring accurate results. ASQ Pro gives you automated scoring and questionnaire selection, customizable letters to parents, individual child and program reports, and much more.

US$149.95** • Stock #: BA-70380 • ISBN 978-1-59857-038-0

ASQ Enterprise* FOR MULTISITE PROGRAMS

Online Data Management

Developed to meet the needs of multisite programs, ASQ Enterprise gives you all the data management features of ASQ Pro plus advanced rights management and aggregate reporting.

US$499.95** • Stock #: BA-70397 • ISBN 978-1-59857-039-7

**To use ASQ Pro or Enterprise, each site must own print versions of ASQ-3™ and/or ASQ:SE-2™ questionnaires that will be managed in the system.*

***Price is for annual subscription—does not include quarterly billing based on screening volume. For cost per screen, see www.agesandstages.com*

ASQ Family Access

Online Questionnaire Completion

Save time and postage with a secure, customizable website where parents complete questionnaires and you access the results electronically. (Available for purchase when you buy ASQ Pro or Enterprise.)

US$349.95 for annual subscription • Stock #: BA-70403
ISBN 978-1-59857-040-3

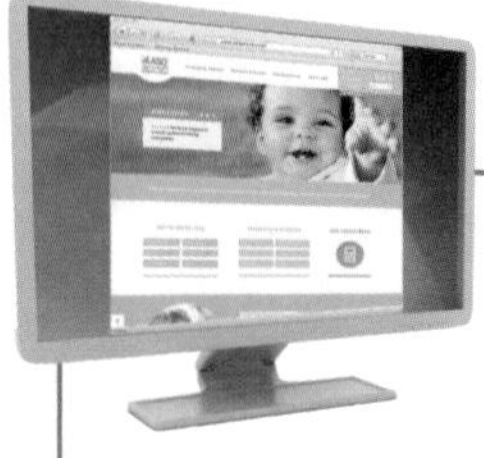

VISIT
www.agesandstages.com
for more on ASQ, including:

- ASQ resources tailored for you—whether you're a clinician, an educator, a child care professional, or a parent
- Interactive database of free resources, such as research articles, sample questionnaires, PowerPoints, and webinars on using ASQ effectively
- Brief videos that give you an inside look at ASQ Pro, ASQ Enterprise, and ASQ Family Access
- A calculator that includes questionnaire interval selection for both ASQ-3™ and ASQ:SE-2™

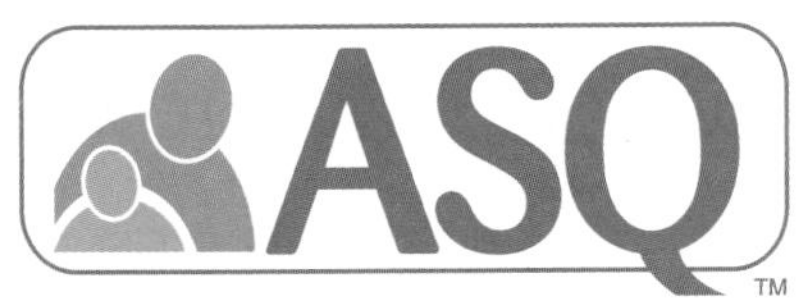

More ASQ Essentials

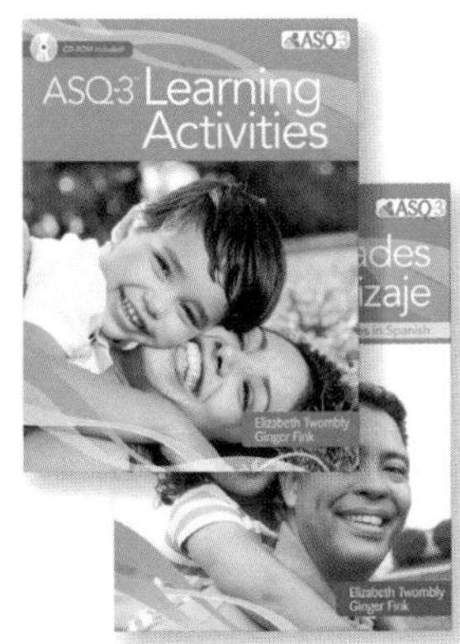

ASQ-3™ Learning Activities

After an ASQ screening, help parents promote children's growth and development with the 400+ fun, creative, and inexpensive learning activities in these books. Available in English and Spanish, the Learning Activities encourage progress in all five key developmental areas screened with ASQ-3™. You can photocopy them from the book, print them from the CD-ROM, or email them to parents for quick, effective ways to boost development between screenings.

English—US$49.95 • Stock #: BA-72469
2013 • 160 pages • ISBN 978-1-59857-246-9

Spanish—US$49.95 • Stock #: BA-72476
2013 • 160 pages • ISBN 978-1-59857-247-6

Sign up for our newsletters!

Looking for tips, information, and news you can use on the job? Sign up for our newsletters and get exclusive practical content like:

- Q&As with expert authors
- free downloads
- original articles
- research-based tips and strategies
- news about our latest products
- training opportunities

Subscribe to ASQ News & Updates and our topic-specific newsletters on Early Childhood, Disabilities, Autism, and more! Easy signup at www.brookespublishing.com.

Connect with us online:

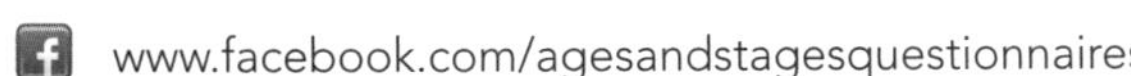

www.facebook.com/agesandstagesquestionnaires
@BrookesASQ
www.pinterest.com/ASQScreener/

ASQ Training DVDs

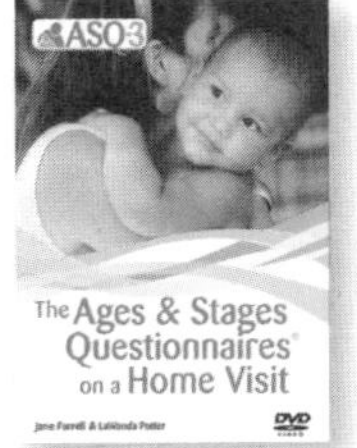

The Ages & Stages Questionnaires® on a Home Visit (Training DVD)

Get a rare inside look at ASQ as a home visitor guides a family with three children through the items on a questionnaire.

US$49.95 • Stock #: BA-69711 • 1995
20 minutes • ISBN 978-1-55766-971-1

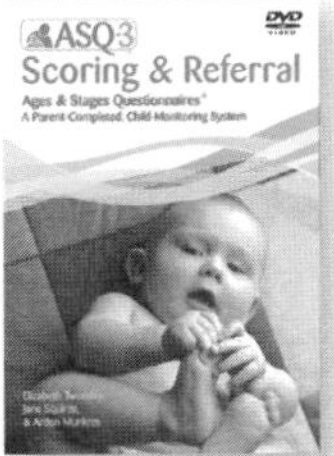

ASQ-3™ Scoring & Referral (Training DVD)

Through footage of ASQ-3™ tasks and close-ups of sample questions and scores, learn how to score the questionnaires accurately and decide if a referral for further assessment is needed.

US$49.95 • Stock #: BA-70250 • 2004, 2009
16 minutes • ISBN 978-1-59857-025-0

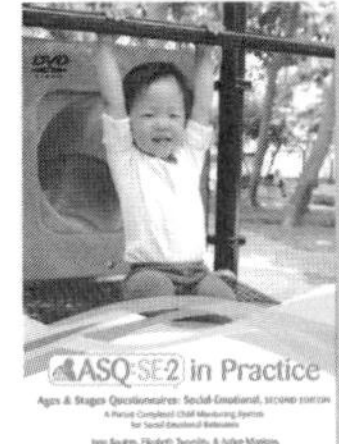

ASQ:SE-2™ in Practice (Training DVD)

Watch a home visitor use ASQ:SE-2™ with the family of a 4-year-old boy. See how parents complete the questionnaires and learn key success factors for working with families.

US$49.95 • Stock #: BA-51608 • 2004, 2016
ISBN 978-1-68125-160-8 *Coming in Fall 2016*

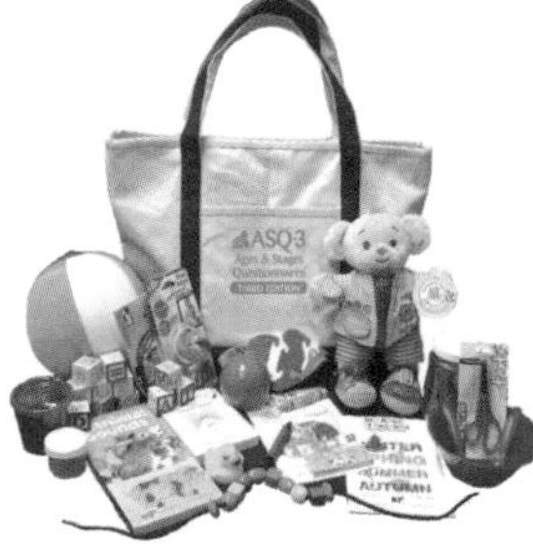

ASQ-3™ Materials Kit

Get quick, convenient access to all the items you need during screening! With more than 20 engaging toys, books, and other items packed in a convenient tote bag, this kit will encourage child participation and support accurate ASQ administration.

US$295.00 • Stock #: BA-70274 • ISBN 978-1-59857-027-4

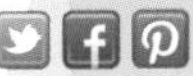